The Complete Self-Care Guide to Homeopathy, Herbal Remedies and Nutritional Supplements

Please Note

This book is a reference tool only and is not to be used as a substitute for professional medical advice, diagnosis or treatment. Always consult a physician or other qualified health care professionals with any questions you may have regarding a medical condition before making any decisions pertaining to illness, health and wellness.

The Complete Self-Care Guide to Homeopathy, Herbal Remedies and Nutritional Supplements

Everything You Need to Know About These Essential Natural Alternatives for Health

Ellen Feingold, M.D.

Whitston Publishing Company, Inc.
Albany, New York
2008

Library of Congress Control Number 2007923048

ISBN 978-0-87875-563-9

Printed in the United States of America

For Michael my Husband and my Best Friend

TABLE OF CONTENTS

Introduction
How to Use This Book

Chapter 1
The New Medicine

PART ONE
HOMEOPATHIC REMEDIES

Chapter 2
Basic Homeopathy

Chapter 3
Homeopathic Remedies for Traumatic Injuries

Ailment/Disorder/Symptom	Homeopathic Remedy
First aid, traumatic injuries, scrapes, bumps, bruises, abrasions, sprains	*Arnica montana*
First aid, traumatic injuries	*Traumeel*
Muscle aches and pains, sprains	*Arniflora*
Skin wounds	*Wound-Care*
Traumatic injuries, anxiety, fears, panic, shock	*Aconitum napellus*
Nerve pains and nerve injuries	*Hypericum perforatum*
Penetrating wounds, puncture wounds	*Ledum palustre*
Broken bones, bone pain, tendon injuries	*Ruta graveolens*
Head injuries, concussions	*Natrum sulphuricum*
Broken bones	*Symphytum officinalis*
Joint pains and stiffness, muscles aches and pains	*Rhus toxicodendron*
Burning, stinging pains, insect bites, allergic hives	*Apis mellifica*
Insect bites	*Sssssting Stop*
Aches and pains with the slightest movement	*Bryonia alba*
Severe nerve pains, lacerations, surgical incisions	*Staphysagria*
Bruising of internal organs, soft tissue pains	*Bellis perennis*
Aches and pains in muscles and joints after sports	*Sports Gel*

Homeopathic Remedies for Traumatic Injuries Associated with Surgery

Ailment/Disorder/Symptom	Homeopathic Remedy
Physical shock and trauma after surgery	*Arnica montana*
Physical and emotional shock after surgery	*Aconitum napellus*
Bright red bleeding from any body opening	*Phosphorus*
Surgical incision pains	*Staphysagria*
Surgical nerve injury pains	*Hypericum perforatum*
Post-surgical tissue swelling and throbbing	*Ferrum phosphoricum*
Dark red bleeding, blood does not clot	*Crotalus horridus*
Physical and emotional shock before and after surgery	*Rescue Remedy*
Pre-dental trauma	*Pre-Dental Procedure*
Post-dental trauma	*Post-Dental Procedure*
Pre-cosmetic surgery trauma	*Pre-Cosmetic Procedure*
Post-cosmetic surgery trauma	*Post-Cosmetic Procedure*
Pre-orthopedic surgery trauma	*Pre-Orthopedic Procedure*
Post-orthopedic surgery trauma	*Orthopedic Post-Op*

Homeopathic Remedies for Burns

Ailment/Disorder/Symptom	Homeopathic Remedy
Infections, inflammation, pain and swelling	*Calendula officinalis*
Post-burns	*Aloe vera*
Inflammation, shock	*Rescue Remedy Cream*
Blistering and burning of the skin and urinary tract infections	*Cantharis*
Scalds and sunburns	*Urtica urens*
Dry, cracking scabs	*Causticum*
Burning pains with restlessness and anxiety	*Arsenicum album*
Thickened, hardened scars	*Graphites*

Chapter 4
Homeopathic Remedies for Fever

Ailment/Disorder/Symptom	Homeopathic Remedy
Sudden, very high, violent fevers	*Belladonna*
Moderately high fevers	*Chamomila*
Low-grade fevers	*Ferrum phosphoricum*
Fevers, teething, pains	*Camilia*
Sudden, high fevers with anxiety	*Aconitum napellus*

Chapter 5
Homeopathic Remedies for Upper Respiratory Infections: Colds, Flu, Coughs, Sore Throats, Laryngitis, Ear Infections, Eye Infections, Sinus Infections

Ailment/Disorder/Symptom	Homeopathic Remedy
Upper respiratory infections	*Aconitum napellus*
Infection with influenza (flu)	*Oscillococcinum*
Infection with influenza (flu)	*Influenzinum*

Ailment/Disorder/Symptom	Homeopathic Remedy
Muscle aches and pains, low-grade fever	*Ferrum phosphoricum*
High fevers with throbbing headache and sudden onset	*Belladonna*
Flu that comes on slowly with heavy feeling	*Gelsemium sempervirens*
Yellow-green mucus discharges in coughs and colds	*Pulsatilla nigricans*
Watery nasal and eye discharges in upper respiratory infections	*Allium cepa*
Burning discharges from nose and eyes, with anxiety and fears	*Arsenicum album*
Colds accompanied by nausea, vomiting, and diarrhea	*Nux vomica*
Colds accompanied by achy, bruised feeling	*Baptisia*
Colds accompanied by severe aches and pains in muscles and bones	*Eupatorium perfoliatum*
Symptoms of upper respiratory infections	*Umcka ColdCare*
Sore throat and congestion	*Echinacea Compound*

Ailment/Disorder/Symptom	Homeopathic Remedy
Heaviness of limbs, thirstlessness, never been well since sick with flu	*Gelsemium sempervirens*
Exhaustion and depression after being sick with flu	*Kali phosphoricum*

Ailment/Disorder/Symptom	Homeopathic Remedy
Coughing brought on by slightest movement	*Bryonia alba*
Thick, yellow-green mucus with cough	*Pulsatilla*
Dry cough after exposure to cold	*Aconitum napellus*
Spasmodic cough in croup, asthma, laryngitis	*Spongia tosta*
Spasmodic, barking coughs	*Drosera rotundifolia*
Dry cough at night after exposure to cold	*Rumex crispus*
Coughs with stringy mucus	*Kali bichromicum*
Coughs due to upper respiratory infections and allergies	*Chestal*

Ailment/Disorder/Symptom	Homeopathic Remedy
Sore throats after exposure to cold weather	*Aconitum napellus*
Sore throats with pus on the tonsils	*Hepar sulphuris calcareum*
Infections and ulcers of the mouth, teeth, gums, and sinuses	*Mercurius solubilis*
Colds, sore throats, hoarseness, laryngitis, and nasal congestion with nosebleeds	*Phosphorus*
Colds and coughs after exposure to damp weather	*Dulcamara*
Hoarseness and laryngitis	*Causticum*
Cold sores and fever sores	*Erpace*
Sore throats and hoarseness	*Echina-Spray*

Chapter 6
Homeopathic Remedies for Allergies and Asthma

Chapter 7
Homeopathic Remedies for Infections

Chapter 8
Homeopathic Remedies for Emotional Problems

Chapter 9
Homeopathic Remedies for Constitutional Problems in Infants, Children, and Adolescents

Ailment/Disorder/Symptom	Homeopathic Remedy
Inferiority, lack of self-confidence, memory difficulties	*Anacardium*
Fears, anxieties, and worries	*Arsenicum album*
Delayed development, shyness	*Baryta carbonica*
Placidity, clumsiness, obesity, flabbiness, lethargy	*Calcarea carbonica*
Rigid thinking, over-empathetic	*Causticum*
Fidgety, impulsivity, thinness	*Iodum*
Domineering, bossiness, controlling	*Lycopodium*
Hyperactivity, self-centeredness	*Medorrhinum*
Pervasive sense of sadness	*Natrum muriaticum*
Creativity, excitability, optimism, easily frightened	*Phosphorus*
Shyness, timidity, insecurity, submissiveness	*Pulsatilla*
Lack of physical stamina	*Silicea*
Suppression of anger leading to rage	*Staphysagria*
Nightmares, night terrors, impulsivity, post-traumatic stress disorder	*Stramonium*
Domineering, selfishness	*Sulphur*
Complications from immunization	*Thuja*
Hyperactivity, impulsivity, difficulties with concentration	*Tuberculinum*
Hyperactivity, restlessness	*Zincum metallicum*
Teething, colic, restlessness, irritability	*Viburcol*
Common ailments in children	*Children's Kit*

Chapter 10
Homeopathic Remedies for Disorders of Menstruation, Fertility, Pregnancy, Labor, Childbirth, Lactation, and Menopause

Ailment/Disorder/Symptom	Homeopathic Remedy
Menstrual pains accompanied by extreme anger	*Chamomilla*

Heavy menstrual bleeding with exhaustion	*China*
Bearing down pains and feeling worn-down	*Sepia*
Bright red menstrual bleeding	*Phosphorus*
Weepiness, sulkiness, and moodiness at the onset of menstruation	*Pulsatilla*
Cramping pains	*Magnesia phosphorica*
Premenstrual syndrome symptoms	*Lachesis*
Swollen, tender breasts before menstruation	*Lac caninum*
Severe abdominal cramping pains on the first day of menstruation	*Colocynthis*
Menstrual cramping associated with back pains	*Cimicifuga racemosa*
General PMS symptoms (pains, bloating, irritability)	*Cyclease PMS*
Menstrual cramps	*Cyclease CRAMP*
Bloating, headaches, tender or swollen breasts, irritability, and mood swings	*PMS Relief*

Ailment/Disorder/Symptom	**Homeopathic Remedy**
Absence of menstrual cycles after severe emotional shock	*Ignatia*
Infertility from scarring of the Fallopian tubes	*Medorrhinum*
Overwhelming grief and sadness from not conceiving	*Natrum muriaticum*
Indifference to childbearing	*Sepia*

Ailment/Disorder/Symptom	**Homeopathic Remedy**
Constant nausea and vomiting during early pregnancy	*Ipecac*
Nausea and vomiting during pregnancy	*Tabacum*
Nausea and vomiting during pregnancy with exhaustion	*Cocculus indicus*
Nausea with frequent spasms of vomiting	*Nux vomica*
Pressure and pain in the uterus or groin	*Bellis perennis*
Nausea of pregnancy	*Pulsatilla*
Nausea at the sight and smell of food	*Sepia*
Great anxiety about health during pregnancy	*Arsenicum album*
Pregnancy with lower back pains	*Kali carbonicum*

Ailment/Disorder/Symptom	**Homeopathic Remedy**
Physical trauma of labor	*Arnica montana*
Emotional trauma of labor	*Aconitum napellus*
Labor not progressing	*Caulophyllum*
Labor with great crying and screaming	*Coffea*
Labor with ineffective contractions	*Nux vomica*
Prolonged labor with weepiness	*Pulsatilla*
Labor facilitation	*Birth Ease*

Ailment/Disorder/Symptom	**Homeopathic Remedy**
Physical trauma of labor	*Arnica montana*
Emotional trauma of labor	*Aconitum napellus*

Ailment/Disorder/Symptom	**Homeopathic Remedy**
Sudden, violent, throbbing breast inflammation	*Belladonna*
Painful, cracked nipples	*Chamomilla*
Hard nodules of the breast	*Conium*
Breast inflammations and infections (mastitis)	*Phytolacca*

Chapter 11
Homeopathy for Digestive Tract Ailments

Chapter 12
Homeopathy for Urinary Tract Ailments

Chapter 13
Homeopathy for Elderly Persons

Chapter 14
Homeopathy for Problems in Joints, Bones and Muscles

Chapter 15
Homeopathy for Eating Disorders and Weight Control

Chapter 16
Homeopathy for Neurologic Disorders

Chapter 17
Homeopathy for Persons with Cancer

Ailment/Disorder/Symptom	**Homeopathic Remedy**
Cancer with family history	*Carcinosin*
Stony hard cancers	*Scirrhinum*
Terminal cancer with pain	*Arsenicum album*
Cancer with bone metastases	*Conium*
Cancerous tumors	*Thuja*

Chapter 18
Homeopathic Constitutional Remedies

Ailment/Disorder/Symptom	**Homeopathic Remedy**
Fastidiousness, perfectionism, chilliness, fearfulness	*Arsenicum album*
Slowness, sluggishness, chilliness, fearfulness	*Calcarea carbonicum*
Jealousy, talkativeness, clairvoyance, menopausal women	*Lachesis*
Insecurity, arrogance, depression	*Lycopodium*
Silent grief, abandoned	*Natrum muriaticum*
Workaholism, perfectionism, chilliness, prone to addictions	*Nux vomica*
Sensitivity, needs company of others, expressivity	*Phosphorus*
Emotional lability with weepiness, self-pitying	*Pulsatilla*
Overwhelmed by responsibilities, apathy	*Sepia*
Eccentricity, hoarding, argumentativeness	*Sulphur*

PART TWO
HERBAL REMEDIES

Chapter 19
Introduction to Herbal Medicine

Chapter 20
Herbs You Need to Know

Ailment/Disorder/Symptom	Herbal Remedy
Upper respiratory infections, influenza	Echinacea
Upper respiratory infections, fungal infections	Goldenseal
Immune system stimulation	Astragalus
Immune system stimulation, anti-cancer activity	Cat's Claw
Migraine prevention	Feverfew
Anti-bacterial agent, cholesterol, blood pressure	Garlic
Cognitive and memory functions of the brain	Ginkgo biloba
Enhance libido, sexual function, and ability to cope with stress	Ginseng
Powerful antioxidant, weight control	Green Tea
Heart disease	Hawthorn
Liver disease, liver cell regeneration	Milk Thistle
Dietary fiber, irritable bowel syndrome, ulcerative colitis	Psyllium
Benign prostatic hypertrophy	Saw Palmetto
Depression	St. John's Wort
Anti-fungal topical	Tea Tree
Insomnia	Valerian

Chapter 21
Herbal Remedies for Women's Health

Ailment/Disorder/Symptom	Herbal Remedy
Menopause, hot flashes	Black Cohosh
Premenstrual syndrome	Chasteberry
Urinary tract infection	Cranberry
Menstrual complaints	Dong quai
Breast tenderness, eczema, ADD/ADHD	Evening Primrose Oil

PART THREE
NUTRITIONAL SUPPLEMENTS

Chapter 22
Introduction to Nutritional Supplements

Chapter 23
Vitamins and Minerals

Ailment/Disorder/Symptom	Nutritional Supplement
Eye health, fetal development, bones, skin, blood	*Vitamin A*
Brain health, muscles (including heart muscle) and nerves	*B Vitamins*
Antioxidant, anti-cancer, anti-ageing activity	*Vitamin C*
Bone health, anti-cancer activity	*Vitamin D*
Skin, heart, nervous and immune systems, oxidative damage repair	*Vitamin E*
Blood clotting (coagulation)	*Vitamin K*
Bone health, teeth, heart, muscles, nerves, and blood clotting	*Calcium*
Glucose metabolism regulation	*Chromium*
Thyroid gland function	*Iodine*
Red blood cell formation and function	*Iron*
Muscle contraction (including the heart muscle), nerve conduction, blood pressure and bone metabolism	*Magnesium*
Bone health	*Manganese*

Chapter 24
Antioxidant Phytochemicals: Natural Anti-Aging Remedies

Ailment/Disorder/Symptom	Nutritional Supplement
Antioxidant and anti-aging activity	*Alpha-lipoic Acid*
Anti-inflammatory activity	*Carotenoids*
Heart function, anti-cancer activity	*Beta-carotene*
Eye function	*Lutein* and *zeaxanthin*
Prostate cancer prevention	*Lycopene*
Blood clotting	*Polyphenols*
Heart, cholesterol, blood vessel function	*Flavonoids*
Cardiovascular system	*Anthocyanins* and *proanthocyanidins*
Heart and blood pressure, anti-cancer and anti-inflammatory activity	*Quercetin*
Immune system	*Glutathione*
Metabolic Detoxification	*Isothiocyanates*
Anti-cancer and antioxidant activity	*Sulphoraphane*
Phytoestrogens	*Lignans*
Anti-cancer and anti-inflammatory activity	*Resveratrol*

Chapter 25
Heart Healthy Nutritional Supplements

Ailment/Disorder/Symptom	Nutritional Supplement
Heart attacks and strokes	*Alcoholic beverages*
Congestive heart failure, high blood pressure	*Amino acids*
Anti-aging activity in heart muscle	*L-carnitine*
Heart muscle contraction	*Coenzyme Q10*
Anti-inflammatory activity	*Enzymes*
Cardiovascular disease and cholesterol	*Fiber*
LDL ("bad") cholesterol lowering while raising HDL ("good") cholesterol	*Guggulipid*
Capillaries and veins, varicose veins	*Horse chestnut*
Total and LDL ("bad") cholesterol lowering	*Phytosterols*
Total and LDL cholesterol, and triglycerides Lowering while raising HDL cholesterol	*Policosanol*

Chapter 28
Nutritional Supplements for Diseases of Joints, Bones and Muscles

Ailment/Disorder/Symptom	Nutritional Supplement
Anti-inflammatory and analgesic (pain relief) activity	*Cetyl myristoleate (CMO)*
Pain relief and joint function	*Chondroitin*
Pain relief and joint function	*Glucosamine*
Anti-inflammatory and analgesic activity	*Devil's claw*
Anti-inflammatory activity	*Enzymes*
Immune system regulation	*Green foods*
Joints, skin, and hair	*Methylsulfonylmethane (MSM)*
Pain relief and joint function, depression	*S-adenosylmethionine (SAMe)*
Pain relief and joint function	*Stinging nettle*

Chapter 29
Nutritional Supplements for Neurologic Disorders

Ailment/Disorder/Symptom	Nutritional Supplement
Memory and thinking	*Dimethylaminoethanol (DMAE)*
Epilepsy	*Gamma-aminobutyric acid (GABA)*
Speech and seizures in autistic children	*Dimethylglycine (DMG)*
Depression	*5-Hydroxytryptophan (5-HTP)*
Memory and concentration	*Huperzine*
Memory, thinking, and muscle activity	*Lecithin*
Memory, learning, and thinking	*Phosphatidylserine*
Brain circulation and stroke prevention	*Vinpocetine*

Chapter 30
Prebiotics and Probiotics

Ailment/Disorder/Symptom	Nutritional Supplement
Immune system function, digestion, diarrhea	*Acidophilus*
Digestion	*Inulin*

Chapter 31
Oils and Fats

Ailment/Disorder/Symptom	**Nutritional Supplement**
Skin, brain, heart, ADD/ADHD, anti-inflammator activity	*Omega-3 fatty acids*
Monounsaturated fat source	*Olive oil*
Monounsaturated fat source	*Canola oil*
LDL ("bad") cholesterol	*Walnut oil*

Appendix

Introduction

How to Use This Book

Putting together homeopathy, herbal remedies, and nutritional supplements for self-care
How to use this book
A short account of the author's personal journey towards alternative medicine
Acknowledgements
About the Author

Putting Together Homeopathy, Herbal Remedies, and Nutritional Supplements for Self-Care

Much of the time that I spend in my clinical practice of alternative medicine, I spend teaching patients how to care for themselves using a combination of **good health practices**:
  —no smoking, moderate alcohol, nutritionally healthy diet, adequate daily physical exercise, adequate sleep, time for daily relaxation techniques, seeking humor and love in everyday life, engaging in activities for intellectual stimulation, doing things for other people, and participating in preventive health testing

and **essential alternative health practices**, namely:
  —homeopathy, herbal remedies, and nutritional supplements.

After all, upon those cornerstones, **good health practices** and **essential alternative health practices,** lay the fundamentals of health care for the majority of illnesses for both men and women throughout the life cycle from the fetus to the very elderly. This book teaches the essential alternative health practices, assuming that you have already mastered many, if not all, of the good health practices for yourself and your family.

This book teaches and preaches self-care. It will help you to integrate homeopathic remedies, herbal remedies, and nutritional supplements for many common conditions during the life cycle, including pregnancy, lactation, infancy, childhood, adolescence, adulthood, and the elderly.

First, within each of those three essential alternative health care practices you will learn the basics. Then you will learn the specifics. You do not have to memorize anything. You can make notes in the margins of the book and use the **Index** to help you to find sections that are meaningful to you and to your family's health. This book will help you to decide which homeopathic remedies, herbal remedies, and nutritional supplements are appropriate to treat or to prevent the ailments that concern you and your family.

Most importantly, you will learn when to consult your homeopath or your Western medicine health care provider by paying strict attention to the **Guidelines for Consulting Your Health Care Provider**, found at the end of each chapter.

> **Note:** The idea for the Guidelines Section came to me after reading Kathi Kemper's book "The Holistic Pediatrician" (2nd Edition). I modeled my Guidelines Section after hers in that book.

> **Note:** Do not discontinue taking any pharmaceutical medication that has been prescribed by your health care provider unless you or your family member is under the supervision of a physician.

When undertaking self-care for yourself or others, it is important to learn to recognize your own inner signals indicating discomfort with something you are doing. Whenever you perceive those signals, whenever you have surpassed your comfort level, get help, even though you may not have exceeded the limits outlined in the **Guidelines for Consulting Your Health Care Provider**. Learn to trust your instincts. It is never wrong to ask for help or advice from your health care provider. It is always better to seek help earlier rather than later.

At the end of most chapters you will also find a section called **Putting It All Together**. This section will help you to integrate the **essential natural alternatives**, namely homeopathy, herbal remedies, and nutritional supplements. It will guide you to the specific chapters in this book that you will need to consult to make a well-rounded decision on self-care.

If you want to learn about medical conditions and diseases in greater depth, you need to seek out reliable, user-friendly, and up-to-date information. The primary source that I go to first is the *Merck Manual*, available at www.merck.com. The site is searchable and you can trust the medical information.

> **Note:** Here are some other reliable online resources:

Family Medicine Net Guide at www.fmnetguide.com

Web MD at www.webmd.com

Aetna's Intelihealth at www.intelihealth.com

American Academy of Family Physicians at www.familydoctor.org

National Institutes of Health at www.nih.gov

National Cancer Institute at www.nci.nih.gov

The Mayo Clinic at www.mayohealth.org/home

Infant's and children's health at www.cdc.gov/health/infantsmenu.htm

Columbia Medical School's Go Ask Alice www.goaskalice.columbia.edu is a reliable site for health information for teens.

The Office on Women's Health at www.4Girls.gov has health information aimed at 10-16 year-old girls.

www.kidsgrowth.com is designed for parents.

www.healthtalk.com and www.mdadvice.com have interactive broadcasts.

Discovery Health's pregnancy center at www.discoveryhealth.com

www.nfam.org is the website for the National Foundation for Alternative Medicine.

www.drugs.com and www.rxlist.com and www.drugdigest.org are reliable sites for interactions between prescription pharmaceutical medicines, side effects, dosage, and precautions. These sites may help you to determine if the prescription drugs your doctor prescribed are safe for you or your family member to take. Remember, however, that these sites will not give you drug-herb interactions. This is essential to know before taking herbal remedies if you are taking prescription pharmaceuticals.

If you want to learn about your prescription pharmaceuticals in greater depth, you may access these free online resources:

www.pdrhealth.com/drug_info/index.html (from the Physician's Desk Reference (PDR)) and

www.safemedication.com (from the American Society of Healthy-system Pharmacists.

When patients in my office ask me questions regarding medical tests that have been prescribed for them or someone in their families, we often read together excerpts from *The Johns Hopkins Consumer Guide to Medical Tests* edited by Simeon Margolis, M.D. This is a good reference book geared to health care consumers, explaining medical laboratory tests and diagnostic procedures in great detail that you may have to undergo in order to arrive at a diagnosis. This diagnostic work-up process is an essential underpinning for both Western and alternative medicine.

Why do I use these particular essential alternative health care practices, namely, homeopathy, herbal remedies, and nutritional supplements?
The answer is that it works! The majority of my patients tend to improve. And my patients generally tend to be able to continue onwards with some measure of self-care. There are many ailments for which I recommend treatment in just one or maybe two out of the three alternative health care practices. For example, in most first aid situations a homeopathic remedy alone will restore health.

However, there are certain ailments where combining all three **essential alternative health practices** together will lead to a healthier person. I will teach you how to combine all three to make a difference in long-term health.

For example:
A menopausal female may benefit from *Black cohosh*, an herbal remedy commonly used to treat hot flashes. But, she is likely to be much healthier in the long run if I encourage her to take the recommended daily dose of calcium and Vitamin D to help prevent osteoporosis. It is likely that I would also recommend

other minerals and vitamins as well as antioxidants. In addition, I would strongly recommend that she take the homeopathic remedy *Lachesis* which is likely to give her relief from many of the other symptoms of menopause such as hot flashes, insomnia, depression, and moodiness. You will learn how to do all this from this book.

You will learn that homeopathy is the safest of the three **essential alternative health care practices** because it has no significant side effects or interactions with prescription medications. I suggest that you start first with homeopathy to treat or prevent the ailment you are interested in. Then you may add the appropriate nutritional supplements to augment the homeopathic remedies and to attain a higher level of health. Then, you may investigate the use of herbal remedies to treat or prevent the ailments that concern you.

But, remember you cannot expect to erase the effects of nicotine addiction, or a diet high in saturated fats, or a sedentary lifestyle by taking homeopathic remedies and nutritional supplements. You and the members of your family must practice the **good health practices** (please see the first paragraph in this chapter) at the same time that you institute the **essential alternative health practices**.

Many, but not all, of the recommendations for homeopathy, herbal remedies, and nutritional supplements, the three **essential alternative health care** practices, are based on sound medical research evidence. I will tell you which ones have been proven safe and effective and for which ones the jury is still out.

This book is mostly about my personal product recommendations for treating or preventing a whole host of ailments. I do not make any recommendation without my having had clinical experience with the product with my own patients in the *Homeopathy Center of Delaware*.

Note: You can visit me on the web at www.drellenfeingold.com.

This book will not teach you to use many other health care practices which have been proven safe and effective, such as acupuncture, massage,

guided imagery, meditation, and many other techniques. You may wish to incorporate some of these health care practices into your program for self-care by investigating them using reliable online websites and books. However, I have not found the addition of any other techniques to be necessary to achieve and sustain good health under most circumstances.

How to Use This Book

There are several ways you can use this book. One way is to read this book from cover to cover, learning the basics and the specifics of homeopathy, herbal remedies, and nutritional supplements. Along the way, you would make notes in the margins so that you could quickly and efficiently find the information of importance to you and your family's health concerns. Whenever you decide on a pathway towards self-care for yourself and your family, remember to utilize the **Guidelines for Consulting Your Health Care Practitioner** at the end of each chapter.

Another way to use this book is to look up the ailment, condition, or disease that you need to treat or prevent in the **Table of Contents** and the **Index**. Read the information and my recommendations under all three alternative health care practices, homeopathy, herbal remedies, and nutritional supplements. The section, **Putting It All Together**, at the end of most chapters will help you to incorporate all the necessary elements. Then you would exercise your own preferences in designing a program of health for yourself and your family, always remembering to pay strict attention to the **Guidelines for Consulting Your Health Care Practitioner** at the end of each chapter.

The measure of self-care attainable for yourself and your family is based on your level of motivation and the extent to which you begin learning about homeopathy, herbal remedies, and nutritional supplements. You can do it. You can learn to become confidently self-reliant in most health care matters. Using this book is a good beginning.

> **Remember:** Keep good medical records for yourself and every member of your family. If you accept that you are

responsible for your health and the health of your family, then you will need an ongoing medical "chart" or folder for each person under your care. Ask for copies of laboratory and medical imaging results. It is your right to have those copies.

Remember: When visiting your homeopath or health care provider, always bring along a list of all the remedies you or your family member is taking, including homeopathy, herbal remedies, and nutritional supplements.

A short account of the author's personal journey towards alternative medicine

I had been a practicing pediatrician and adolescent gynecologist for decades before it became clear to me that my practice was, essentially, a revolving door. Many of my patients did not actually get cured. They got better, yes. But, then they got worse again.

The pharmaceutical drugs that I was prescribing in ever-increasing strength and toxicity did not seem to make a whole lot of difference in the long run. Kids still came down with ear infections, relapsing all winter long, whether or not they drank the antibiotics that I prescribed.

Mothers in my practice were whispering about something else. And I started to learn about that something else. I am indebted to the group of mothers in my practice in Jerusalem in the 1980s and early1990s who taught me so much. When I began my formal education in homeopathy, I knew I had found the answer to cure. Not only does homeopathy have the ability to cure chronic relapsing conditions that Western medicine cannot, but it does so in the gentlest manner, without any discernable side effects.

Homeopathy amazed me. It will amaze you too.

When I started practicing homeopathy, I realized that it alone was not the whole story, either. I saw that I needed to put it together with herbal remedies and nutritional supplements to effect a deep healing in most cases.

And then a few years later, I realized that most of what I was doing in my practice of homeopathy, herbal remedies, and nutritional supplements, was possible to do without me, the physician. I realized that the most profound answer to the conundrum of Western medicine was the educated woman and mother, the keeper of the family's health.

Acknowledgements

This book was written as a labor of love, but it could not have been completed without the help of these people:

My husband Michael who encouraged me every step of the way;

My daughter Felicia Marjorie, my most successful patient, who taught me so much about healthy living and who inspired me to keep learning and keep writing;

My son Barnett who bought me just the books I needed to fill in the gaps in my knowledge;

My son Daniel, the surgeon, who gave me his New England Journal of Medicine issues with articles on herbal medicine;

My son Joseph, the brain scientist, and my most compliant patient;

My daughter-in-law Shiri who uses homeopathy, and as a newly minted western medical doctor, gives me great hope for young doctors; my other daughters-in-law, Tonja and Jessica, and my son-in-law Oz, all of whom helped me in innumerable ways;

My grandchildren Judah, Ethan, Noa, Lev, Lily, Max, Ravit, Yoav, Leo, and Reuben who responded so well to the remedies in this book;

To Ms. Patti Berk, our office manager, without whose labors this book would not have been published;

Mr. Richard Replogle, Representative of the Boiron Institute, maker of homeopathic pharmaceuticals, supplied me with books about homeopathy and Boiron's products;

To the representatives from many homeopathic, herbal, and nutritional supplements companies who helped me over several years with information and samples to evaluate their products with my patients;

To my teachers of homeopathy, Drs. Yoav Kamcagi and Daniel Greilsammer. They opened my eyes to the gentle healing of homeopathy as I will try to do for you.

And to Paul Laddin and Jill Wolcott of Whitston Publishing, without whose wisdom and guidance there would be no book at all.

Please Note

You will notice that throughout this book I recommend many different homeopathic, herbal, and nutritional products, specific manufacturers, books, newsletters, and online resources. I have no financial interest in any item that I recommend in this book. All recommendations are based solely on my clinical experience.

About the Author

Dr. Ellen Feingold, M.D. has been a physician for thirty-five years, most of that time practicing pediatrics and adolescent medicine. While living and working in Jerusalem, Israel, she took the Masters in Public Health degree at Hebrew University-Hadassah Medical School where she learned how to evaluate medical evidence from research studies. In 1994, she began her studies in homeopathy at the Israel Medical College of Homeopathy, graduating in 1996. Currently, she is the Director of the Homeopathy Center of Delaware where she practices homeopathy, herbal medicine, and nutritional therapies exclusively, treating persons of all ages. Although she treats the entire spectrum of human diseases, her clinical interests are cancer, emotional ailments, eating disorders, and obesity. She has always been interested in empowering men and women to practice self-care for many common ailments, safely and effectively.

Dr. Feingold recommends many books, health products and pharmaceutical manufacturers in the pages of this book based on her own clinical experience. She has no financial interest in any product or pharmaceutical manufacturer mentioned in this book.

You may contact Dr. Feingold via her website www.drellenfeingold.com.

Chapter 1

The New Medicine

What is complementary and alternative medicine (CAM)?
What is integrative medicine?
What is holistic medicine?
What are the essential natural alternative remedies?
Putting It All Together

What is complementary and alternative medicine (CAM)?

Complementary and alternative medicine, often abbreviated as CAM, refers to therapies that are not used in mainstream or conventional Western medicine.

Nation-wide, a bit more than one-third of all the households surveyed used one or more CAM modalities during 1997-2002 (representing 72 million adults in this country). The CAM modality most commonly used was herbal medicine but many used homeopathic remedies and nutritional supplements.

Names for CAM	Names for Western Medicine
Complementary	Orthodox
Alternative	Conservative
Integrative	Allopathic
Holistic	Western
Natural Medicine	Conventional, mainstream

Note: This **Table** lists names for CAM on the left-hand side and the names for Western medicine on the right. The names down each side of the two columns once had very different meanings but the differences between them have become blurred so that each has become mostly interchangeable.

Note: The *Institute of Medicine* (*IOM*) acts as an adviser to the federal government on controversial issues of medical research and health of the American people. In 2005, the *IOM* issued a special report on complementary and alternative medicine (CAM) in the United States. The 300-page report evaluated CAM usage, CAM research methods, CAM health delivery, and CAM medical education and issued recommendations. Perhaps the report's most far-reaching recommendation is that *all* health profession schools include CAM information in medical, dental, and nursing curricula.

Note: The *National Center for Complementary and Alternative Medicine* (*NCCAM*) is part of the *National Institutes of Health* (*NIH*). NCCAM recommends that scientifically proven CAM modalities be integrated into conventional medicine. Contact *NCCAM* at www.nccam.nih.gov or 1-888-644-6226 (the *NCCAM* Clearinghouse).

What is integrative medicine?

Despite the interchangeability of nomenclature, there is still a special meaning for the term "integrative medicine." Integrative medicine is a term first used by Dr. Andrew Weil who teaches that some CAM therapies should be included, or integrated into Western medicine. Just as there are proven successful therapies in Western medicine, there are some in certain forms of CAM. Dr. Weil teaches that we should no longer separate those therapies that have been shown to be safe and effective on either side of the therapy fence.

Integrative medicine is essentially mainstreaming unconventional therapies into Western medicine. Integrative medicine takes the best of both worlds and offers it to the patient. Integrative medicine is concerned with the individual, the whole person.

This book, *The Complete Self-Care Guide to Homeopathy, Herbal Remedies, and Nutritional Supplements*, takes the **integrative medicine** approach to treating most of the conditions and diseases that afflict persons in Western society.

Throughout this book you will be encouraged to use the tools of homeopathy, herbal remedies, and nutritional supplements, and at the same time to check the **Guidelines for Consulting Your Health Care Practitioner** at the end of each chapter. The **Guidelines for Consulting Your Health Care Practitioner** are based on Western medicine. Failing to check the **Guidelines for Consulting Your Health Care Practitioner** at the end of each chapter may be dangerous to your health and the health of your family members.

> **Note:** Do not discontinue taking any pharmaceutical medication that has been prescribed by your health care provider unless you or your family member is under the supervision of a physician.

For more information on integrative medicine, take a look at Dr. Weil's monthly newsletter called *Self-Healing* at www.drweilselfhealing.com.

What is holistic medicine?

The approach to health care which includes all parts of a patient's self, the physical, emotional, mental (or intellectual), sexual, and spiritual parts, is called **holistic**, indicating wholeness. Homeopathy is a system of medicine that operates on the holistic model, along a mind-body-spirit continuum. Western medicine, on the other hand, does not.

What are the essential natural alternative remedies?

The essential natural alternative remedies that I will teach you to use are **homeopathy, herbal remedies, and nutritional supplements**. These are the health care practices that I use with my patients in my clinic, *The Homeopathy Center of Delaware*, where I have been practicing since 1998. Before then, I practiced a combination of pediatrics, adolescent medicine, and public health along with alternative medicine for more than thirty years, in both New York and Jerusalem, Israel.

I consider these three health care practices, homeopathy, herbal remedies, and nutritional supplements to be "essential" because these are the treatments that will likely help you to treat or prevent most of the ailments that beset you and your family members. You will learn how to combine all three for some ailments and how to use one or two of them for others.

Many, but not all, of the recommendations for homeopathy, herbal remedies, and nutritional supplements are based on sound medical research evidence. As you read this book you will find that I tell you which ones have been proven safe and effective and which ones have not.

Self-care with the essential natural alternatives that I recommend in this book may help to keep you and your family members out of harm's way. Keeping away from hospitals and the invasive procedures that are often done there may actually save your life! This is because there are so many "medical mistakes" caused every year in our hospitals. A recent article* published in the prestigious *Journal of the American Medical Association* reported on 250,000 deaths from errors and mistakes *every year* in the U.S. These deaths include 12,000 from unnecessary surgery, 7,000 from medication errors in hospitals, 20,000 from other fatal errors in hospitals, 80,000 from infections in hospitals, and 106,000 from side effects of pharmaceuticals.

> *Starfield B, Is U.S. Health Really the Best in the World?, *Journal of the American Medical Association*, 2000 July 26; 284(4):483-485.

This book will not teach you to use many other health care practices which have been proven safe and effective, such as acupuncture, massage, guided imagery, meditation, and many other techniques. You may wish to incorporate some of these health care practices into your program for self-care by investigating them using reliable online websites and books. However, I have not found the addition of any other techniques to be necessary to achieve and sustain good health under most circumstances.

This book will give you the tools to select those essential health care options from a wide array of homeopathic remedies, herbal remedies, and nutritional supplements to design a program of self-care for yourself and your family. This book will also help you to recognize when self-care is not appropriate. Every chapter has a section, **Guidelines for Consulting Your Health Care Practitioner**. Please pay strict attention to that section when making your selections and designing your self-care program.

Putting It All Together

At the end of most chapters you will also find a section called **Putting It All Together**. You know that to take charge of your and your family's health, you must use a combination of **good health practices,** namely:

—no smoking, moderate alcohol, nutritionally healthy diet, adequate daily physical exercise, adequate sleep, time for daily relaxation techniques, seeking humor and love in everyday life, engaging in activities for intellectual stimulation, doing things for other people, and participating in preventive health testing

along with **essential alternative health practices,** namely:

—homeopathy, herbal remedies, and nutritional supplements.

After all, **good health practices** and **essential alternative health practices,** are the fundamentals of health care for the majority of illnesses for both men and women throughout the life cycle from the fetus to the very elderly.

The **Putting It All Together** section will help you to integrate the **essential natural alternatives,** namely homeopathy, herbal remedies, and nutritional supplements into a comprehensive treatment plan. It will guide you to the specific chapters in this book that you will need to consult in order to make well-rounded decisions on self-care. This isn't a cookbook so if you expect to achieve relief from serious, chronic disorders, you will need to make some informed decisions. You probably realize that self-care requires that you make a series of complicated choices. It's not easy to take responsibility for your health care or that of your family's. You've also realized that the more you read and learn, the more independent, or at the very least, self-directed, your health care can be.

This book will teach you that homeopathic remedies are the least dangerous of the **essential alternative health practices.** And, in fact, homeopathic remedies carry no side effects and do not interfere with the action of conventional pharmaceutical medications. So, you will learn to choose

homeopathy as first-line remedies for self-care for yourself and your family.

But, even though homeopathy is a safe choice, you will learn to pay strict attention to the **Guidelines for Consulting Your Health Care Provider,** found at the end of each chapter. The **Guidelines** tell you when you must consult your homeopath or your Western medicine health care provider.

You will learn never to discontinue taking any pharmaceutical medication that has been prescribed by your health care provider unless you or your family member is under the supervision of a physician.

You will learn to look for the nutritional supplements or the ailment you want to treat or prevent after you've checked out the homeopathic remedies. And then, after that, in case you still need help treating or preventing, you will learn to look for herbal remedies.

You will learn to consult **ConsumerLab.com**'s product reviews for herbal remedies and nutritional supplements. You may read the results by subscribing to **www.ConsumerLab.com** or buy their book, *ConsumerLab.com's Guide to Buying Vitamins and Supplements, What's Really in the Bottle?*

For example:
Let's say your father is 88 years old and has been living with you and your family for the past 5 years, ever since your mother died. You have instituted most (no one's perfect) of the **good health practices** in your household so he's had the benefit of a healthy lifestyle.

But lately, you and your children have commented that his memory has been slipping. His forgetfulness resonates with one of your big worries that soon you won't be able to leave him alone in the house for fear he'd wander off and not find his way back.

You've taken him to a neurologist and she made the diagnosis that your father suffers from the early stages of Alzheimer's disease. She prescribed a new medication that could prolong the early stage longer than if he didn't take it. But, you are concerned that he may have side effects since he's been known in the past to be very sensitive to pharmaceutical medications. So, you've determined to try the **essential alternative health practices** first before plunging into pharmaceuticals.

You will need to read the **Introduction, Chapter 1: The New Medicine** and **Chapter 2: Basic Homeopathy.** Then you will read **Chapter 13: Homeopathy for Elderly Persons.**

Then you take a look at **Chapter 16: Homeopathy for Neurologic Disorders** because you are certain that your father has a neurologic disorder.

Then you read **Chapter 18: Homeopathic Constitutional Remedies** because you realize that a constitutional remedy might benefit your father in other ways. It's not just about his forgetfulness, but also about his anxieties and increasing fears, his loss of appetite and progressive weakness.

Throughout all of this, you will determine which homeopathic remedy or remedies are likely to benefit your father by following the **keynote** symptoms.

Then let us say that your father has been taking homeopathy for the past 8 weeks with some slight improvement in appetite, fears and anxieties, but no real change in memory. You now decide that it's time to add those vitamins and minerals uniquely involved in neurologic function, so you check out **Chapter 23: Vitamins and Minerals.**

Then you begin a study of **Chapter 29: Nutritional Supplements for Neurologic Disorders** and decide on which supplement or supplements are indicated for people with your father's symptoms. And you pay strict attention to the **Guidelines for Consulting Your Health Care Provider,** found at the end of each chapter.

You notice while reading **Chapter 29: Nutritional Supplements for Neuro-**logic Disorders that it's a good idea to investigate *omega-3 fatty acids* for brain health and so at this point you read **Chapter 31: Oils and Fats.**

You recognize that herbal remedies are the third kind of **essential alternative health practices.** So you check out **Chapter 20: Herbs You Need to Know.** After paying strict attention to the **Guidelines for Consulting Your Health Care Provider,** found at the end of the chapter, you study the list of drug interactions carefully before you decide on adding *Ginkgo biloba* to your father's daily remedies and supplements.

You realize that it is a good idea to check with your health care provider if your family member is very old because herbal remedies and nutritional supplements given injudiciously may overwhelm the body's defenses in that age group. So, you make an appointment with your father's health care provider to go over the growing list of homeopathic remedies, herbal remedies, and nutritional supplements your father is poised to take.

Once again you marvel at the complicated choices you've had to make. Taking responsibility for your father's health care isn't simple. You've had to read a lot and make some tough choices.

But, in the process, you've learned a lot and your health and the health of your family have improved. And you believe you are doing everything you can to help prevent the onset of chronic, destructive ailments. Best of all, you took the initiative and you're in charge.

Another example:
Let's say you, a healthy 55-year-old female, just had your yearly gynecologic check-up, getting a Pap smear and breast examination. Your annual mammogram was done a few weeks ago so your doctor had those results (no pathological findings) as well. You tell

her you have not had your monthly menstrual cycle for just about a year. She then solemnly pronounced that you have entered menopause. She gives you some advice about taking enough calcium and getting your first bone density study. You discuss your symptoms of hot flashes, night sweats, and difficulties sleeping with her but she does not suggest any of the *essential natural alternatives* (homeopathy, herbal medicines, and nutritional supplements).

Let us say that you've been reading *The Complete Self-Care Guide to Homeopathy, Herbal Remedies, and Nutritional Supplements* ever since your husband developed high cholesterol last year. So, you've already digested the **Introduction, Chapter 1: The New Medicine** and **Chapter 2: Basic Homeopathy**. And you've conquered **Chapter 22: Introduction to Nutri-tional Supplements** and **Chapter 19: Introduction to Herbal Medicine** as well.

Since you've done some preliminary reading, you feel prepared to venture forth in matters of your own health. So you begin your odyssey for good health for your senior years. Your goal is to decrease the hot flashes, night sweats, and difficulties sleeping you have been experiencing as well as to make plans for preventive health maintenance for the important decades coming along.

First, you focus on homeopathic remedies for menopause by reading the section on menopause in **Chapter 10: Homeopathic Remedies for Disorders of Menstruation, Fertility, Pregnancy, Labor, Childbirth, Lactation, and Menopause,** paying strict attention to the **Guidelines for Consulting Your Health Care Provider,** found at the end of the chapter.

Next, you read **Chapter 18: Homeopathic Constitutional Remedies.** Your symptoms are very close to the **keynote** symptoms described for the homeopathic constitutional remedy *Lachesis.* Once again you pay strict attention to the **Guidelines for Consulting Your Health Care Provider,** found at the end of the chapter. You order *Lachesis* from one of the *Homeopathic Remedy Supply Houses* found in the **Appendix** at the end of the book.

After finding some relief from your hot flashes, night sweats, and difficulties sleeping, you prepare to augment the effects of *Lachesis* by adding herbal remedies and nutritional supplements.

You start by adding those vitamins and minerals uniquely suited to the menopause, so you check out **Chapter 23: Vitamins and Minerals.** You decide to begin an iron-free multivitamin-multimineral supplement along with extra calcium, Vitamin D, and magnesium, in an effort to prevent osteoporosis in your later years.

Then you become interested in trying to prevent cataracts and age-related macular degeneration ten or twenty years down the road, so you read about *lutein* and *zeaxanthin* in **Chapter 24: Antioxidant Phytochemicals.** You pay strict attention to the **Guidelines for Consulting Your Health Care Provider,** found at the end of both those chapters.

Even though your hot flashes, night sweats, and difficulties sleeping have been decreased, they have not been eliminated. So, you decide to read about *Black Cohosh* in **Chapter 21: Herbal Remedies for Women's Health.** While reading that chapter, you resolve to eat *soy*-based foods two or three times a week. You pay attention to the side effects and interactions of *Black Cohosh* and *Soy* found in those sections. You check out the **Guidelines for Consulting Your Health Care Provider,** found at the end of that chapter.

The last step before you order nutritional supplements and herbal remedies is to call your gynecologist and ask her whether she has any objections.

You realize you've gained ten pounds since beginning the menopause, so you read the *Introduction* to **Chapter 26: Nutritional Supplements for Healthy Weight Control**. The advice on diet and exercise prepares you to make some changes in lifestyle to follow the **good health practices**, that you've been thinking about for awhile to help your whole family become healthier. You realize that it doesn't make good sense to begin nutritional supplements for your weight problem before making some important changes, like cutting out white flour and added sugar. And you resolve to stop eating fast foods as much as possible. In fact, you will stop buying prepared foods so you can monitor the salt content in the foods you and your family consume.

This leads you to realize that in the months and years ahead you will need to be making more lifestyle changes, in the hopes of preventing the onset of chronic, relapsing destructive diseases like diabetes, cardiovascular disease, cancer, and arthritis.

You look back on your journey into menopause so far with satisfaction. You've taken some important first steps towards good health for yourself and your family. Your health and sense of well-being have improved. Your confidence in the future has increased. You've helped your whole family in its quest towards healthy living. And best of all, you're in charge of your health and yourself.

PART ONE

Homeopathic Remedies

Chapter 2

Basic Homeopathy

This Book in General

Reading and "digesting" this chapter will give you an understanding of homeopathy and how it does its healing work in the human body. But, in order to learn how to use homeopathic remedies, it is not essential that you read it first, or ever, unless you find it difficult to use remedies that you do not understand. If you prefer to understand the medical system that brings you and your family healing remedies, then go ahead and read this chapter.

Or you may start by first giving a remedy recommended in this book and then becoming astonished at its gentle, curative powers, only to then become motivated to find out more about homeopathy. Then you may wish to read this chapter.

This chapter is an introduction to the entire field of homeopathy. You do not have to read the whole chapter at one time. You can choose the parts which pertain to the questions you are trying to answer or the ailment you are trying to treat, and come back to the rest at another time.

If after reading this chapter, you prefer to work with a homeopath, please visit www.homeopathyusa.org/onlinedirectory or www.nationalcenterforhomeopathy.org to search for a practitioner near you.

What is homeopathy?

Homeopathy is a whole system of medicine. Other whole systems of medicine include Ayurvedic medicine, Traditional Chinese medicine, and Western medicine. Homeopathy is an alternative to Western medicine. Homeopathy employs very, very dilute amounts of natural substances from plants, animals, and minerals, to stimulate the sick person's body to overcome his or her own illness. In contrast, Western medicine employs very, very concentrated amounts of either natural or synthetic substances to counteract a sick person's illness. For more differences between homeopathy and Western medicine, please see **Homeopathy vs. Western medicine** at the end of this chapter.

How did homeopathy get started?

Homeopathy was discovered by Dr. Samuel Hahnemann, a German physician, chemist, linguist, and translator of medical works. He was born in 1755 and died in 1843. Most homeopathic physicians consider him to be a genius. He rejected the medical therapies of his day, such as bloodletting (using leeches) and purging, believing them to cause the sick person to become even sicker, either in the short or long run.

Today, we know that he was right.

Instead, he developed the revolutionary idea that:

> If a healthy person takes an undiluted full-strength substance into his body, that substance can cause a whole complex of symptoms.
>
> If a sick person takes that same substance into his body in very, very, very dilute amounts, then that form of the substance can cure those same symptoms.
>
> The diluted form of a substance cures the same symptoms that the undiluted form causes.

The Law of Similars

That is what is called the **Law of Similars**. It is the first and foremost principle upon which homeopathy is based. The principle is sometimes called Like Cures Like, or in Latin, Similia Similibus Curantur.

It's a good idea to go back to the definition of the first principle of homeopathy, the **Law of Similars**, and read it again and again, until you understand it. The idea may sound so peculiar to people steeped in Western medicine, that it may be difficult to grasp at first.

If the **Law of Similars** is starting to sound to you like the principle of immunization, then you've caught on. The principle of Like Cures Like is a difficult concept to absorb, but once you see its similarities to immunization, you'll be able to better understand the rest of the chapter. Although homeopathy and immunization are not exactly the same, they are similar, and you can understand homeopathy if you keep in mind what you know about immunizations.

Interesting Note:
The word "**homeopathy**" is derived from the Greek roots, **homeo** meaning the same, and **pathy** meaning treatment of. Western medicine doctors practice **allopathy**, which comes from the Greek roots, **allo** meaning other, and **pathy** meaning treatment of.

Interesting Note:
Dr. Samuel Hahnemann wrote six editions of *The Organon of Medicine*, which are still considered the homeopath's most treasured books. In it, he expounds upon his philosophy of homeopathic diagnosis and treatment. The sixth edition was completed in 1842, just one year before he died, but it was not published until 1920.

How to distinguish herbal medicine from homeopathy: Here we should note three profound differences between herbal medicine and homeopathy that will help you to distinguish one from the other.

The first difference is that herbal medicine uses undiluted natural plants as medicines, which can have side effects just like Western medicines. Homeopathy uses only extremely dilute natural substances, which do not have side effects and are safe for all people, even including pregnant women, newborn babies, and the very elderly.

The second difference is that herbal remedies use only plant substances whereas homeopathic remedies use materials from all three kingdoms, plant, animal, and mineral.

The third difference is that herbal remedies are prescribed on the basis of Western medicine principles, for example, using an anti-diarrheal herbal remedy to treat diarrhea. Homeopathic remedies are prescribed on the basis of the principle of Like Cures Like, for example, using an extremely dilute remedy that would cause diarrhea (if given in full strength) to treat diarrhea.

We will learn about homeopathy and herbal medicines in this book because in order to be able to take care of yourself and your family, you will need to know how and when to use remedies in both systems of medicine, along with nutritional supplements.

An illustration of the principle of Like Cures Like: What does your baby's pediatrician tell you to do when you suspect your baby swallowed something toxic that she shouldn't have eaten?

Your pediatrician may tell you to give your baby a dose of full strength *Ipecac*, a natural plant called *Ipecacuanha* that causes vomiting. Within about twenty minutes of taking Ipecac, your baby will vomit, probably several times, thereby emptying her stomach almost completely, which can save her life.

Homeopaths often prescribe homeopathic *Ipecac* in extremely dilute amounts to **treat** vomiting. In homeopathy, what causes vomiting can be used to treat vomiting. Homeopaths use *Ipecac* to treat vomiting from many causes: morning sickness, motion sickness, vertigo, and others.

The Law of Potency

Another principle upon which homeopathy is based is the **Law of Potency**. This states that the more a substance is diluted, the *greater* is the potency. In different words, the remedy actually becomes stronger the more dilute it is. Yes, less is more in homeopathy. This is counterintuitive to people whose frame of reference is Western medicine where more is more.

How are homeopathic remedies prepared?

Homeopathic remedies are prepared by homeopathic pharmaceutical companies according to rigorous standards. The first step is the extraction of the substance, either plant, animal, or mineral, by alcohol. This is called the **Mother Tincture**, meaning it is undiluted. The undiluted substance is usually toxic if taken internally.

Then one drop of the Mother Tincture is diluted with 99 drops of double-distilled-purified water. This is the first dilution. The substance has been diluted to 10^2, which means it has been diluted 100 times. This is called 1C, or the first centesimal potency.

Now comes the most important step. It is the step that probably gives homeopathic remedies their unusually strong yet gentle power in the human body. The process is called **succussion**. It means that the newly diluted solution is energetically shaken by a machine or by hand in a certain standardized manner. Succussion actually potentiates the action of the substance so that this step is called **potentization**.

To make the second dilution we take one drop of the first dilution with 99 drops of double-distilled-purified water. Now the original substance has been diluted to 10^4, which means it has been diluted 10,000 times. This is called 2C, or the second centesimal potency. Now, the machine performs the all-important succussion in exactly the same manner as before.

The same procedure is repeated until the desired potency is achieved. Many homeopaths prescribe remedies in the 12C, 30C or 200C potency. This means that the Mother Tincture has been diluted to 10^{24}, or 10^{60}, or 10^{400}, respectively. To get an idea of how dilute 200C (a very commonly used potency) is, it would mean that the Mother Tincture has been diluted to ten with 399 zeros!

This is so dilute that it is statistically impossible that any, not even one, molecule is left from the original Mother Tincture. How can this be? Then how does homeopathy work? We will attempt to answer this question in the section called, **the physics of water**. In the meantime, let us first talk about molecules and Avogadro's number.

The big sticking point: Avogadro's number

Avogadro's number is 6.02×10^{23}. That is the number of molecules that would be found in one mole of any substance. This is hard to understand if you don't remember basic chemistry. But, it essentially means that if something is diluted above 10^{23} (this corresponds to 12C, a rather low potency in homeopathy) then statistically speaking, no atoms of the original substance are likely to be left.

This is the big sticking point with Western med-

icine doctors. This is the main reason why conventional doctors find it difficult to accept homeopathy. Many doctors of Western medicine cannot conceptualize how a substance diluted beyond Avogadro's number can have any power in the human body beyond placebo. After all, they say, there are no atoms left to perform the chemical work of healing.

Homeopathy has long recognized this point. Homeopaths have been able to make the leap from an atomic explanation of how chemicals work to an energy explanation of how homeopathic remedies work. And this explanation involves the **physics of water**.

Interesting Note:
Homeopathic medical research has proven beyond a shadow of a doubt that when homeopathic remedies and placebos* are compared, homeopathic remedies are more effective against diseases than placebo. This means that homeopathic remedies cause a real and measurable effect in the human body. This medical research has been published in peer-reviewed mainstream medical journals like *British Medical Journal* and *The Lancet* and *Pediatrics*. But no one has yet proven *how* homeopathic remedies actually work in the body, although we think we may be on the right track by trying to understand the physics of water.

*A placebo is a dummy medicine that is usually simply lactose, milk sugar, with no active ingredients in it.

The physics of water

What is it?
The human body is composed mostly of it. It bathes every cell in the body. There are thousands more molecules of it than there are of protein in the human body. It is essential for life on our planet. It is of course, **water**, perhaps the most important biological molecule on our planet.

As important as water is, we know comparatively little about it, from a physical-chemical point of view. Physical chemists, on the cutting edge of physics research, are just now researching the properties of water. One of those properties is the "**memory of water.**"

When a substance is dissolved in water, it makes an electromagnetic "imprint" on the water molecules. No two substances make the same imprint. Basically, every substance has an energy signature in the form of a specific energy radiation, called electromagnetic radiation, created by the electrons in the molecule. This energy signature is transferred to the water molecules, which in turn transmits that exact energy signature to every cell in the body, because, as you remember, water bathes every cell, thereby communicating in electrical-chemical terms the energy information of that substance. Water molecules "remember" the unique energy signature that has been impressed upon it. No wonder homeopathy can effect such deep healing! Researchers theorize that is what may happen with homeopathic dilutions above Avogadro's number.

Interesting Note:
Water, H_2O, is the most common liquid on earth and one of the commonest compounds in the universe, but it behaves in notoriously peculiar ways (at certain limits of density and temperature and diffusivity). The properties of water are not as yet understood by earthling scientists. Understanding the arrangement of molecules in water, the structure of water, may explain the relationship between structure and behavior. Thus, we may come closer to understanding how homeopathic dilutions behave in a water medium.

For more information:
www.digibio.com

The Provings

When homeopaths want to know what a plant, animal, or mineral substance can cure, they first find out what that substance can cause, if given full-strength to healthy persons. This is called a **proving**.

All the information of all the provings are gathered together into a book called the **Materia Medica**. This is a listing of what each substance can cause (and thereby cure). The listing for each substance is categorized in a standardized form, according to the various parts of the body. The mind is the first section in every Materia Medica, because in homeopathy, the mind is considered a part of the body. This is why homeopathy is considered to be a "**holistic**" system of medicine. Homeopathy does not separate the mind from the physical body, something that Western medicine does do.

Most of our information from provings was systematically catalogued many years ago with the provings of the great homeopaths of the 19th and early 20th centuries. However, provings are still going on today with new substances entering our Materia Medica all the time.

The first proving was accomplished by Dr. Samuel Hahnemann in 1790. Dr. Hahnemann was working as a translator at that time, translating a popular medical book by Dr. William Cullen into German. While translating, he noted that Dr. Cullen stated that quinine (a substance that came from the bark of the cinchona tree) worked to treat malaria because of its astringent properties. Dr. Hahnemann's chemistry training did not allow him to overlook this incongruity. After all, many other substances had even greater astringent properties and were not recommended as treatments for malaria. Therefore, there had to be something else at work.

Dr. Hahnemann took a dose of quinine and recorded every symptom that he experienced in the most minute detail. He realized that he was developing symptoms of malaria! He would develop the malaria symptoms whenever he took a dose of quinine. He grasped the revolutionary idea that quinine caused the symptoms it could cure. In that moment, he created a new system of medicine.

Since the first proving, homeopaths have collected and collated information from provings on approximately 3,000 substances. For each substance, the proving gives a "picture" of the remedy, or a compilation of all the physical, emotional, mental (sometimes called intellectual), sexual, and spiritual symptoms that that substance can cause, and therefore, when transformed into a remedy, can cure.

The Vital Force

In homeopathy, the force of life that is within every biological organism, residing within every living cell, is known as the **Vital Force**. It is an ancient concept that has had many names throughout the ages. The Chinese call it Chi or Qi. The Hindu name for it is Prana. The Hebrew word is Ruach. The Christian word is Soul or Spirit. It is that force which pushes living organisms towards life and towards health. It is the force that supports self-healing.

The Vital Force is that energy in every living cell that homeopathic remedies effect. The homeopathic remedy stimulates the Vital Force in every cell to produce a generalized healing effect throughout the entire organism so that the body, in essence, heals itself. This is how the sick person overcomes his or her own illness once the proper homeopathic remedy is taken internally.

> **Note:** To help you gain a deeper grounding in homeopathy and a better understanding of its philosophy, you may want to explore some of the books on homeopathy in the **Appendix** as well as some of the articles at the following websites:
> www.homeoint.org is the French Homeopathe Internationale (choose the English language option)
> www.homeopathyhome.com
> www.simillimum.com
> www.simillibus.com
>
> Free online courses in homeopathy are available at:
> www.homeopathyworld.com
> www.hpathy.com
> www.1800homeopathy.com
> www.homeopathyworks.com
> These sites will help you learn the basics of self-care with homeopathy.

The best way for an individual to support homeopathy is to become a member of the *National Center for Homeopathy (NCH)* at www.nationalcenterforhomeopathy.org. The *NCH* monthly magazine, *Homeopathy Today*, is worth the $55 it costs per year to be a member. The *NCH* advocates on behalf of homeopathy. And subscribe to homeopathy's e-magazine www.hpathy.com.

The elements of the homeopathic interview

Homeopathy unites all the aspects of the self: the physical, emotional, mental (intellectual), sexual, and spiritual parts of a person. The homeopath needs to understand all those parts of a person in order to prescribe homeopathic remedies for serious, chronic, relapsing ailments, such as emotional disorders, heart ailments such as hypertension (high blood pressure), diabetes, arthritis, and many others. Homeopathic prescribing for this level of seriousness is generally best done by a homeopath. But, you may attempt a homeopathic prescription for yourself or for a family member even for serious ailments, as long as you follow the **Guidelines for Consulting Your Health Care Provider** at the end of every chapter.

> *Internet Resources:*
> You may investigate the database of the *National Center for Homeopathy (NCH)* online directory at www.nationalcenterforhomeopathy.org for a listing of practitioners.
>
> The *NCH* online site can also help you locate other learning activities, participate in Chat rooms, and otherwise get involved in homeopathy, the world's gentlest medicine. Become a member and get the monthly *Homeopathy Today*, geared to beginners in homeopathy and clinicians alike.
>
> You may explore the *American Institute of Homeopathy*'s listing of MD homeopaths at www.homeopathyusa.org.

You will find more web addresses for important homeopathic organizations under **Homeopathy Internet Resources** in the **Appendix**.

There is much that you can do with homeopathy for yourself and for your family, to prevent and even to treat serious disorders. The mission of this book is to teach you how. The most important thing you have to know is when to consult with your health care provider. You should follow the **Guidelines for Consulting Your Health Care Provider**, found at the end of every chapter.

During the homeopathic interview the patient has the opportunity to express in his or her own words the entire complex of symptoms for which he or she is seeking help. The homeopath tries to understand every facet of every symptom. The homeopath will usually leave ample time for this exercise because the prescription of the **simillimum** is based upon this interview.

The **simillimum** is the "most similar" remedy that most closely fits the entire complex of symptoms that the patient expresses to the doctor. You already understand that the homeopath chooses a remedy that causes these same symptoms (if given undiluted) and therefore, that cures these symptoms (if given as a very, very, very diluted homeopathic remedy).

Remember that different people with the same disease may each receive a different homeopathic remedy because the totality of each person's symptoms is unique to that person. Finding the homeopathic remedy that "covers" the totality of a person's symptoms is called finding the **simillimum**.

How does the homeopath choose the remedy?

First the homeopath orders the symptoms into a prioritized listing, according to which she considers most important, which is second, etc. Then she consults a book (or software program) called a **Repertory**. The **Repertory** is an index of symptoms listing the remedies that have been documented during a proving to cause those symptoms. It is

organized in the same manner as the **Materia Medica**, that is, along the same body-part subdivisions. This is the procedure that the homeopath follows to discover the patient's simillimum.

Interesting Note:
Homeopaths have developed their body of evidence about each substance not only from provings but also from clinical observations on persons who suffered toxic reactions to substances.

For example, homeopaths learned much about the curative properties of mercury during the days when Western physicians prescribed mercury to treat syphilis. They observed the toxic effects of undiluted mercury on the human body and this gave them the understanding of what homeopathic dilutions of mercury can cure.

Interesting Note:
The listings in the **Materia Medica** are by remedy whereas the listings in the **Repertory** are by symptom. Both books are subdivided by body-part.

A homeopath will look up a substance (remedy) in the **Materia Medica** (see page 23). She will look up a symptom in the **Repertory** (see page 24).

Important Note:
It is not possible in homeopathy to give "Remedy X" for "Disease Y," as is the standard procedure in Western medicine. Homeopathy must individualize treatment because every person is unique.

Modalities

Part of the Homeopathic Interview consists of questions about those factors that make a patient feel better or worse. Something that causes a patient to feel better or worse is called a **modality**. It is something that modulates the intensity or frequency of a symptom.

ARSENICUM SULPHURATUM RUBRUM   (ARS-S-R.)
no Unique remedy rubic,   11 Common rubrics
COMMON RUBRICS
Activity[54] [124] coff.[5] iod.[5] lach.[5] op.[5] phos.[5] stann.[5] valer.[5]
    increased excessively[54] [16] *bell.*[54] *cinnb.*[54] *coff-t.*[54] coff.[54] op.[54] *phos.*[54]
Dreams; vivid[54] [198]
Fear; death, of[54] [152]   ACON.[122] ARS.[122]
Irritability[54] [441]
Morose, cross fretful, ill-humor, peevish[54] [332]
Restlessness, nervousness; heat; with[58] [71]   ars. puls. rhus-t.
Sadness, despondency, dejection, mental depression, gloom, melancholy[54] [499]
Smiling[38] [15]   hyos.[54] *verat.*[54]
Talk, talking, talks; indisposed to, desire to be silent, taciturn[54] [251]   NUX-V.[122]
Work; aversion to mental; eating, after[54]   anac.[36] dig.[36]

ARSENICUM ALBUM   (ARS.)
146 Unique remedy rubrics, 1121 Common rubrics
UNIQUE REMEDY RUBRICS
Anger, irascibility; eat, when obliged to[1]
    himself, with; day, all[54]
    recovery, if one spoke of her complete[36]
Anguish; evening; pressing in head, during[36]
    constricted, as if everything became[36]
    indescribable; metritis, pericarditis, cholera asiatica, in[54]
    mania, during[36]
    palpitation, with; lie on back, cannot, agg. ascending stairs[54]
    respiration, preventing[36]
    tossing about, with; catarrh of chest, in[54]
Anxiety; night; rheumatism, with[54]
    midnight; after; one am.; until two am.[58]
    continued, in anasarca[54]
    expected of him, when anything is
    health, about; despair of getting well[54]
    hypochondriacal; originate in upper part of chest, seems to[54]
    murdered someone, as if he had; mania, in[54]
    nausea; with; weakness, and, recurring periodically[102]
    others, for; some persons, about[36]
    paroxysms, attacks of; night agg.[54]
    stomach; in; night, rising upwards
        periodically, returns with weakness[102]
    suffocation, with[54]
    swelling of; skin, dropsy, with[54]
    syncope, with[10]
Aversion; persons, to; those around
Biting; tumblers, edge of, when trying to drink[36]
Carried; desires to be; fast; dentition, during[102]
Company; aversion to, agg.; friends, of intimate; offended them, while he thinks he has
    desire for; dysmenorrhea, in, after vexation[54]
Complaining; pitiful[54]
Conversation; aversion to; morning, in bed[36]

The Complete Materia Medica Mind©   201, with permission

Heli O. Retzek, *The Complete Materia Medica Mind*, based on Roger van Zandvoort's *The Complete Repertory Mind*, The Netherlands: Institute for Research in Homeopathic Information and Symptomatology, 1995, page 201.

MIND

ANXIETY; night; agg. (cont.)
  pulsating in chest, from undulating: aster.
  remain in bed, cannot: rhus-t.
  rheumatism, with: *ars*.
  starting out of sleep, on: samb.
  storm, during: nat-m.
  typhoid, in: *canth*.
  visions, with frightful: *camph*.
  waking [G4]: aesc. alum. arg-n. ars. carb-v.
    carbn-o. caust. chel. chin. cina con. dros.
    graph. kali-ar. kali-s. lac-ac. lyc. nat-c.
    nat-m. nit-ac. phos. plat. psor. puls. rat.
    sep. sil. sulph. zinc.
  and on [K5, S1-61, G4]: *aesc. alum.* arg-n. *ars*.
    carb-v. carbn-o. chel. *cina* con. *dros*. graph.
    kali-ar. kali-s. lac-ac. lyc. nat-c. *nat-m*.
    nit-ac. *phos*. plat. psor. *puls*. rat. sep. sil.
    SULPH. zinc.
  heat, with: *sulph*.
  every two or three hours: nat-m.
  frightful dreams, from: chin.
  amel. [S1-60]: quas.
midnight:
  before [K5, S1-61, G4]: am-c. ambr. androc. ars.
    bar-c. bar-s. bor. *bry. carb-v. carbn-s*.
    caust. cocc. ferr. gels. *graph. hep*. kali-c.
    laur. *lyc. mag-c*. mag-m. merc. *mur-ac*.
    nat-c. *nat-m*. nat-p. nat-s. nat-sil. nux-v.
    phos. *puls*. ruta sabin. sil. stront-c. *sulph*.
    tub. verat.
  10 P.M.:
    lying down, after: hep.
    until midnight: androc.
  11 P.M. [K5, S1-61, G4]: bor. ruta
  sleep, in: merc.
  waking, on [S1-61]: caust. sil.
    amel. on rising [K5, S1-61, G4]: caust. sil.
  about: sil. tub.
    rising, on, amel.: sil.
    waking, on: sil.
  after [K5, S1-61, G4]: acon. alum. ant-c. **ARS**. calc.
    camph. carb-an. cast. *cench*. chin. coc-c.
    colch. con. dulc. graph. hep. ign. lyc.
    m-arct. mang. nat-m. **NUX-V**. ph-ac.
    psor. quas. rat. *rhus-t*. sil. **SPONG**.
    squil. verat.
  1 A.M.:
    waking, on: quas. squil.
    2 A.M., until: ars.
    3 A.M., until [K5, S1-62, G4]: hep.
  2 a.m. [K5, S1-62, G4]: carb-an. chin. coc-c.
    graph. nat-m.
    until [K5, S1-62, G4]: carb-an.

    4 A.M., until [S1-62]: COC-C.
  3 A.M. [K5, S1-62, G4]: acon. ant-c. **ARS**. camph.
    rhus-t. sil. verat.
    after [K5, S1-62, G4]: *ars*. rhus-t.verat.
    5 A.M., until [S1-62, G4]: ant-c.
  4 A.M. [K5, S1-62, G4]: alum. *coc-c*.
  5 A.M. [S1-62]: nat-m. **psor**.
    5 P.M., until: psor.
  waking, on [S1-62, G4]: calc. con. ign. lyc. ph-ac.
    half waking, on [S1-62, G4]: con.
abdomen:
  arising from [K43, G34]: asaf. dig.
  in [K541, S1-477, G461]: acon. agar. aloe alum.
    am-m. ambr. anac. androc. ant-c.
    ANT-T. apoc. argn-n. arn. **ARS**. ars-s-f.
    asaf. aur. bar-c. bell. bry. calc. calc-p.
    calen. carb-an. carb-v. carl. cast-eq.
    cham. colch. con. **CUPR**. dig. dios. dros.
    euph. gran. grat. hydr. ign. inul. *kali-c*.
    lach. laur. lept. lyc. mag-m. mag-p.
    merc. merc-c. *mez. mosch*. mur-ac. naja
    nat-m. nat-p. nit-ac. nux-v. olnd. ozone
    petr. ph-ac. phel. phos. pic-ac. plat. plb.
    podo. rhod. rhus-t. seneg. sep. spig.
    squil. staph. stram. sul-ac. *sulph. tarent*.
    thuj. tub. verat. vesp.
    • ABDOMEN; Anxiety • ABDOMEN; Ap-
    prehension
  morning [K541, G461]: ign. nat-m. sul-ac.
    bed, in [K541, G461]: sul-ac.
    breakfast, after [K541, G461]: *ign*.
  forenoon: cast-eq.
  evening [K541, G461]: cham. tarent.
  night [K541, G461]: nit-ac.
  adhere to chest, as if abdomen would: mez.
  burst, as if it would, amel. during sleep:
    am-m.
  colic, with, in children: *calc-p*.
  convulsive, spasmodic, contracting, cutting:
    plb.
  cramp, as from: lyc.
  distension in, with [S1-62, G4]: mag-m.
  eating, after [G461]: bar-c.
  flatus amel. [K541, G461]: mur-ac.
  griping, as if intestines would be constricted:
    spig.
  pain in, with: *cham*. mag-p.
  puffed, after parturition: *ambr*.
  restlessness, with anxious: alum.
  rigid, as if would become: *mez*.
  stool:
  agg.:
    before [K541, G461]: calc. merc.

24, with permission

Roger van Zandvoort, *The Complete Repertory Mind-Generalities*, The Netherlands:
Institute for Research in Homeopathic Information and Symptomatology, 1994, page 24.

Dimensions of a symptom

The homeopath is searching for striking or singular symptoms in her patient. This is what leads the homeopath to the proper prescription. One of the ways a homeopath proceeds is to ask questions about the four dimensions of every symptom.

The four **dimensions of a symptom** are:
1) The "which" type modalities which describe **sensations**, or which type of pain (such as a migraine headache that is throbbing or pressing).
2) The "where and when" type modalities which describe the **location and timing** of the symptom (such as a migraine headache on the right side above the eye and that appears at 4 o'clock every day).
3) The "what else" type modalities which describe **concomitants**, or other symptoms that accompany the main symptoms (such as a migraine headache coming on after vomiting)
4) The modalities which describe any factor that makes the symptom either **better or worse**, amelioration or aggravation, (such as light having an aggravating effect on a migraine headache).

> *Let's take a look at that patient who has a migraine headache:*
> If that patient were to consult her Western medicine health care practitioner, it would be unlikely that the doctor would be interested in this degree of detail.
> After all, in Western medicine, migraine headaches are migraine headaches and they are all treated with the same medicines. Individuality of symptom expression does not matter because in this system of medicine, it does not exist.
> But if that patient were to consult her homeopathy practitioner, it would be essential that she describe her migraine headache in great detail. Each patient's migraine headache is different, unique. The difference is what counts in homeopathy.

In homeopathy, it is essential to grasp each person's individual expression of symptoms.

In homeopathy, each person expresses his or her disease in a unique way.

In homeopathy, the best remedy to fit each person's expression of his or her illness is sought. It might be any of the more than 3,000 remedies in the **Materia Medica**.

In homeopathy, the person's unique expression of disease determines the remedy.

Keynotes

A homeopathic remedy usually has certain characteristic symptoms associated with it that determine its use. When a patient describes those very characteristic symptoms, "**keynote**" symptoms, he is actually pointing the homeopath towards prescribing the remedy that fits those "**keynote**" symptoms.

> *For example:*
> A sick person comes to the homeopath and describes hot, burning pains in his feet, which are worse from 4 a.m. until 8 a.m. The patient goes on to describe his tendency to have skin rashes that are worse with bathing in hot water. These symptoms are the **keynotes** of the homeopathic remedy, *Sulphur*, which we will study in greater detail in **Chapter 18: Homeopathic Constitutional Remedies**. These characteristic **keynote** symptoms may lead the homeopath to prescribe *Sulphur*.

Polychrests

Some homeopathic remedies have been found during the provings to have an effect on every (or almost every) tissue of the body. These remedies are called "**polychrests**" (an alternative spelling is "**polycrest**"). They are the broad-spectrum remedies that have multiple uses and many pronounced **keynotes**.

Note: We will study most of the important polychrests in **Chapter 18: Homeopathic Constitutional Remedies**, **Chapter 8: Homeopathic Remedies for Emotional Problems** and **Chapter 9: Homeopathic Remedies for Constitutional Problems in Infants, Children and Adolescents**.

Polychrest remedies tend to be used as **constitutional** remedies for chronic, relapsing conditions. A constitutional remedy is one that treats a person's distinguishing features, the person's total being, welding together the physical, emotional, mental (intellectual), sexual, and spiritual realms. It is often contrasted with an **acute** remedy, which treats a minor part of a person's total being, such as a muscle ache or an earache. For more information please see **Acute prescribing vs. constitutional prescribing**.

Kingdoms

All homeopathic remedies are members of one of the three kingdoms: Plants (by far the most numerous), Animal (by far the least numerous), and Mineral (an intermediate number). All plants have been categorized into botanical families. Categorizing remedies into Kingdoms and Families helps us to see patterns within our **Materia Medica**. Plant remedies that are members of the same botanical family may have similar homeopathic effects in the body.

Miasms

Remedies tend to fall into classes called **miasms**. A miasm is a disease predisposition, a tendency to fall ill with a certain constellation of symptoms. Most miasms are genetic or familial, which is why homeopaths ask questions about patients' family histories.

A person who always breaks out into skin rashes after a particularly stressful day at work is said to belong to a specific miasm. That person would likely require a constitutional remedy that is associated with that particular miasm. When the homeopath wants a deeper understanding of her patient, she will often try to understand the miasm to which her patient belongs. This level of understanding often helps to determine the proper remedy for the patient. When homeopaths treat on a miasmatic basis they give their patients the opportunity to heal on the deepest level possible. Indeed, taking the miasmatic remedy may prevent those miasmatic diseases that would have been expected by inheritance.

Interesting Note:
Homeopathy has the ability to overcome a deep-seated miasm that has plagued a patient for decades. Its powerful remedies have the ability to overcome even genetic factors. The genetic factors that can be overcome are those that are modifiable by changing one's lifestyle, such as an inherited tendency towards obesity. Homeopathy can help a person overcome obesity, even on a genetic basis, provided he makes the crucial lifestyle changes in nutrition and physical exercise.

Genetic diseases that are not modifiable, such as cystic fibrosis or sickle cell anemia, will not be changed by homeopathy. However, the onerous complications of such genetic diseases can be helped with homeopathy.

Homeopaths often disagree on the existence of certain miasms especially those that have been proposed in recent years. However, homeopaths agree on the existence of the four miasms, three of which were described by Dr. Samuel Hahnemann.

Homeopathic Miasm Formulas are available from *Professional Complementary Health Formulas, Inc.* However, you will need your homeopath to diagnose your particular miasm and to order your *Miasm Formula* for you.

Homeopathy is moving towards a fuller understanding of miasms of which a total of nine have been described so far. When you master the theory and practice of homeopathy in this book, then I recommend that you advance to the study of miasms.

The **Table of Miasm**s gives you the names of the more common Miasms, the General Condition that they signify, and the organs most commonly affected.

Table of Miasms

Miasm	General Condition	Organs involved
Psora	Deficiency	Intestines, skin
Sycosis	Excess, growths	Genitalia, warts, kidney, liver, lung, heart, blood
Syphilinum (Luetic)	Ulceration, destruction	Brain, spine, peripheral nerves, teeth, bone
Tuberculinism	Reduction, discharges	Muscles, bone, lung
Carcinosin	Growths with destruction	Organs in Sycosis and Syphilis combined

Begin by reading some books on homeopathy that particularly interest you. You will find a listing of recommended books in **Book Resources for Homeopathy**, in the **Appendix**. The first step is calling or emailing to order a catalogue from *Homeopathic Educational Services*, or *Homeopathy for Health* or *WholeHealthNow*. You will be dazzled by the number and quality of books, tapes, software, and homeopathic products. For specific information on miasms you may visit www.radicalhealing.com.

Different forms of homeopathy

Homeopathy may be practiced in different ways. In "**classical homeopathy**" the homeopath determines, based upon the extensive and intensive homeopathic interview, which **single remedy** best fits the totality of the patient's symptoms. The homeopath tries to determine the simillimum. Classical homeopathy often follows **constitutional prescribing**, meaning that the remedy, most often a polychrest, suits a patient because the patient falls into a certain constitutional type that is best expressed by a certain remedy.

One of the joys of homeopathy is coming to understand your own and your close family members' constitutional types. Once you are able to do so, you will have a powerful tool, the constitutional remedy, at your disposal to help both prevent and treat many ailments that beset people as they go through life. Usually, constitutional prescribing will be in the higher potencies, 200C and higher. Remember that with homeopathic remedies, the more dilute they are, the more powerful. Constitutional prescribing with single remedies in high potency is most often appropriate for chronic, relapsing conditions.

However, single remedies can sometimes be used for acute ailments as well. Sometimes a single-remedy is known to affect a certain condition and does not require an extensive homeopathic interview to match the patient's entire picture to the remedy. This time, prescribing single remedies in homeopathy is much like prescribing a drug in Western medicine. Single remedy prescribing is effective for many conditions in homeopathy, for example, *Cantharis* for bladder infections (cystitis), *Aconite* for fear and anxiety, and *Rhus toxicodendron* for arthritic aches and pains. We will learn about many single remedies in the following chapters. I hope you will begin to feel comfortable using certain single remedies for specific ailments for yourself and for your family members.

At the same time, you will learn about **combination remedie**s. In **combination homeopathy**, several homeopathic remedies, in lower potencies, usually ranging from 2X to 6C, are combined into one solution. It is the shotgun approach to healing, and it is often successful. Combination remedies usually treat acute, self-limited conditions. They usually have names like *Earache*, or *Fever*, or *Cough*, or *Teething*. These remedies are suitable for you to learn about and have on hand in case you need a gentle, harmless approach to a non-life-threatening ailment for yourself or a family member. It is highly unlikely that a combination remedy will have any side effects whatsoever. It is also unlikely that a homeopathic aggravation, also called a healing crisis, will occur when using a combination remedy.

That is because the potencies of the individual remedies are too low to cause an aggravation.

> **Note:** You may want to order a catalogue of homeopathic combination remedies from King Bio, Washington Homeopathic Products, and Hyland's. You'll find their listings under **Homeopathic Remedies Supply Houses** in the **Appendix**.

Single acute remedies and combination remedies are short cuts in homeopathy which are utilized in the hopes that the time-consuming homeopathic interview may be eliminated (along with the homeopath!). Using single acute remedies and combination remedies are safe and often effective.

It is my hope that while using this book as your primary resource, you will become proficient in using both single and combination homeopathic remedies. There is much that you can do with homeopathy for yourself and for your family, to prevent and even to treat both minor and serious disorders. The mission of this book is to teach you how. The most important thing you have to know is when to consult with your health care provider. You should follow the **Guidelines for Consulting Your Health Care Provider**, found at the end of every chapter.

Acute prescribing vs. constitutional prescribing

Matching the totality of an individual to the proper remedy is called constitutional prescribing. It is generally used for severe, serious, chronic, relapsing conditions. The disease conditions treated by constitutional prescribing generally require a MD or DO physician in order to make the correct **diagnosis** of the disease. Making the correct diagnosis is step one in both systems of medicine, homeopathy and Western.

Once you have a definite diagnosis, you may consult with a homeopath for treatment options, or depending on the nature of the diagnosis, you may choose to try homeopathic treatment yourself.

Once the diagnosis is made, it is your choice how to treat it. You may choose to integrate both Western medicines and alternative modalities like homeopathy, herbal remedies, and nutritional supplements. Or you may choose to use only one system of medicine. The choice is yours. However, whatever your choice, always remember to consult and follow the **Guidelines for Consulting Your Health Care Provider**, at the end of every chapter.

Acute prescribing matches the disease or condition to a remedy. This is reminiscent of the way Western medicine physicians choose a drug. Acute prescribing is generally used for acute, self-limited conditions that are not chronic or recurring. These conditions often do not require a MD or DO physician to diagnose or prescribe treatment. The trick is to follow the **Guidelines for Consulting Your Health Care Provider**, at the end of every chapter.

Detoxification The Gentle Way

Homeopathy is the gentle and yet effective way to achieve detoxification from environmental poisons, such as pesticides, herbicides, insecticides, fungicides, pollutants, nicotine addiction, substances of abuse, alcohol addiction, and prescription pharmaceuticals.

> **Note:** Please do not consider other methods of detoxification, such as fasting, purging, chelation or colonic irrigation. These methods are likely to be harmful, dangerous, and invasive. They surely are unnatural and they all come with side effects. Homeopathic detoxification does not.

For detoxification purposes, you may want to consider the homeopathic combination remedy called *Ubichinon Compositum*, which is a manufactured by Heel, Inc., a homeopathic supply house.

> **Note:** You will find more information on *Ubichinon Compositum* in **Chapter 13: Homeopathy for Elderly Persons**.

Another homeopathic detoxification remedy is the *Detox-Kit*, also manufactured by Heel, Inc. It consists of 3 components, *Lymphomyosot, Berberis*

Homaccord and *Nux vomica Homaccord*, each in a 50 ml bottle. *Lymphomyosot* detoxifies the lymphatic system; *Berberis*, the excretory organs, specifically the kidneys, skin, and liver; and *Nux vomica*, the digestive system and liver. Thus, the *Detox-Kit* provides for the elimination of diverse toxins from most sources. The directions for use are to put 30 drops of each of the three solutions into one quart of water and drink it during the day.

Bach Flower Remedies

The homeopathic physician, Dr. Edward Bach, discovered what came to be called **Bach Flower Remedies**. The 38 flower remedies are made by extracting each blossom in water, thereby producing a flower essence. Flower remedies are not prepared by standardized homeopathic dilutions with potentization. Although flower remedies are often utilized by homeopaths, they are not, strictly speaking, homeopathic remedies. Other than one very specific flower remedy called *Rescue Remedy* (in liquid drops or spray and cream), I do not utilize *Bach Flower Remedies* in my practice of alternative medicine.

If you master the principles in this book, learning to use homeopathy, herbal remedies, and nutritional supplements, you may find that you do not need *Bach Flower Remedies* to prevent and treat most ailments. If you wish to learn about *Bach Flower Remedies* and how to use them to treat various ailments, I recommend that you investigate the *Rescue Remedy* website www.rescueremedy.com. As for books, I recommend reading *The Complete Book of Flower Essences* by Rhonda PallasDowney or *Rescue Remedy, the Healing Power of Bach Flower Rescue Remedy* by Gregory Vlamis.

Safety and effectiveness of homeopathic remedies

Homeopathic remedies are considered to be both safe (see *Interesting Note* below for more about safety) and effective (please see *Interesting Note* under **Avogadro's number** for more about the effectiveness of homeopathic remedies).

They do not have side effects the way Western drugs do. However, homeopathic remedies may cause what is called a "**homeopathic aggravation,**" also called a healing crisis. This is a short-lived, generally mild, aggravation in symptoms. The homeopath considers the homeopathic aggravation to be a sign that the correct remedy has been chosen. A homeopathic aggravation usually heralds a complete healing.

Interesting Note:
Homeopathic remedies come either in **C dilutions**, which are diluted a hundred-fold each time, or in **X dilutions** which are diluted ten-fold each time.* A homeopathic remedy whose potency is labeled as 30C has been diluted to 10^{60} whereas one whose potency is labeled as 30X has been diluted to 10^{30}.

Homeopathic remedies which are labeled as 6X (diluted to 10^6) or greater are considered to be safe for anyone to take, including pregnant and lactating women, and for all ages, including newborns and the very elderly. Remedies which are below the 3X potency may not be safe, and in fact may be toxic, because too much of the Mother Tincture may still be present.

> **Remember:** Many homeopathic remedies start out as toxic substances and become gentle healers through the processes of dilution and potentization.

> **Note:** *This is a good place to think about the similarities and differences between homeopathic remedies and immunizations.*

*Homeopathic remedies also come in **M and LM dilutions**, which are diluted 1000-50,000-fold each time. It is unlikely that you will use M or LM dilutions because their great potency generally requires the supervision of a professional homeopath.

Interesting Note:
The father of American Homeopathy, Dr. Constantine Hering, developed **Hering's Laws of Cure**. These laws dictate that healing begins with the current symptoms first, then going on to heal the deeper layers of illness as well. These deeper layers are present as a result of former ailments that were not treated successfully or were "suppressed" with conventional drugs. In addition, Hering's Laws of Cure tells homeopaths in what order to expect healing.

Potency and frequency

General guidelines to treat acute, self-limited ailments include treating with single homeopathic remedies at potencies of 15C or 30C. They may be administered every 1-2 hours, or more or less frequently depending on the severity of the acute situation. The potency is not as important as giving the correct remedy. So, if you have a certain indicated remedy at a 6C potency, but my recommendation calls for 30C, please go ahead and give the 6C, although you may have to give it more frequently.

When combination homeopathic remedies are used for acute conditions, the potencies of the contained remedies are usually in the very low potency range, from 2X to 6C. The combination remedy may be administered 3 or 4 times daily, or more or less often depending on the severity of the acute situation.

In general, when using the lower potencies, frequency of administration is not crucial. Lower potency remedies, such as 30C and below, are usually repeated often, every $\frac{1}{2}$ to 4 hours. You should notice improvement in symptoms after just one to perhaps a few repetitions. If you do not see improvement, it is wise to stop the remedy and try a different one, guiding yourself by the **keynote** symptoms. You may use different remedies together or you may try a combination remedy.

General guidelines to treat serious, chronic, relapsing ailments (including emotional disorders) are to use single remedies at potencies of 200C. These are generally administered once weekly to

once monthly, but they may be used once or twice daily at first if the condition warrants it, quickly decreasing the frequency as you see improvement. Do not continue giving the remedy if it becomes apparent that it is not working. You may always stop one remedy and choose to administer another remedy on the basis of the **keynote** symptoms of the new remedy. In addition, you may administer more than one remedy at a time.

Different homeopaths have developed different regulations for potency and frequency of administration of homeopathic remedies. Following the recommendations in this book is a safe way to begin to amass your own experiences with prevention and treatment using homeopathic remedies.

This book does not discuss giving potencies that are higher than 200C because very high potency remedies are more likely to produce a "homeopathic aggravation," also called a "healing crisis." Not being a trained homeopath, you may find it difficult to distinguish between a patient's condition getting worse and a patient going through a healing crisis. The potency of your homeopathic remedies are not decreased or changed in any way after the expiration date on the label of the vial, given proper storage of your remedies.

How to take homeopathic remedies

You should take homeopathic pellets, granules, or liquid on (or under) a *"clean tongue."* That means that you should drink and eat **nothing** for 20 minutes before taking the remedy and for 20 minutes afterwards. Empty out the pellets or granules directly on (or under) a *"clean tongue"* from the remedy tube or bottle. Do not touch the pellets or granules. If the pellets or granules are handled they are rendered inactive. It is a good idea to give pellets (or granules) to children older than 3 years, adolescents, and adults and to give liquid drops to children younger than 3 years. If you only have pellets available, you may dissolve 2 pellets in 2 teaspoons of bottled water (tap water has impurities that may interfere with the remedy) and give 3-5 drops of the resulting remedy as a dose. However, this method may not result in the potency you want, so it is much better to have the liquid drops on hand. Usually, younger children chew their pellets rather than allowing them to dissolve. In my experience this does not adversely impact the action of the remedy.

The number of pellets or granules or drops is not considered to be important in homeopathy. I generally recommend 3 drops for infants and young children, 5 drops or pellets or granules for older children and adults. Some homeopaths prescribe one drop or one pellet.

The most important thing is choosing the correct remedy. The second most important thing is choosing the proper potency. My advice is not to worry too much about frequency of administration or number of pellets or drops.

Substances that interfere with the action of homeopathic remedies

The prevailing opinion in homeopathy is that many substances particularly those with strong odors and tastes interfere with the action of homeopathic remedies. This is called antidoting. Do not drink coffee or tea (decaffeinated or regular), mentholated cough drops (or menthol in any form), or use mint toothpaste (or mint in any form, including spearmint and peppermint) for 20 minutes before taking the remedy and for 20 minutes afterwards.

The only products that I believe should not be used during the entire duration of the homeopathic treatment are camphor-containing products. Homeopaths will occasionally use camphor-containing products (such as Vicks VapoRub or other deep heat linaments) to antidote a remedy if the remedy has caused a significant aggravation. Consequently, be sure not to use any camphor-containing product when you are using homeopathic remedies.

> **Note:** Some homeopaths include other substances on the "beware of interference" list, like eucalyptus, and *Tea tree oil* (on the skin). And there are some practitioners who believe that electric blankets and x-ray machines may cause homeopathic remedies to be antidoted despite evidence to the contrary.

Storage of homeopathic remedies

Homeopathic remedies must be stored away from sunlight and away from all strong odors, such as perfumes, nail polish, and hair sprays (to mention just a few), products containing mint or menthol, and camphor and camphor-containing products. It is a good idea to keep your homeopathic remedies in a kitchen cabinet rather than in the bathroom medicine cabinet. Never replace pellets that have fallen out of a remedy vial or bottle. Discard them.

Over-the-counter remedies

Homeopathic remedies are regulated by Federal Drug Administration (FDA) according to the Federal Food, Drug, and Cosmetic Act of 1938. Homeopathic remedies are sold over-the-counter (OTC). In order to comply with FDA regulations, all drugs (and the FDA includes homeopathic remedies under drugs) that are sold OTC must have an indication on the label, such as cough, nausea, or some other non-life-threatening condition, but may not name a disease as a labeled indication.

Remember that in homeopathy, the sick person is matched to a remedy, so that any one of the 3,000 homeopathic remedies potentially may be the best match for a certain patient. Another patient with the "same" illness (in Western medical terms) would likely match to a different remedy, because her unique expression of the illness would be different.

Unfortunately, the FDA does not take this into account with labeling of homeopathic remedies. So, we are stuck with nonsense labeling.

> *For example:*
> You may purchase the homeopathic remedy *Arsenicum album* 200C to prevent and treat your child's asthma. You may become confused if you read the label on the vial which will say, "for exhaustion." The indication on the label may very likely have nothing to do with the reason you have purchased that remedy. It is printed on the label in order to comply with FDA regulations for OTC drugs.

Homeopathic remedies will also be labeled with an **expiration date**, which I believe is not useful. Homeopathic remedies do not expire. It is not necessary to discard your homeopathic remedies after the expiration date on the vial.

One of the advantages of homeopathic remedies being available OTC is that they are not costly and probably cost less than if they would be sold by prescription only. The cost for a vial of homeopathic remedy at 30C and 200C potencies varies from about $7 to about $9. Liquid drops usually cost somewhat more.

Homeopathic Remedy-Prescription Drug Interactions

Homeopathic remedies may be taken along with your prescription pharmaceuticals without diluting the effectiveness of those drugs. And in fact, your homeopathic remedy may help your prescription drug to work better and you may become healthy sooner. But, certain prescription drugs may interfere with the effectiveness of your homeopathic remedies. Certain drugs in Western medicine block the action of homeopathic remedies. The standout example is steroid medications. *Any steroid* (and steroids come with so many names and so many types), whether taken internally, applied to the skin, or inhaled into your airways, is likely to render your homeopathic remedy less effective, and in some cases, useless.

Sometimes steroids are life saving and I certainly have no argument with taking them in that case. However, steroid medications are often prescribed indiscriminately. If your doctor wants to prescribe a steroid medication for you (either orally, topically, or by inhalation), you should ask him/her what is likely to happen with your condition if you do not take it. Even short courses of steroids may have unhealthy side effects and may be dangerous. Before you decide to take steroids, you may wish to read about treating your condition with homeopathy, herbal remedies, and nutritional supplements instead.

Homeopathy vs. Western Medicine
A comparison of homeopathy and Western medicine is found in the following chart:

Comparison	Homeopathy	Western Medicine
Symptoms*	body's attempt to activate the vital force towards cure	body's announcement that there is sickness that needs to be cured
The interview	goal to find the individual's unique symptom picture in the illness	based on the general symptoms of the illness
Treatment*	different remedies for different patients' expressions of the disease	same treatment for most patients
Approach	no magic bullet exists	magic bullet exists for each disease (pharmaceutical approach)
Goal of treatment*	health without the use of medications	health with continued use of medicines
Health*	physical, emotional, mental, and spiritual well-being	the absence of disease

(Continued)

Comparison	Homeopathy	Western Medicine
Satisfaction	the health care consumer is generally satisfied	the health care consumer is often dissatisfied
Cost	low cost for practitioner and remedies	high cost for practitioner and medicines
Technology	low tech	high tech
Theory of disease causation	the body's vital force is disturbed	no unified theory—differs by body system
Mechanism of action	"memory of water," cutting-edge physics of water	concrete mechanism of action based on the atomic theory
Focus	on the whole person (holistic)	on the disease
Practitioner	generalist, all ages	subspecialty care, by system, by age group
Outcome	cure often occurs	chronic, relapsing conditions
Toxicity of treatments	non-toxic, gentle, non-addictive	may be toxic, may be addictive
Potency	less is more (the more a remedy is diluted and succussed, the more the curative power is increased while simultaneously decreasing toxicity)	more is more (the more potent the medicine, the more drug it contains, and the more toxic it becomes, with increasing side effects)
Suppression	no suppression—deep cure on cellular level	suppression—the disease disappears if the symptoms disappear
Laws of treatment	The Law of Similars	The Law of Contraries
Drug experimentation	matching people (provers) to people (patients)	matching animals to people (patients)
Side effects	absent to minor (occasional short-lived homeopathic aggravation before cure)	generally long list of possibly serious side effects

* Based on Table in Sollars, D, *The Complete Idiot's Guide to Homeopathy*, 2001, pp. 276.

Note: Do not discontinue taking any pharmaceutical medication that has been prescribed by your health care provider unless you or your family member is under the supervision of a physician.

Chapter 3

Homeopathic Remedies for Traumatic Injuries

Traumatic Injuries in General

Ailment/Disorder/Symptom	Homeopathic Remedy
First aid, traumatic injuries, scrapes, bumps, bruises, abrasions, sprains	*Arnica montana*
First aid, traumatic injuries	*Traumeel*
Muscle aches and pains, sprains	*Arniflora*
Skin wounds	*Wound-Care*
Traumatic injuries, anxiety, fears, panic, shock	*Aconitum napellus*
Nerve pains and nerve injuries	*Hypericum perforatum*
Penetrating wounds, puncture wounds	*Ledum palustre*
Broken bones, bone pain, tendon injuries	*Ruta graveolens*
Head injuries, concussions	*Natrum sulphuricum*
Broken bones	*Symphytum officinalis*
Joint pains and stiffness, muscles aches and pains	*Rhus toxicodendron*
Burning, stinging pains, insect bites, allergic hives	*Apis mellifica*
Insect bites	*Ssssting Stop*
Aches and pains with the slightest movement	*Bryonia alba*
Severe nerve pains, lacerations, surgical incisions	*Staphysagria*
Bruising of internal organs, soft tissue pains	*Bellis perennis*
Aches and pains in muscles and joints after sports	*Sports Gel*

Homeopathic Remedies for Traumatic Injuries Associated with Surgery

Surgical Injuries in General

Ailment/Disorder/Symptom	Homeopathic Remedy
Physical shock and trauma after surgery	*Arnica montana*
Physical and emotional shock after surgery	*Aconitum napellus*
Bright red bleeding from any body opening	*Phosphorus*
Surgical incision pains	*Staphysagria*
Surgical nerve injury pains	*Hypericum perforatum*
Post-surgical tissue swelling and throbbing	*Ferrum phosphoricum*
Dark red bleeding, blood does not clot	*Crotalus horridus*

Physical and emotional shock before and after surgery	*Rescue Remedy*
Pre-dental trauma	*Pre-Dental Procedure*
Post-dental trauma	*Post-Dental Procedure*
Pre-cosmetic surgery trauma	*Pre-Cosmetic Procedure*
Post-cosmetic surgery trauma	*Post-Cosmetic Procedure*
Pre-orthopedic surgery trauma	*Pre-Orthopedic Procedure*
Post-orthopedic surgery trauma	*Orthopedic Post-Op*

Homeopathic Remedies for Burns

Burns in General

<u>Ailment/Disorder/Symptom</u>	<u>Homeopathic Remedy</u>
Infections, inflammation, pain and swelling	*Calendula officinalis*
Post-burns	*Aloe vera*
Inflammation, shock	*Rescue Remedy Cream*
Blistering and burning of the skin and urinary tract infections	*Cantharis*
Scalds and sunburns	*Urtica urens*
Dry, cracking scabs	*Causticum*
Burning pains with restlessness and anxiety	*Arsenicum album*
Thickened, hardened scars	*Graphites*

Guidelines for Consulting Your Health Care Provider
Putting It All Together

Traumatic Injuries in General

Homeopathic remedies are ideally suited to the "First Aid" treatment of accidental traumatic injuries. We will learn to use single remedies and combination remedies to treat a long list of accidental injuries. This includes any injury to the soft tissues of the body: bruising, bleeding, strains, sprains, muscle aches and pains, muscle cramps, swelling after injury, sports injuries, overexertion, and sore muscles.

Traumatic injuries are often accompanied by emotional shock. We will learn how to deal with the emotional shock resulting from trauma (including concussion) as well as the emotional shock resulting from bereavement. In addition to all of that, we will learn how to *prevent* trauma before scheduled surgery, labor, childbirth, and dental work.

The best first step for bumps on the head, or anyplace on the body when a lump or a swelling appears is to apply an *ice pack*. A product called *Colpac* contains a silicate gel filing. *Colpac* is useful because it is stored in the freezer and so is readily available when you require an *ice pack*.

The best second step is usually to take a homeopathic remedy right away. You can go ahead and give homeopathic remedies according to their **keynote** symptoms while the *ice packs* are doing their work. In addition, you may give homeopathic remedies together with *acetaminophen* or *ibuprofen*.

The best first step for minor cuts, bruises, and abrasions that have broken the skin is to wash them out well with soap and water. Then use a topical disinfectant such as hydrogen peroxide or *witch hazel*. *Witch hazel* is a liquid extract of the herb *Hamamelis virginiana*. It is not only a first class disinfectant but also an anti-irritant useful to relieve the itching from insect stings and bites, and a topical anti-inflammatory for muscle aches and pains.

It is important to prepare your household before a traumatic injury by having *latex-free* bandaids on hand. More and more people are becoming allergic to latex, showing symptoms ranging from cough and congestion to asthma. You can help to prevent an allergic reaction to latex by decreasing exposure, especially when the skin has been broken and the body more vulnerable to immune system reactivity. Stock up on *latex-free* fabric bandaids.

As with any and all medical conditions, when dealing with traumatic injuries you must pay strict attention to the **Guidelines for Consulting Your Health Care Provider** at the end of this chapter. Just after that, you will find **Recommendations for Homeopathic First Aid Remedy Kit**. You may want to refer to the last section **Putting It All Together** for ideas on how to integrate the essential natural alternatives, homeopathy, herbal remedies, and nutritional supplements.

Arnica montana

What is it? Perhaps the most important homeopathic remedy to have in your homeopathic first aid kit is the plant *Arnica montana*, common name *Leopard's bane*, a member of the *Compositae* botanical family. This remarkable homeopathic remedy is used both internally in the form of pellets (or granules) and liquid for infants and children, and externally on sore muscles or bruised skin as creams, ointments, gels, and spray. Do not use the creams, ointments, gels, or spray on broken skin because it may cause a rash.

An extraction of the whole flowering plant is used to produce the remedy. The creams and gels are actually herbal remedies, meaning that an extract of the full-strength plant is used. The pellets and liquid are homeopathic remedies produced according to strict standards of dilution and potentization, rendering it a gentle yet powerful healing remedy.

When should you use it? Ideally, *Arnica* should be taken as soon after an injury as possible in order to help with the healing process. In fact, giving *Arnica* immediately after a fall or a bruise could prevent bruising from developing. But, if ailments persist as a result of a traumatic injury, it can be taken at any time to relieve those ailments, even years later. *Arnica* helps injured people to cope, physically and emotionally, with the stress of the injury. *Arnica* is homeopathy's painkiller much as acetaminophen or ibuprofen is in Western medicine.

The **keynote** symptom leading you to use *Arnica* is that the injured person denies that anything is wrong, saying, "Leave me alone, I'm okay." However, it is perfectly clear to those around him that he has been injured, perhaps severely, although he characteristically refuses to get help from a doctor. However, I strongly urge you to consider using *Arnica* whenever there is an injury from any cause, even without the characteristic **keynote** symptom. *Arnica* is useful when the injured patient awakens suddenly in the middle of the night from dreaming of the accident, one of the prominent symptoms of post-traumatic stress disorder. So think of *Arnica* whenever PTSD occurs, even long after the accident itself.

Homeopathy is replete with reports in its medical literature on the benefits of using *Arnica*. There are no reports of side effects when *Arnica* is used in homeopathic dilution. A recent report in the peer-reviewed medical journal *Alternative Therapies in Health and Medicine* on the "Use of *Arnica* to Relieve Pain After Carpal-Tunnel Release Surgery" reported a greater decrease in the pain 2 weeks after surgery in the group using *Arnica* than in the placebo group.

Using *Arnica* on yourself or on a family member who has been injured is a particularly satisfying way to start using homeopathic remedies.

How should you use it? If you wish to purchase *Arnica* for your beginner's **Homeopathic First Aid Remedy Kit**, then I advise *Arnica* 30C in pellets (or granules) and liquid drops. You would give 3-5 pellets to an adolescent or adult and 3-5 drops to an infant or child, repeating the dose every $\frac{1}{2}$-2 hours, as needed at first, then decreasing to 3-4 times daily. Decrease the frequency of giving the remedy when the injured person begins to feel better and stop using the remedy when complaints taper off considerably. You may always return to the remedy. It is next to impossible to overuse the remedy when there is an acute injury situation.

Arnica may be the most commonly used homeopathic remedy for trauma and injuries, but you can always use *Arnica* with one or more of the remedies discussed below, each given according to their **keynote** symptoms. *Arnica* is particularly useful before and during labor and delivery because of its effects on decreasing both the physical and emotional toll of trauma.

Arnica may well be the first remedy with which you begin your homeopathic odyssey. It will not disappoint you. I recommend that you have it readily available to you to be at the ready whenever you or your family may experience an injury.

Traumeel

What is it? *Traumeel*, made by Heel, Inc., a German homeopathic pharmaceutical supply house selling remedies in the United States is a combination remedy specifically designed to treat many different kinds of traumatic injuries.

When should you use it? *Traumeel* contains *Arnica* as well as 13 other homeopathic remedies, all in low potency, all suited to treating traumatic injuries. You may think of *Traumeel* as a broad-spectrum *Arnica*.

How should you use it? *Traumeel* comes in tablet, liquid drop, gel, and ointment forms. *Traumeel* is not to be used for children younger than 12 years because of the low potencies of the remedies. Remember that the more dilute a homeopathic remedy, the stronger and less toxic it is. Give children 12 years of age and older 3-10 drops of the liquid, or $\frac{1}{2}$ to 1 tablet, depending on age. You may repeat this several times daily, depending on need. The ointment and gel are not to be used on broken skin.

Arniflora

What is it? *Arniflora Gel* and *Arniflora Cream* are produced by Boericke & Tafel, a homeopathic pharmaceutical supply house. It consists of *Arnica montana* 1X (only diluted 10 times) in a concentration of 8% in a witch hazel base.

When should you use it? The **keynote** symptoms leading you towards using *Arniflora Gel* or *Arniflora Cream* are bruises and sprains with muscle aches and pains, as long as the skin is not broken.

How should you use it? *Arniflora Gel* and *Arniflora Cream* are indicated for adults and children 2 years and older. Apply *Arniflora Gel* or *Arniflora Cream* 1-4 times daily.

Wound-Care

What is it? *Wound-Care* is a combination homeopathic remedy (as an ointment) produced by Weleda, a homeopathic supply house. The ingredients are: *Mercurialis perennis, Balsamum peruvianum* and *Calendula officinalis*. Since their potency is the

Mother Tincture, this preparation is technically herbal in nature. The other ingredients are: *Peanut Oil, Lanolin, Cod Liver Oil* and *Beeswax*. Persons with allergies to peanuts should not use this.

When should you use it? The **keynote** symptoms indicating the usefulness of *Wound-Care* are minor skin wounds consisting of abrasions and cuts in order to promote healing.

How should you use it? Cleanse the wound first with soap and water or hydrogen peroxide. Then apply a thin layer of *Wound-Care* with or without a dressing. You may use twice daily.

Aconitum napellus

What is it? This homeopathic remedy, called in shorthand *Aconite*, is made from the plant commonly called *monkshood* or *wolfsbane*, a member of the *Ranunculaceae* botanical family. The whole plant just before flowering is used to make the remedy. The plant is highly toxic so the homeopathic remedy is never used below the 3X potency.

When should you use it? *Aconite* is the homeopathic substitute for *Valium*, because of its calming effect on anxiety. The **keynote** symptoms leading you to use *Aconite* are fear and restless agitation with a sudden onset. *Aconite* is useful for treating the emotional shock or fright after a traumatic injury. It is often used along with *Arnica* to control the pain and shock from trauma and to speed the healing process. *Aconite* is used to treat panic attacks, fear of death during labor, and fear of dying when sick. Fear, anxiety, pains and restlessness are worse after midnight. *Aconite* is also useful during bereavement to ease the emotional shock of death of a loved one.

The sudden onset part of the picture is especially useful for people who have been exposed to abrupt changes in the environment. I recommend that you immediately take *Aconite* as soon as you feel stressed from being cold or wet, or from leaving an air-conditioned environment (such as an airplane), or from exposure to cold, dry winds. Using the sudden onset **keynote** symptom as your guide, you may prevent many colds and coughs as well as earaches from taking a hold of yourself or your family members by giving a dose or two of *Aconite* as soon after the exposure as possible. *Aconite* is an indispensable accompaniment to air travel.

How should you use it? You should have *Aconite* 30C and 200C in pellets and *Aconite* 30C in liquid drops in your **Homeopathic First Aid Remedy Kit**. Give 3-5 pellets or drops of *Aconite* 30C every ½-2 hours as needed. The use of *Aconite* 200C is indicted for adolescents and adults when anxiety and shock have come under control and the patient can graduate to once daily or once weekly administration. You may give *Aconite* 200C once daily, decreasing the frequency as the fear and anxiety improves, and stopping when the condition is under control.

If you were to decide to start your homeopathic adventure with only one remedy, you would probably choose *Arnica*, but if you wish to extend *Arnica's* usefulness into every part of the human being, physical, emotional, mental, sexual, and spiritual, you would administer *Aconite* along with it. I recommend that you have both *Arnica* and *Aconite* readily available at all times.

Hypericum perforatum

What is it? This is the homeopathic remedy of the plant *St. John's Wort*, a member of the *Hypericaceae* botanical family. We will study the herbal preparation of *St. John's Wort* as a remedy for depression in **Chapter 20: Herbs You Need to Know**. For the homeopathic remedy, the whole plant in flower is used.

When should you use it? The **keynote** symptoms that lead you to use *Hypericum* are severe shooting pains that are characteristic of nerve pain or nerve injury. *Hypericum* is especially helpful when a body part rich in nerve endings has been injured, such as fingers, toes, eye, lips, and any part of the nervous system like the head and the spine, as well as puncture wounds and burns. *Hypericum* has a profound effect on nerves.

How should you use it? I advise you to have *Hypericum* 30C in pellets and liquid drops on hand in your **Homeopathic First Aid Remedy Kit** as well as either the ointment or spray. You would give 3-5 pellets to an adolescent or adult and 3-5 drops to an infant or child, repeating the dose every ½-2 hours, as needed at first, then decreasing to 3-4 times daily. Decrease the frequency of giving the remedy when the injured person begins to feel better and stop using the remedy when complaints taper off considerably. You may always return to the remedy. It is next to impossible to overuse the remedy when there is an acute injury situation.

Ledum palustre

What is it? This common name for this plant is *wild rosemary*, a member of the *Ericaceae* botanical family. The homeopathic remedy is made from the dried twigs.

When should you use it? The **keynote** symptom leading you to use *Ledum* is that there is a penetrating wound, such as a puncture wound or an insect sting, especially with a lot of bruising with swollen, purple-colored skin. *Ledum* is especially indicated for an injury that has produced black eyes.

How should you use it? You should have *Ledum* 30C in pellets and liquid drops in your **Homeopathic First Aid Remedy Kit**. You would give 3-5 pellets to an adolescent or adult and 3-5 drops to an infant or child, repeating the dose every $\frac{1}{2}$-2 hours, as needed at first, then decreasing to 3-4 times daily. Decrease the frequency of giving the remedy when the injured person begins to feel better and stop using the remedy when complaints taper off considerably. You may always return to the remedy. It is next to impossible to overuse the remedy when there is an acute injury situation.

Ruta graveolens

What is it? This common name for this plant is *Rue*, a member of the *Rutaceae* botanical family. During the Middle Ages it was believed that *Rue* sprinkled around indoor rooms would keep the plague at bay. This was based on its ability to kill fleas and other insects. The plant used as the herbal remedy tends to improve the eyesight, especially after eye strain. The whole plant gives off a disagreeable odor. An extract of the whole plant before flowering is used to produce the homeopathic remedy.

When should you use it? The **keynote** symptom leading you to use *Ruta* is deep aching pains, usually as a result of bruising of the bone's outer covering, called the periosteum, or due to tendon injuries.

Injury of the bones, including broken bones, can be very painful. *Ruta* shares with one of our powerful remedies for joint problems *Rhus toxicodendron*, the peculiar symptom of pain being worse on first movement but better on continued movement.

How should you use it? You should have *Ruta* 30C in pellets and liquid drops in your **Homeopathic First Aid Remedy Kit**. You would give 3-5 pellets to an adolescent or adult and 3-5 drops to an infant or child, repeating the dose every $\frac{1}{2}$-2 hours, as needed at first, then decreasing to 3-4 times daily. Decrease the frequency of giving the remedy when the injured person begins to feel better and stop using the remedy when complaints taper off considerably. You may always return to the remedy. It is next to impossible to overuse the remedy when there is an acute injury situation.

Natrum sulphuricum

What is it? This is the non-metallic chemical compound sodium sulphate, a naturally occurring salt in the body.

When should you use it? The **keynote** symptom leading you to use *Natrum sulphuricum* is head injury, including concussion with or without loss of consciousness. To prevent damage from head injury, *Natrum sulphuricum* should be used as soon as possible after the injury. However, it may be useful for residual problems long after the injury, such as for headaches that occur after a concussion, or for the depression that may accompany head trauma.

How should you use it? You should have *Natrum sulphuricum* 30C in pellets and liquid drops in your **Homeopathic First Aid Remedy Kit**. You would give 3-5 pellets to an adolescent or adult and 3-5 drops to an infant or child, repeating the dose every $\frac{1}{2}$-2 hours, as needed at first, then decreasing to 3-4 times daily. Decrease the frequency of giving the remedy when the injured person begins to feel better and stop using the remedy when complaints taper off considerably. You may always return to the remedy. It is next to impossible to overuse the remedy when there is an acute injury situation.

Symphytum officinalis

What is it? The common name for this plant is *comfrey* or *knitbone*, a member of the *Boraginaceae* botanical family. The herbal preparation has been used to treat wounds. The active ingredient allantoin encourages new cells to grow. The herbal preparation of comfrey is used externally only because ingesting the herb may be toxic to the liver. The homeopathic remedy is not toxic.

When should you use it? The **keynote** of this remedy is broken parts. It is effective in bringing parts together. It is useful to promote healing of broken bones that have not yet knit and for bone pain that continues after the fracture has healed. It also helps to prevent refracture at the same site, such as a rib or ankle bone.

How should you use it? You should have *Symphytum officinalis* 30C in pellets and liquid drops in your **Homeopathic First Aid Remedy Kit.** You would give 3-5 pellets to an adolescent or adult and 3-5 drops to an infant or child, repeating the dose every ½ -2 hours, as needed at first, then decreasing to 3-4 times daily. Decrease the frequency of giving the remedy when the injured person begins to feel better and stop using the remedy when complaints taper off considerably. You may always return to the remedy. It is next to impossible to overuse the remedy when there is an acute injury situation.

Rhus toxicodendron

What is it? The botanical name for this plant is *Rhus toxicodendron*, a member of the *Anacardiaceae* botanical family. The common name for this plant is *poison ivy*. The homeopathic remedy is usually abbreviated as *Rhus tox*. The homeopathic remedy is prepared from the leaves before the plant comes into flower.

When should you use it? The **keynote** symptoms leading you to consider using *Rhus tox* is joint and muscle pain and stiffness which is worse on first starting to move but improves on continues movement. *Rhus tox* is considered for use on the basis of its modalities, those factors that make symptoms better or worse. Think of giving *Rhus tox* when the patient's condition is worse at the first movement and better at continued movement. The joint and muscle pains are often due to sprains and strains, but can also be due to osteoarthritis and rheumatic arthritis.

Rhus tox is not only used for joint and muscle pains, but also for skin complaints. The **keynote** symptoms leading you to use *Rhus tox* for skin problems are itchy, red, scaly skin with burning pains and blisters. These are the kind of symptoms that you would likely get if you touched *poison ivy* in your garden. According to the **Law of Similars** what *Rhus tox* can cause, it can cure, once it is transformed into the gentle yet powerful homeopathic remedy. The skin problems that may be helped and perhaps cured with *Rhus tox* include eczema, herpes, chickenpox, diaper rash, any contact dermatitis, and of course poison ivy.

There are two other **keynote** symptoms that may help you to choose *Rhus tox*. The first is the red-tipped tongue. You may try *Rhus tox* whenever you notice that the triangular tip of the tongue is reddened. The second is the person's extreme sensitivity to cold and damp, making the joint, muscle, or skin problems worse.

How should you use it? The instructions for use of *Rhus tox*, either for joint and muscle or skin problems, are different from the others in this chapter. It is my experience that *Rhus tox* works best in the 200C potency, even for acute conditions. You should have *Rhus tox* 200C in pellets and liquid drops in your **Homeopathic First Aid Remedy Kit.** You may give *Rhus tox* 200C 1-3 times daily, decreasing the frequency as the condition improves, and stopping when the condition is under control.

Apis mellifica

What is it? This is a homeopathic remedy from the animal kingdom, made from the whole, crushed *honeybee*. If you already understand the first and foremost homeopathic principle, the **Law of Similars**, you will instinctively recognize that *Apis* is used to treat bee bites.

When should you use it? The **keynote** symptoms leading you to consider using *Apis* are burning, stinging pains that come on suddenly, along with puffiness or swelling (edema), blisters, and itch. The pains are made much worse from touch. Heat makes everything worse. This kind of pain can be found in bladder infections (cystitis) and eye infections (conjunctivitis), as well as in many skin ailments, such as stings, bites, and allergic hives (urticaria). *Apis* particularly fits people who tend to be busy all the time ("busy bees"). They may be restless, fidgety, and awkward. *Apis* is an indispensable remedy.

How should you use it? You should have *Apis mellifica* 30C in pellets and liquid drops in your **Homeopathic First Aid Remedy Kit**. You would give 3-5 pellets to an adolescent or adult and 3-5 drops to an infant or child, repeating the dose every $\frac{1}{2}$-2 hours, as needed at first, then decreasing to 3-4 times daily. Decrease the frequency of giving the remedy when the injured person begins to feel better and stop using the remedy when complaints taper off considerably. You may always return to the remedy. It is next to impossible to overuse the remedy when there is an acute injury situation. You may administer *Apis* along with *Arnica* for bee stings, if you wish, but in my experience, it is usually not necessary.

Sssssting Stop

What is it? *Sssssting Stop* is a topical combination homeopathic remedy manufactured by Boericke & Tafel. It contains *Echinacea angustifolia*, *Ledum palustre* and *Urtica dioica*, in very low potencies along with Citronella and Eucalyptus oils in a water gel base. It does not contain hydrocortisone or antihistamines.

When should you use it? The **keynote** symptoms for use of *Sssssting Stop* is itching, pain, and redness at the sit of an insect bite (mosquitoes, bees, wasps). It is also effective on cold sores.

How should you use it? Apply *Sssssting Stop* topically on the skin (for external use only). You may reapply as frequently as necessary. It is usually effective in just a few moments.

Bryonia alba

What is it? The common name for the plant *Bryonia alba* is *wild hops*, a member of the *Cucurbitaceae* botanical family. The homeopathic remedy is prepared from the root of the plant before it flowers.

When should you use it? The **keynote** symptoms for use of the homeopathic remedy *Bryonia* are pain with the slightest movement and the patient feels better lying on the affected side, or applying pressure to the part. Patients who need *Bryonia* are reluctant to move. Conditions for which *Bryonia* should be considered are those which develop very slowly, like a bruised rib, severe headaches, pneumonia with pain on coughing from inflamed lining of the lung (pleurisy), and joint inflammation of arthritis.

How should you use it? This is a remedy which does not need to be in your **Homeopathic First Aid Remedy Kit** because it is used after you realize that the condition is developing slowly, giving you enough time to buy *Bryonia* at a health food store or to order it from one of the **Homeopathic Remedy Supply Houses** found in the **Appendix**. *Bryonia* is used in 30C pellets or liquid drops. You would give 3-5 pellets to an adolescent or adult and 3-5 drops to an infant or child, repeating the dose every $\frac{1}{2}$-2 hours, as needed at first, then decreasing to 3-4 times daily. Decrease the frequency of giving the remedy when the injured person begins to feel better and stop using the remedy when complaints taper off considerably. You may always return to the remedy. It is next to impossible to overuse the remedy when there is an acute injury situation.

Staphysagria

What is it? The botanical name of this remedy is *Delphinium staphysagria*, common name *stavesacre* or *larkspur*, a member of the *Ranunculaceae* botanical family. The seeds are extremely poisonous. The homeopathic remedy is non-poisonous.

When should you use it? The **keynote** symptoms of *Staphysagria* are severe nerve pains, especially from lacerated tissues, with extreme sensitivity to touch, in those who are seething with suppressed rage. *Staphysagria* will speed the healing of lacerated tissues. *Staphysagria* is indicated before surgery to prevent pain from the incision, which is understood by the body to be a laceration.

How should you use it? This remedy is not required for your **Homeopathic First Aid Remedy Kit** because you will have advance notice when to purchase it when needed. *Staphysagria* is used in

30C pellets or liquid drops. You would give 3-5 pellets to an adolescent or adult and 3-5 drops to an infant or child, repeating the dose every ½-2 hours, as needed at first, then decreasing to 3-4 times daily. Decrease the frequency of giving the remedy when the injured person begins to feel better and stop using the remedy when complaints taper off considerably. You may always return to the remedy. It is next to impossible to overuse the remedy when there is an acute injury situation.

Bellis perennis

What is it? This is the homeopathic remedy made from the plant *Bellis perennis* whose common name is *daisy* or *bruisewort*, a member of the *Compositae* botanical family.

When should you use it? The **keynote** symptoms of *Bellis perennis* are bruising of soft tissues and internal organs with soreness and pain such as after childbirth.

How should you use it? This remedy is not required for your **Homeopathic First Aid Remedy Kit** because you will have advance notice when to purchase it when needed. *Bellis perennis* is used in 30C pellets or liquid drops. You would give 3-5 pellets to an adolescent or adult and 3-5 drops to an infant or child, repeating the dose every ½-2 hours, as needed at first, then decreasing to 3-4 times daily. Decrease the frequency of giving the remedy when the injured person begins to feel better and stop using the remedy when complaints taper off considerably. You may always return to the remedy. It is next to impossible to overuse the remedy when there is an acute injury situation.

Sports Gel

What is it? *Sports Gel* is a topical gel produced by Boericke & Tafel, a homeopathic pharmaceutical supply house. It consists of the following homeopathic remedies in very low potency: *Bellis perennis*, *Hypericum perforatum*, *Rhus toxicodendron* and *Ruta graveolens*.

When should you use it? The **keynote** symptoms indicating the usefulness of *Sports Gel* are muscle and joint pains after playing sports or exercising.

This includes back pain, nerve and bone injuries, as well as sprains and strains from over-use.

How should you use it? This gel is indicated for adults and children over the age of 6 years. Apply 1-4 times daily to the affected area. Care should be taken not to allow ingestion of this product because since the remedies are present in such low potency they may still retain some of their toxicity from the herbal form.

Homeopathic Remedies for Traumatic Injuries Associated with Surgery

Surgical Injuries in General

Certain homeopathic remedies are uniquely suited to **prevent** the trauma and shock of surgery in the patient who is scheduled to undergo a surgical procedure. These same homeopathic remedies are also used in the **treatment** of patients who have already had surgery to overcome the physical and emotional stresses of such a traumatic procedure. You will find a **Pre-Surgery Prescription** at the end of this chapter.

As with any and all medical conditions, when dealing with post-surgical conditions you must pay strict attention to the **Guidelines for Consulting Your Health Care Provider** at the end of this chapter.

Arnica montana

What is it? Perhaps the most important homeopathic remedy to have in your homeopathic first aid kit is the plant *Arnica montana*, common name *Leopard's bane*, a member of the *Compositae* botanical family.

When should you use it? It is not surprising that the first and foremost homeopathic remedy for traumatic injuries, *Arnica montana*, would also be first on the list for preventing and treating surgical trauma. *Arnica* facilitates the healing process, no matter the source of the trauma.

Arnica, in the case of surgical trauma, is a broad-spectrum healer, often given even without the **keynote** indication, "Leave me alone, I'm okay."

Arnica is most effective given prior to surgery, because it is always easier to succeed with prevention rather than waiting until a condition has developed and then trying to treat it.

How should you use it? So, if you have the choice, start giving *Arnica* 30C pellets or liquid drops once or twice daily for each day starting three days before the scheduled surgery. Then give *Arnica* 30C 1-4 times just after surgery, for one or two days, until the pain of the bruised tissues is alleviated. *Arnica* is an important remedy in the **Pre-Surgery Prescription**.

Aconitum napellus

What is it? This homeopathic remedy, called in shorthand *Aconite*, is made from the plant commonly called *monkshood* or *wolfsbane*, a member of the *Ranunculaceae* botanical family.

When should you use it? This is the homeopathic remedy whose **keynote** symptom is fear and restless agitation often from physical or emotional (or combined) shock. Its gentle action is optimized when given prior to surgery to alleviate the anxiety associated with a surgical procedure, but it can be used afterwards as well. *Aconite* is often given together with *Arnica*. Together they make up two of the three remedies of the **Pre-Surgery Prescription**.

How should you use it? Use *Aconite* 30C pellets or liquid drops. Start giving *Aconite* 30C pellets or liquid drops once or twice daily for each day starting three days before the scheduled surgery. Then give *Aconite* 30C 1-4 times just after surgery, for one or two days, until the pain of the bruised tissues is alleviated. *Aconite* is an important remedy in the **Pre-Surgery Prescription**.

Phosphorus

What is it? This is the homeopathic remedy that is made from the non-metallic chemical element *Phosphorus*. It is one of the commonest elements in the human body because it makes up part of ATP (adenosine triphosphate), the chemical that stores our energy.

When should you use it? The **keynote** symptom for homeopathic *Phosphorus* is bright red bleeding from any site in the body, from nosebleeds to cut finger to bleeding from surgery. Homeopathic *Phosphorus* is sometimes called the "homeopathic bandaid." *Phosphorus* is also very useful to prevent side effects from the anesthetics that are used during surgery. The person needing *Phosphorus* will likely have a strong need for the presence of others, called a need for company, and will feel better from being touched or from massage.

Phosphorus is most effective when used prior to surgery, much the same as *Arnica* and *Aconite*. In fact, *Arnica*, *Aconite* and *Phosphorus* are three of the four remedies that comprise the **Pre-Surgery Prescription**.

How should you use it? Give *Phosphorus* 30C pellets or liquid drops once or twice daily for each day starting three days before the scheduled surgery. Then give *Phosphorus* 30C every $\frac{1}{2}$-2 hours just after surgery to decrease the possibility of post-operative bleeding. Then you may decrease the frequency of administration depending on whether the bleeding is under control or the threat of bleeding has passed.

Staphysagria

What is it? This homeopathic remedy prepared from *Delphinum staphysagria*, is the best choice for healing the pain of the surgical incision.

When should you use it? The **keynote** symptom of *Staphysagria* is pain from lacerations. This remedy is commonly used a week or so post-surgery, after the incision would have been thought to have healed, but the patient is still suffering from pain. At this point, *Staphysagria* should be given.

How should you use it? *Staphysagria* is used in 30C pellets or liquid drops. Start giving *Staphysagria* 30C pellets or liquid drops once or twice daily for each day starting three days before the scheduled surgery. Then give *Staphysagria* 30C 1-4 times just after surgery, for one or two days, until the pain of the bruised tissues is alleviated. *Staphysagria* is an important remedy in the **Pre-Surgery Prescription**.

Hypericum perforatum

What is it? This homeopathic remedy prepared from *St. John's Wort*, is especially indicated after surgery of nerve-rich tissues, such as lips, fingers, toes, anus, genitals, eyes, or any part of the nervous system.

When should you use it? The **keynote** symptom of *Hypericum perforatum* is shooting, electrical-type pains that are typical of nerve injury. *Hypericum perforatum* should be considered for use whenever the surgery is in an area of the body rich in nerve endings. For this reason, *Hypericum perforatum* is useful after circumcision.

How should you use it? *Hypericum* 30C is used in pellets and liquid drops. It is also available in ointment or spray. Start giving *Hypericum* 30C pellets or liquid drops once or twice daily for each day starting three days before the scheduled surgery. Then give *Hypericum* 30C 1-4 times just after surgery, for one or two days, until the pain of the bruised tissues is alleviated. *Hypericum* is an important remedy in the **Pre-Surgery Prescription**.

Ferrum phosphoricum

What is it? This is the homeopathic form of iron phosphate salt found in many tissues of the body. *Ferrum phos* (as it is called for short) is used to remove congestion from blood vessels.

When should you use it? The **keynote** symptom of *Ferrum phos* is post-surgical swelling with throbbing. It is also useful for bright red bleeding, especially nosebleeds. *Ferrum phos* also has a role in the homeopathic treatment of fever.

How should you use it? Give *Ferrum phos* 30C pellets or liquid drops post-operatively every $\frac{1}{2}$-2 hours until the swelling and throbbing are diminished. Then decrease the frequency and stop when the symptoms have ceased.

Crotalus horridus

What is it? This is an animal homeopathic remedy made from the venom of the rattlesnake.

When should you use it? The **keynote** symptom of *Crotalus horridus* is bleeding whenever the blood does not clot and the blood is dark and thin. Think of *Crotalus* whenever the bleeding seems to seep, rather than pump actively.

How should you use it? Give *Crotalus* 30C pellets or liquid drops every $\frac{1}{2}$-2 hours after a surgical wound has caused dark, thin bleeding that seeps into the bandage. Decrease the frequency of administration depending on control of the bleeding.

Rescue Remedy

What is it? This is a combination *Bach Flower Remedy* that is, strictly speaking, not homeopathic. *Rescue Remedy* is a combination of five flower essences.

When should you use it? It is very useful for the **keynote** symptoms of stress and anxiety. Whenever you or one of your family members is confronted with a sudden, unexpected threat to emotional health, from an accident, to surgery, to childbirth, it is worthwhile to give a few doses of *Rescue Remedy* to restore calm and a sense of well being.

Rescue Remedy is also available as a skin cream. This should become your first-line cream to calm any skin irritation or inflammation instead of steroid ointments, no matter the diagnosis. It both moisturizes and calms inflammation, speeding the healing process.

How should you use it? Give *Rescue Remedy* as the liquid drops, 4 drops or as the spray, 2 sprays every $\frac{1}{2}$-1 hour for as long as the oppressive feelings of stress and anxiety persist. Decrease the frequency of administration depending on control of the symptoms. *Rescue Remedy* skin cream is to be used readily and repeatedly without fear of side effects, whenever you need to treat a skin lesion, whether from accidental trauma (cuts and burns), eczema, dermatitis, or diaper rash.

Pre-Dental Procedure

What is it? This is a homeopathic combination remedy produced by Standard Homeopathic Company for Arrowroot, a homeopathic supply house. The ingredients are: *Arnica, Ruta, Aconite, Gelsemium,*

Ledum, Phosphorus and *Hypericum,* all in low (30X) potency.

When should you use it? Use *Pre-Dental Procedure* before a dental procedure. It is designed to help your body prepare for a dental procedure including dental surgery.

How should you use it? Allow 2 tablets to dissolve in the mouth 4 times the day before the procedure and 4 times the day of the procedure.

Post-Dental Procedure

What is it? This is a homeopathic combination remedy produced by Standard Homeopathic Company for Arrowroot, a homeopathic supply house. The ingredients are: *Arnica, Ruta, Apis mellifica, Phosphorus, Hypericum, Ledum, Hamamelis, Hepar sulph* and *Staphysagria,* all in low (30X) potency.

When should you use it? Take *Post-Dental Procedure* to help your body cope with the trauma of dental procedures and dental surgery.

How should you use it? Allow 2 tablets to dissolve in the mouth every 4 hours starting immediately after the procedure and stopping when there is improvement.

Pre-Cosmetic Procedure

What is it? This is a homeopathic combination remedy produced by Standard Homeopathic Company for Arrowroot, a homeopathic supply house. The ingredients are: *Arnica, Hamamelis, Aconite, Gelsemium, Ruta, Ledum* and *Ignatia,* all in low (30X) potency.

When should you use it? Use *Pre-Cosmetic Procedure* when you want to prepare your body for the trauma of cosmetic surgery.

How should you use it? Allow 2 tablets to dissolve in the mouth 4 times the day before the procedure and 4 times the day of the procedure.

Post-Cosmetic Procedure

What is it? This is a homeopathic combination remedy produced by Standard Homeopathic Company for Arrowroot, a homeopathic supply house. The ingredients are: *Arnica, Ruta, Staphysagria, Symphytum, Hamamelis, Hypericum, Apis mellifica, Ledum, Thiosinaminum* and *Hepar sulph,* all in low (30X) potency.

When should you use it? Use *Post-Cosmetic Procedure* when you want to help your body cope with the after effects of cosmetic surgery.

How should you use it? Allow 2 tablets to dissolve in the mouth every 4 hours starting immediately after the procedure and stopping when there is improvement.

Pre-Orthopedic Procedure

What is it? This is a homeopathic combination remedy produced by Standard Homeopathic Company for Arrowroot, a homeopathic supply house. The ingredients are: *Aconite, Arnica, Gelsemium, Phosphorus, Ruta, Hypericum, Apis mellifica* and *Ledum,* all in low (30X) potency.

When should you use it? Use *Pre-Orthopedic Procedure* when you want to prepare your body to cope with the trauma of an orthopedic procedure or orthopedic surgery.

How should you use it? Allow 2 tablets to dissolve in the mouth 4 times the day before the procedure and 4 times the day of the procedure.

Orthopedic Post-Op

What is it? This is a homeopathic combination remedy produced by Standard Homeopathic Company for Arrowroot, a homeopathic supply house. The ingredients are: *Arnica, Ruta, Staphysagria, Symphytum, Hamamelis, Hypericum, Apis mellifica, Ledum, Thiosinaminum* and *Hepar sulph,* all in low (30X) potency.

When should you use it? Use *Orthopedic Post-Op* when you want to help your body to copy with recovery from an orthopedic procedure or orthopedic surgery.

How should you use it? Allow 2 tablets to dissolve in the mouth every 4 hours starting immediately after the procedure and stopping when there is improvement.

Homeopathic Remedies for Burns

Burn Injuries in General

The homeopathic treatment of burns, or any condition, is based on the symptoms that the patient describes. The homeopathic remedies discussed below are all recommended for your **Homeopathic First Aid Remedy Kit for Burns** because, as with most traumatic injuries or accidents, the sooner burns are treated the faster the relief from pain and the faster the body's response towards healing can begin. The homeopathic burn remedies, pellets, liquid drops, skin ointments, and gels should be readily available.

First degree burns cause a pinking to reddening of the skin. They are painful but there is no blistering. Sunburns and scald burns from hot water are usually first degree burns. Most sunburns can be prevented by using sunblock lotion with Sun Protection Factor (SPF) 30. The lotion contains chemicals which block out ultraviolet B rays, responsible for sunburn.

Second degree burns cause a reddening of the skin along with blisters and they are very painful. You may see serum ooze or seep from the burn. Third degree burns are not painful because the nerve endings in the skin are no longer functioning properly. The color of a third degree burn is often white but parts of it may be red or blackened.

According to Western medicine, the first step in the first aid treatment of minor burns is to apply *cold water*. According to Western medicine, *cold water* acts to lessen the pain and decreases the thermal injury itself.

But according to homeopathic medicine, the first step in the first aid treatment of minor burns is to apply *warm water*! Why warm water? This is a direct application of the Law of Similars upon which everything in homeopathy is based. The **Law of Similars** states that *like cures like*. Warm water is like, or *similar*, to the hotness of a burn. Hot water would be the *same* as a burn, and cold water would be *opposite* to a burn (the Western medicine way). Try soaking the part in *warm water* the next time that you or your family member experiences a burn.

After applying *warm water* to the burn, go ahead and consider giving some of the remedies below according to their **keynote** symptoms.

Along with the remedies specific for burns, you may always consider giving *Arnica* for soft tissue injury and *Aconite* for the physical and emotional shock associated with the burn.

As with any and all medical conditions, when dealing with burns you must pay strict attention to the **Guidelines for Consulting Your Health Care Provider** at the end of this chapter.

Calendula officinalis

What is it? This is the plant *Calendula officinalis*, common name *marigold*, a member of the *Compositae* botanical family. The leaves and orange flowers are used to prepare the tincture of *Calendula* and from that, the ointments and creams are made. Since it does not go through the dilutions and successions that are necessary to make the homeopathic remedy, it is technically speaking, used as an herbal remedy. *Califlora Gel* is a topical gel produced by Boericke & Tafel, a homeopathic pharmaceutical supply house. *Califlora Gel* is *Calendula officinalis* in very low potency (1X), as a 10% concentration.

> **Note:** Boiron and Weleda also produce *Calendula* ointment. Weleda *Calendula Oil* contains organic sesame oil and is used for infants' massage.

When should you use it? *Calendula* is applied to the burned skin to reduce the pain and swelling as well as an antiseptic to prevent infection. In fact, you may use *Calendula* cream or ointment or gel on cuts and abrasions to reduce the tendency to infection. *Califlora Gel* is particularly useful for sunburned skin because the gel is cooling and soothing.

How should you use it? Apply *Calendula* cream, ointment or *Califlora Gel* liberally to the skin every $\frac{1}{2}$-2 hours as soon as the burned area is dried from the application of cold water. You may reapply *Calendula* as often as necessary. *Califlora Gel* is not recommended for children under the age of 2 years because *Calendula officinalis* is in such low potency that it may be toxic to youngsters.

You may use *Calendula Essence*, a homeopathic remedy of mother tincture of *Calendula officinalis* by Weleda as a compress (2 teaspoons in one cup of warm water) on bruised, but intact, skin. You may use *Calendula Essence* as a localized bath for diaper rash (diaper dermatitis). Weleda also makes *Calendula Baby Cream* and *Calendula Baby Oil* (both containing *Calendula* extract).

Aloe vera

What is it? This plant, *Aloe barbadenis*, the *desert lily*, is a member of the *Liliaceae* botanical family. The *Aloe vera* remedy is made from the liquid that is exuded when the broad, fleshy leaves are cut across.

When should you use it? Here too the tincture is used so that the remedy is not technically homeopathic, but herbal instead. *Aloe vera* is used to speed healing especially after sunburns, although it can be used to soothe any skin irritation. It comes in many different preparations, but the gel is cooling to burnt skin.

How should you use it? Apply *Aloe vera* cream, ointment liberally to the skin every ½-2 hours as soon as the burned area is dried from the application of cold water. You may reapply *Aloe vera* as often as necessary.

> **Note:** You may apply *Aloe vera* skin cream to cold sores on lips. It probably inactivates the herpes virus that is the cause of cold sores while it speeds healing. I recommend that you grow your own *Aloe vera* plant so you can cut one of the leaves and squeeze the juice directly onto the cold sore, or onto any skin irritation.

Rescue Remedy Cream

What is it? This is the *Bach Flower Remedy* that is composed of five different flower essences.

When should you use it? They act together to calm inflammation and reduce soreness. The moisturizing ability of the cream acts to stem further serum seepage from the burn site.

How should you use it? Apply *Rescue Remedy* cream, ointment liberally to the skin every ½-2 hours as soon as the burned area is dried from the application of cold water. You may reapply *Rescue Remedy* as often as necessary.

Cantharis

What is it? This is the homeopathic remedy made from the whole insect, the *Spanish fly, Cantharis vesicatoria*.

When should you use it? The **keynote** symptoms leading you to give *Cantharis* are burning pains with blistering, which worsens on being touched, along with restless activity. *Cantharis* is useful to treat burning pains of the skin and urinary tract. The pain of sunburn may disappear very quickly after taking *Cantharis* by mouth.

How should you use it? Give *Cantharis* 30C pellets or liquid drops every ½-2 hours. When the burning pains and blistering have lessened you may decrease the frequency of administration. You may stop giving *Cantharis* when there has been substantial relief.

Urtica urens

What is it? This plant is the *stinging nettle*, a member of the *Urticaceae* botanical family

When should you use it? The **keynote** symptom leading you to give *Urtica urens* is stinging pains, very often along with itching, in skin that has suffered a burn but has not blistered. *Urtica urens* is best used for superficial burns such as scalds from hot water and sunburn.

How should you use it? Give *Urtica urens* 30C pellets or liquid drops every ½-2 hours. When the burning pains and blistering have lessened you may decrease the frequency of administration. You may stop giving *Urtica urens* when there has been substantial relief. *Urtica urens* is also available in a cream. Apply *Urtica urens* cream, ointment liberally to the skin every ½-2 hours as soon as the burned area is dried from the application of cold water. You may reapply *Urtica urens* as often as necessary.

Causticum

What is it? The homeopathic remedy is a chemical compound prepared from calcium hydroxide (lime) and potassium bisulphate.

When should you use it? The **keynote** symptoms

leading you to give *Causticum* are burning, tearing pains with dryness leading to cracking. The older burns that need *Causticum* may have already healed and the scabs are dry and cracking.

How should you use it? Give *Causticum* 30C once or twice daily until the condition is improved. You may stop giving *Causticum* when the pains associated with dryness have ceased.

Arsenicum album

What is it? This is the homeopathic remedy made from the chemical compound arsenic oxide which is highly poisonous if not given in homeopathic dilution.

When should you use it? The **keynote** symptoms leading you to choose *Arsenicum album* are burning pains (which surprisingly may be improved with warmth) with great anxiety and restlessness. *Arsenicum album* is often used as a constitutional remedy, for colds and flu, and for asthma. Persons needing *Arsenicum album* usually feel chilly and they may express a fear of death.

How should you use it? Give *Arsenicum album* 30C every ½-2 hours until the burning pains with anxiety are relieved. Then give *Arsenicum album* 200C once or twice daily until improvement. You may stop giving *Arsenicum album* when the situation is under control.

Graphites

What is it? This is the homeopathic remedy made from *graphite*, also called *plumbago* or *black lead*, used to make lead pencils and as a lubricant. It is a naturally occurring soft carbon, a mineral.

When should you use it? The **keynote** symptoms leading you to give *Graphites* are thickened, hard scars under which there may be burning sensations. In addition, *Graphites* is useful to treat skin cracking with the formation of honey-colored fluid forming a thick yellow crust. This is often seen in eczema but it may also occur in a burn.

How should you use it? Give *Graphites* 30C once or twice daily until the hard, thick scarring has become softer and pain-free. You may stop giving *Graphites* when the scar is no longer a problem.

Guidelines for Consulting Your Health Care Provider

You should consult your health care provider if any of the following occurs during a course of treatment for traumatic injuries:

- the wound is not healing the way you think it should (trust your instincts!)
- you suspect a broken bone
- you suspect a limb or a body part has been crushed by something heavy
- you see frank pus in the wound
- you see red lines running from the wound towards the center of the body
- the wound is extremely painful
- the wound continues to bleed
- the patient has a fever higher than 101°F (38.4°C)
- the patient is having trouble breathing or complaining of chest pains or there is mental confusion or lethargy
- the injury was on the head in a very young infant (3 months old or less)
- the injury was on the head with loss of consciousness (concussion)
- there is vomiting with a head injury (even if no loss of consciousness)
- the patient has had a seizure or a convulsion

After Surgery:
You should consult your health care provider if:
- the patient seems to be getting worse in any way (trust your instincts!)
- the surgical wound continues to ooze pus or blood
- the surgical wound has opened
- the patient has difficulty with movement, speech, eating, drinking, sleeping
- the patient is having trouble breathing or complaining of chest pains or there is mental confusion or lethargy
- the patient has a fever higher than 101°F (38.4°C)
- the patient has mental confusion
- the patient has had a seizure or convulsion

Burns:
You should consult your health care provider if:
- the burn's appearance or anything about the burn causes you considerable anxiety (trust your instincts!)
- the area of the burn is larger than the palm of your

hand
- the burn is on the face and you may be concerned with scarring
- the burn is from a caustic chemical or an electrical wire
- the patient is having trouble breathing or complaining of chest pains or there is mental confusion or lethargy
- the burn has areas in the center which are *not* painful
- you suspect a third degree burn
- you are unable to give effective pain control
- you suspect an infection in the burn wound
- the patient has a fever higher than 101°F (38.4°C)
- your young child has changed his or her eating, sleeping, or playing behaviors

> **Note:** Do not discontinue taking any pharmaceutical medication that has been prescribed by your health care provider unless you or your family member is under the supervision of a physician.

Recommendations for Homeopathic First Aid Remedy Kit

Arnica montana 30C—pellets and liquid drops, and either cream, ointment, gel, or spray
Traumeel combination remedy—tablets and drops, and either ointment or gel
Arniflora—gel or cream
Wound-Care—ointment
Aconitum napellus 30C—pellets and liquid drops and *Aconitum napellus* 200C—pellets
Hypericum perforatum 30C—pellets and liquid drops, and either ointment or spray
Ledum palustre 30C—pellets and liquid drops
Ruta graveolens 30C—pellets and liquid drops
Natrum sulphuricum 30C—pellets and liquid drops
Symphytum officinalis 30C—pellets and liquid drops
Rhus toxicodendron 200C—pellets and liquid drops
Apis mellifica 30C—pellets and liquid drops
Sssssting Stop—gel
Sports Gel—gel

> **Note:** Homeopathic Remedy Kits, for first aid and for general use, are available from several of the Homeopathic Remedy Supply Houses listed in the **Appendix**. However, I much prefer you to create your own **Homeopathic First Aid Remedy Kit** so that you can have the liquid drops on hand for infants and children and so that you can administer the remedies in the potencies that I recommend.

Additional Homeopathic Remedies for Traumatic Injuries

Staphysagria 30C—pellets and liquid drops
Bryonia alba 30C—pellets and liquid drops
Bellis perennis 30C—pellets and liquid drops

Pre-Surgery Prescription

Arnica montana 30C—pellets and liquid drops
Aconitum napellus 30C—pellets and liquid drops
Phosphorus 30C—pellets and liquid drops
Hypericum perforatum 30C—pellets and liquid drops
Start giving *Arnica* 30C, *Aconite* 30C, *Phosphorus* 30C and *Hypericum* pellets or liquid drops once or twice daily for each day starting three days before the scheduled surgery. Then give *Arnica*, *Aconite*, *Phosphorus*, and *Hypericum* 1-4 times just after surgery, for one or two days, or until the physical and emotional stress and shock from surgery has passed.

Homeopathic Remedies for Traumatic Injuries Associated with Surgery

Arnica montana 30C—pellets and liquid drops
Aconitum napellus 30C—pellets and liquid drops
Phosphorus 30C—pellets and liquid drops
Staphysagria 30C—pellets and liquid drops
Hypericum perforatum 30C—pellets and liquid drops
Ferrum phosphoricum 30C—pellets and liquid drops
Crotalus horridus 30C—pellets and liquid drops
Rescue Remedy—Bach Flower Remedy—liquid drops, spray, and cream *Pre-Dental Procedure*—tablets
Post-Dental Procedure—tablets
Pre-Cosmetic Procedure—tablets
Post-Cosmetic Procedure—ablets
Pre-Orthopedic Procedure—tablets
Orthopedic Post-Op—tablets

Recommendations for Homeopathic First Aid Remedy Kit for Burns

Calendula officinalis—cream or ointment and *Calendula Essence* for a compress

Aloe vera—gel

Rescue Remedy—liquid drops and cream

Cantharis 30C—pellets and liquid drops

Urtica urens 30C—pellets and liquid drops and cream

Causticum 30C—pellets and liquid drops

Arsenicum album 30C and 200C—pellets and liquid drops

Graphites 30C—pellets and liquid drops

Guidelines for Administration of Homeopathic Remedies

Once you have chosen the homeopathic remedy and the potency that is likely to help you or your family member, you should try to give as few repetitions of the remedy as you can. You start off repeating it more frequently in a severe, acute situation, quickly decreasing the frequency once improvement has begun, stopping the remedy as soon as the problem has resolved.

> **Note:** For more information on *how often* to give the homeopathic remedy please see **Potency and Frequency**, in **Chapter 2: Basic Homeopathy**. For information on *how much* of the homeopathic remedy to give and the importance of a *"clean tongue,"* please see **How to take homeopathic remedies** in the same chapter.

Lower potency remedies, such as 30C and below, are used to treat acute ailments. They are usually repeated often, every ½-2 or ½-4 hours. You should notice improvement in symptoms after just one to perhaps a few repetitions. If you do not see improvement, it is wise to stop the remedy and try a different one, guiding yourself by the **keynote** symptoms. You may use different single remedies together or you may try a combination remedy. And you may use homeopathic remedies together with pharmaceutical prescription and non-prescription drugs without any effect of interference.

General guidelines to treat serious, chronic,

relapsing ailments include using single remedies at potencies of 200C. These are generally administered once weekly to once monthly, but they may be used once or twice daily at first if the condition warrants it, quickly decreasing the frequency as you see improvement. Do not continue giving the remedy if it becomes apparent that it is not working. You may always stop one remedy and choose to administer another remedy on the basis of the **keynote** symptoms of the new remedy. In addition, you may administer more than one remedy at a time.

Putting It All Together

Traumatic injuries, like falls, sprains, abrasions, bruises, bumps, cuts, bites, and burns, are usually acute problems that do not require long-term remedies for treatment. But, even so, it is probably good health practice to make sure that the patient has all the vitamins and minerals necessary to replenish any lost blood and to repair injured tissues (please refer to **Chapter 23: Vitamins and Minerals**) as well as a general antioxidant supplement necessary to facilitate tissue repair (please refer to **Chapter 24: Antioxidant Phytochemicals**). Increased doses of *Vitamin C* may be especially useful to repair wounds.

Infants, toddlers and young children as well as elderly persons are more prone to traumatic injuries than people in other age groups. You may want to take a look at constitutional remedies for youngsters and the elderly. A discussion of constitutional homeopathic remedies are found in **Chapter 9: Homeopathic Remedies for Constitutional Problems in Infants, Children, and Adolescents**, **Chapter 18: Homeopathic Constitutional Remedies** (for adults) and **Chapter 13: Homeopathy for Elderly Persons**.

People who suffer from arthritis may be prone to repeated traumatic injuries. If this is the case, you may benefit from reading **Chapter 14: Homeopathy for Problems in Joints, Bones, and Muscles** and **Chapter 28: Nutritional Supplements for Diseases of Joints, Bones, and Muscles**.

Chapter 4

Homeopathic Remedies for Fever

Fever in General

Ailment/Disorder/Symptom	Homeopathic Remedy
Sudden, very high, violent fevers	*Belladonna*
Moderately high fevers	*Chamomila*
Low-grade fevers	*Ferrum phosphoricum*
Fevers, teething, pains	*Camilia*
Sudden, high fevers with anxiety	*Aconitum napellus*

Guidelines for Consulting Your Health Care Provider
Putting It All Together

Fever in General

The most important thing to know about fever is that it is a normal defense mechanism of the body, a normal response to any of a large number of conditions causing inflammation. Fever does two important things. First, it tells us that the body is coping with some type of inflammation. So it is like a trumpet call, telling us to pay attention, this patient is sick. Many different conditions cause inflammation, such as infections of all kinds, certain types of arthritis, teething, cancer, and becoming overheated.

Second, fever raises the temperature inside the body so that enzymatic chemical reactions can work faster. The enzymes are working faster in order to control the inflammation by increasing the number of chemicals fighting it. This means that we shouldn't interfere with the work that fever is doing to control inflammation.

Homeopaths and pediatricians do not generally recommend giving any remedies for fever if the temperature is less than 101°F (38.4°C). The first step in treating fever is to offer more *fluids* and keep offering them. This is because fever has a tendency to cause dehydration. The more a patient with fever drinks, the gentler fever's effects on the body will be. Once the body temperature has reached 101°F (38.4°C) or more you may go ahead and give one or several of the homeopathic remedies specifically used for fever, according to their **keynote** symptoms. In addition, you may give homeopathic remedies together with acetaminophen or ibuprofen.

At the end of this chapter you will find my Recommendations for **Homeopathic First Aid Remedy Kit for Fever** and **Guidelines for Administration of Homeopathic Remedies**.

As with any and all medical conditions, when dealing with fever you must pay strict attention to the **Guidelines for Consulting Your Health Care Provider** at the end of this chapter. You may want to refer to the last section **Putting It All Together** for ideas on how to integrate the essential natural alternatives, homeopathy, herbal remedies, and nutritional supplements.

Belladonna

What is it? This is the homeopathic remedy made from the plant, *Atropa belladonna*, a member of the *Solanaceae* botanical family. The common name is *deadly nightshade*. The plant and its sweet berries are very poisonous. The toxic chemical is atropine, which dilates the pupils, hence the name *Belladonna*, or *"beautiful lady."* The homeopathic remedy is non-toxic and has no side effects. The homeopathic remedy is made from the whole plant.

When should you use it? The **keynote** symptoms leading you to use *Belladonna* for fever are sudden and violent fevers of close to 104°F (40°C) accompanied by burning heat with redness and a throbbing headache. *Belladonna* is called for when there is a sudden, high fever with skin that is flushed bright red and wide, staring, glassy eyes. Laying a hand on the child's face feels like he is radiating heat. Chills may accompany the fever but there is usually no sweating until the crisis when the fever "breaks." Only then there is much sweating. *Belladonna* suits the intelligent child who is easily excited and agitated.

How should you use it? Give *Belladonna* 30C pellets or liquid drops every ½-2 hours until the fever "breaks" or has been moderated. You may first decrease the frequency of administration and then stop altogether when the temperature is less than 101°F (38.4°C).

Chamomilla

What is it? The homeopathic remedy is made from the plant *Matricaria chamomilla*, common name *Chamomile*, a member of the *Compositae* botanical family. The whole plant in flower is used to produce the remedy. The herbal remedy is used to calm the digestive and nervous systems. *Chamomile* ointments and creams are used to calm irritations and inflammations of the skin.

When should you use it? The homeopathic remedy, *Chamomilla* has its most common use in the treatment of fever. The **keynote** symptoms leading you to give *Chamomilla* are moderately high fever of about 103°F (39.5°C), in angry, screaming children who must be carried in order to stop them from crying. A peculiar symptom strongly indicating the use of *Chamomilla* is when one cheek is pale and the other is red. *Chamomilla* is particularly effective for the pains and irritability of teething and for the fever that sometimes accompanies teething, although in this case the fever will usually be no more than low-grade. *Chamomilla* is also useful to treat colic in infants.

How should you use it? Give *Chamomilla* 30C pellets or liquid drops every ½-2 hours until the fever "breaks" or has been moderated or the teething pains and irritability have decreased. You may first decrease the frequency of administration and then stop altogether when the temperature is less than 101°F (38.4°C).

Ferrum phosphoricum

What is it? This is the homeopathic form of iron phosphate salt found in many tissues of the body. It is often used to help stop bleeding but it also has a place in the treatment of fever.

When should you use it? The **keynote** symptoms leading you to use *Ferrum phos* (as it is called for short) is the earliest stages of an infection or an inflammation that has a slow onset, with a low-grade fever of 101°F (38.4°C) or less.

How should you use it? Give *Ferrum phos* 30C pellets or liquid drops every ½-2 hours until more definite symptoms appear which require different homeopathic remedies. Then you may stop *Ferrum phos*. It is possible that if you start *Ferrum phos* at the first signs of an impending infection, you may be able to prevent the later stages of high fever. The first signs may be simply that you don't like the way your child's eyes look, that she appears to you like she's beginning to get sick. Trust yourself and your intuition. This is the stage to give *Ferrum phos*.

Camilia

What is it? *Camilia* is a combination homeopathic remedy produced by Boiron, a homeopathic pharmaceutical supply house. *Camilia* consists of the following homeopathic remedies in very low potency: *Belladonna*, *Chamomilla* and *Ferrum phosphoricum* in purified water. The drops are sugar-free.

When should you use it? Note that the homeo-pathic ingredients in *Camilia* are the same ones that treat fever (please see the 3 foregoing remedies above). The **keynote** symptoms pointing to the use of *Camilia* are all the symptoms associated with teething, such as: fever, pain, irritability, sleeplessness, and difficulties with feeding, eating and digestion. *Camilia* may also be used to treat fever even if the source is not teething, but rather a viral illness.

How should you use it? *Camilia* comes in single-use doses of liquid drops. You may administer a single-use dose every 15 minutes, depending on the severity of the teething symptoms, rapidly decreasing the frequency as soon there is improvement, stopping when the infant no longer shows those symptoms. Overdosage is not possible. *Camilia* tastes like water.

Aconitum napellus

What is it? This homeopathic remedy, called in shorthand *Aconite*, is made from the plant commonly called *monkshood* or *wolfsbane*, a member of the *Ranunculaceae* botanical family. The whole plant just before flowering is used to make the remedy. The plant is highly toxic so the homeopathic remedy is never used below the 3X potency. *Aconite* is used as a first aid treatment for traumatic injuries and surgical procedures.

When should you use it? *Aconite* has many other uses in homeopathy. One of the most important uses is for sudden high fevers (103°F [39.5°C] to 104°F [40°C]) with great anxiety and fear of dying which are the **keynote** symptoms leading you to use *Aconite*. Other **keynote** symptoms are infections or inflammations that have come on as a result of swift changes in weather conditions, such as being out in a snowstorm. Giving *Aconite* right after the exposure to cold or wind without waiting for symptoms to develop may completely prevent the illness from developing.

How should you use it? You may use *Aconite* 30C every ½-2 hours depending on need for either the fever or the fright indications or both. You may always use *Aconite* along with other homeopathic remedies. As the fever and the fright are decreased, you may decrease the frequency of administration of *Aconite* until stopping it when the temperature is 101°F (38.4°C) or less and the child is no longer frightened.

Table of Homeopathic Remedies for Fever and Their Keynote Characteristics

Remedy	Belladonna	Chamomilla	Ferrum phos	Aconite
Keynote Characteristic				
Onset	sudden, violent		slow	sudden
Fever	high	moderate	low-grade	high
Main symptom	skin flushed red	Irritable, anger, crying	no symptoms yet	great anxiety fear of death
Strange symptom	skin radiating heat, glassy eyes	one cheek red the	none	sensitive to exposure to extremes of weather

Guidelines for Consulting Your Health Care Provider

Fever:
You should consult your health care provider if:
- the patient doesn't look right or act right (trust your instincts!)
- the patient had a seizure with fever (febrile convulsion)
- the patient has a unidentified rash
- the infant is less than three months old and has a fever of 100°F (38°C) or more
- the patient's fevers continue more than 3 days
- the patient is uninterested in eating or drinking or playing
- the patient has not had a wet diaper in the past 12 hours or has had less than 4 wet diapers in the past 24 hours
- the patient has had more than 2 days of vomiting or diarrhea along with fever
- you suspect the patient has fever with dehydration
- the patient is having trouble breathing or complaining of chest pains or there is mental confusion, lethargy, or irritability.

Note: Do not discontinue taking any pharmaceutical medication, which has been prescribed by your health care provider unless you or your family member is under the supervision of a physician.

Note: Washington Homeopathic Products, Inc. manufactures a *Children's Kit* containing 12 different combination homeopathic remedies with indications for 12 different common ailments in children. The ailments treated are: children's tonic, colic, constipation, coughs and colds, diarrhea, earache, fever, hives, insomnia, motion sickness, teething, and tonsillitis. Each combination remedy contains pellets of appropriate homeopathic remedies in low potencies. *Children's Kit* is suitable for travel. *Children's Kit*'s fever contains *Aconitum napellus*, *Belladonna* and *Gelsemium*, all in 6C potency.

Recommendations for Homeopathic First Aid Remedy Kit for Fever
Belladonna 30C—pellets and liquid drops
Chamomila 30C—pellets and liquid drops
Ferrum phosphoricum 30C—pellets and liquid drops
Camilia—combination remedy, single-dose drops
Aconitum napellus 30C—pellets and liquid drops

Guidelines for Administration of Homeopathic Remedies

Once you have chosen the homeopathic remedy and the potency that is likely to help you or your family member, you should try to give as few repetitions of the remedy as you can. You start off repeating it more frequently in a severe, acute situation, quickly decreasing the frequency once improvement has begun, stopping the remedy as soon as the problem has resolved.

> **Note:** For more information on *how often* to give the homeopathic remedy please see **Potency and Frequency**, in **Chapter 2: Basic Homeopathy**. For information on *how much* of the homeopathic remedy to give and the importance of a *"clean tongue,"* please see **How to take homeopathic remedies** in the same chapter.

Lower potency remedies, such as 30C and below, are used to treat acute ailments. They are usually repeated often, every ½-2 or ½-4 hours. You should notice improvement in symptoms after just one to perhaps a few repetitions. If you do not see improvement, it is wise to stop the remedy and try a different one, guiding yourself by the **keynote** symptoms. You may use different single remedies together or you may try a combination remedy. And you may use homeopathic remedies together with pharmaceutical prescription and non-prescription drugs without any effect of interference.

General guidelines to treat serious, chronic, relapsing ailments include using single remedies at potencies of 200C. These are generally administered once weekly to once monthly, but they may be used once or twice daily at first if the condition warrants it, quickly decreasing the frequency as you see improvement. Do not continue giving the remedy if it becomes apparent that it is not working. You may always stop one remedy and choose to administer another remedy on the basis of the **keynote** symptoms of the new remedy. In addition, you may administer more than one remedy at a time.

Putting It All Together

Depending on the chronicity of the fever episodes, you may decide to incorporate certain homeopathic remedies from **Chapter 5: Homeopathic Remedies for Upper Respiratory Infections: Colds, Flu, Coughs, Sore Throats, Laryngitis, Ear Infections, Eye Infections, Sinus Infections** and **Chapter 7: Homeopathic Remedies for Infection**s.

Depending on the source of the fever episodes, it may be a good idea to read **Chapter 11: Homeopathy for Digestive Tract Ailments** and **Chapter 12: Homeopathy for Urinary Tract Ailments**.

People with ailments that cause fever generally require all the vitamins and minerals necessary to repair and replenish tissues (please refer to **Chapter 23: Vitamins and Minerals**) as well as a general antioxidant supplement (please refer to **Chapter 24: Antioxidant Phytochemicals**).

Depending on the chronicity of the fever episodes, you may want to consider learning about nutritional supplements to augment the immune system, especially *medicinal mushrooms* (please refer to **Chapter 27: Nutritional Supplements to Prevent Cancer and Augment Your Immune System**). You will also benefit from reading about *Echinacea*, *Goldenseal* and *Astragalus* in **Chapter 20: Herbs You Need to Know**.

In addition, it is a good idea to consider giving the sick person's homeopathic constitutional remedy (please refer to **Chapter 9: Homeopathic Remedies for Constitutional Problems in Infants, Children, and Adolescents** or to **Chapter 18: Homeopathic Constitutional Remedies** if you are dealing with an adult).

Chapter 5

Homeopathic Remedies for Upper Respiratory Infections:
Colds, Flu, Coughs, Sore Throats, Laryngitis, Ear Infections, Eye Infections, Sinus Infections

Upper Respiratory Infections in General

Colds and Flu Prevention:

Ailment/Disorder/Symptom	Homeopathic Remedy
Upper respiratory infections	*Aconitum napellus*
Infection with influenza (flu)	*Oscillococcinum*
Infection with influenza (flu)	*Influenzinum*

Colds and Flu Treatment:

Ailment/Disorder/Symptom	Homeopathic Remedy
Muscle aches and pains, low-grade fever	*Ferrum phosphoricum*
High fevers with throbbing headache and sudden onset	*Belladonna*
Flu that comes on slowly with heavy feeling	*Gelsemium sempervirens*
Yellow-green mucus discharges in coughs and colds	*Pulsatilla nigricans*
Watery nasal and eye discharges in upper respiratory infections	*Allium cepa*
Burning discharges from nose and eyes, with anxiety and fears	*Arsenicum album*
Colds accompanied by nausea, vomiting, and diarrhea	*Nux vomica*
Colds accompanied by achy, bruised feeling	*Baptisia*
Colds accompanied by severe aches and pains in muscles and bones	*Eupatorium perfoliatum*
Symptoms of upper respiratory infections	*Umcka ColdCare*
Sore throat and congestion	*Echinacea Compound*

After Colds and Flu:

Ailment/Disorder/Symptom	Homeopathic Remedy
Heaviness of limbs, thirstlessness, never been well since sick with flu	*Gelsemium sempervirens*
Exhaustion and depression after being sick with flu	*Kali phosphoricum*

Cough:

Ailment/Disorder/Symptom	Homeopathic Remedy
Coughing brought on by slightest movement	*Bryonia alba*
Thick, yellow-green mucus with cough	*Pulsatilla*
Dry cough after exposure to cold	*Aconitum napellus*
Spasmodic cough in croup, asthma, laryngitis	*Spongia tosta*

Spasmodic, barking coughs	*Drosera rotundifolia*
Dry cough at night after exposure to cold	*Rumex crispus*
Coughs with stringy mucus	*Kali bichromicum*
Coughs due to upper respiratory infections and allergies	*Chestal*

Sore Throats and Laryngitis:

Ailment/Disorder/Symptom	**Homeopathic Remedy**
Sore throats after exposure to cold weather	*Aconitum napellus*
Sore throats with pus on the tonsils	*Hepar sulphuris calcareum*
Infections and ulcers of the mouth, teeth, gums, and sinuses	*Mercurius solubilis*
Colds, sore throats, hoarseness, laryngitis, and nasal congestion with nosebleeds	*Phosphorus*
Colds and coughs after exposure to damp weather	*Dulcamara*
Hoarseness and laryngitis	*Causticum*
Cold sores and fever sores	*Erpace*
Sore throats and hoarseness	*Echina-Spray*

Ear Infections:

Ailment/Disorder/Symptom	**Homeopathic Remedy**
Ear infections with throbbing pain	*Belladonna*
Ear infections with ear very sensitive to touch	*Hepar sulphuris calcareum*
Ear infections with smelly pus leaking out of the ear	*Mercurius solubilis*
Ear infections	*Earache*

Eye Infections:

Ailment/Disorder/Symptom	**Homeopathic Remedy**
Profuse tearing, burning eyes, discharge from eyes	*Euphrasia officinales*
Burning and stinging pains in eyes	*Apis mellifica*
Styes on eyelids	*Staphysagria*

Sinus Infections:

Ailment/Disorder/Symptom	**Homeopathic Remedy**
Sinus infections with stringy mucus	*Kali bichromicum*
Sinus infections with yellow-green mucus	*Pulsatilla*
Severe sinus pain with face sensitive to touch	*Hepar sulphuris calcareum*
Sinus infections with thick, smelly mucus	*Mercurius solubilis*
Recurrent sinus infections	*Sinus Relief*

Guidelines for Consulting Your Health Care Provider
Putting It All Together

Upper Respiratory Infections in General

Upper respiratory infections are caused by viruses, hundreds of different viruses, but they are not the only reason we come down with a cold or the flu. There are certain other equally important factors, which make one person more susceptible to the invading virus than another. One such factor is *stress*, both emotional and psychological stress as well as environmental stress, such as getting wet or being chilled outside in cold weather. The stress itself may not be as damaging as how we react chemically inside our bodies to the stress. This chemical reactivity is probably determined by *genetics*.

A second factor is the status of the person's *immune system*. Children have an immune system that hasn't yet been exposed to a large number of viruses. This will naturally happen just by living into adolescence and adulthood. Until then, the child will tend to become more easily infected with upper respiratory viruses. Adults may have a tendency to become easily infected with upper respiratory viruses due to malfunctioning immune systems. This can happen as a result of many different conditions, such as cancer, AIDS, chronic fatigue syndrome, or smoking.

A third reason why certain people may be vulnerable to infection with upper respiratory viruses is the person's *nutritional status*, which is determined by a combination of the healthfulness of the daily diet and nutritional supplements.

The public health burden of the common cold is enormous. According to a 2003 article in the *Archives of Internal Medicine*, the common cold is responsible for $40 billion every year in the U.S. in expenditures ranging from visits to the physician to prescriptions medicines to the costs that parents incur when they have to stay home to take care of themselves or their sick children. The cost of homeopathic remedies to treat and prevent the common cold and the flu are minimal. The remedies are often effective and they have no side effects. Homeopathic remedies should be utilized as first-line treatment for upper respiratory tract illnesses.

The public health burden of upper respiratory infections is not the only reason why homeopathic remedies should be your first approach. The results of medical research studies are showing that the use of antihistamines, *corticosteroids*, and antibiotics for the treatment of acute otitis media (ear infection) provide no significant benefits. Researchers at the University of Texas found that children who used antihistamines had a prolonged course of fluid in the middle ear when compared to those who did not use antihistamines.

The treatment and prevention of upper respiratory viruses is a good example of how homeopathy, herbal remedies, and nutritional supplements work together to make a person healthier than she would be just using one or two of these alone.

You may prefer to use a *combination homeopathic remedy* to treat colds or coughs, or any of the conditions discussed in this chapter. *Combination remedies* are certainly easier to use than single remedies and are very often effective. You would buy either tablets or liquid with names like, *Cough*, or *Cold*, or *Flu*. Combination remedies will likely include many of the single remedies listed below, but in very low potency. Using combination remedies is like taking a stab in the dark.

However, many people find that combination remedies do not work well enough so it is important to be able to use single remedies according to their **keynote** symptoms. You may always give a remedy, gauge the reaction, and if necessary, give a different remedy. You may use more than one single remedy at one time. You should have on hand those remedies for treating those **keynote** symptoms that tend to recur in you or members of your family.

As with any and all medical conditions, when dealing with infections of the upper respiratory tract such as colds, flu, coughs, sore throats, laryngitis, ear infections, eye infections, and sinus infections you must pay strict attention to the **Guidelines for Consulting Your Health Care Provider** at the end of this chapter. You may want to refer to the last section **Putting It All Together** for ideas on how to integrate the essential natural alternatives, homeopathy, herbal remedies, and nutritional supplements.

Colds and Flu Prevention

Aconitum napellus

What is it? This homeopathic remedy, called in short *Aconite*, is made from the plant commonly called *monkshood* or *wolfsbane*, a member of the *Ranunculaceae* botanical family. The whole plant just before flowering is used to make the remedy. The plant is highly toxic so the homeopathic remedy is never used below the 3X potency. *Aconite* is used as a first aid treatment for traumatic injuries and surgical procedures and for fevers.

When should you use it? The **keynote** symptoms leading you to use *Aconite* for both early prevention and early treatment of colds or flu are sudden onset and a sense of impending illness, especially after being exposed to cold or any extreme weather. In my experience, *Aconite* is suitable to prevent or treat colds and flu after the following environmental conditions: cold and dry winds (such as shoveling snow or sitting in an air-conditioned auditorium); cold and wet weather; extremely hot weather. There may be sudden onset with chills, sweats, and fever. Judiciously administered doses of *Aconite* as soon after the exposure as possible without waiting for symptoms to develop may completely prevent the illness from developing.

How should you use it? You may use *Aconite* 30C every ½-2 hours depending on the sense of impending illness. It is possible that just one dose of *Aconite* 30C will prevent the illness if given early enough just after the exposure or just at the first sense of impending illness. You may always use *Aconite* along with other homeopathic remedies. You may decrease the frequency of administration of *Aconite* and stop it when the patient has either averted the cold or has improved from the infection.

Oscillococcinum

What is it? This homeopathic remedy is made by Boiron from an extract of the liver and heart of the Mallard duck (*Anas barbariae*) which has been infected with the influenza virus, or "flu."

When should you use it? It is the most commonly used treatment for influenza in France and is becoming more widely used in the United States during flu season. *Oscillococcinum* is both a preventive and a treatment for flu, especially when taken at the very first sign of flu. It may be used by homeopaths as an alternative to the influenza vaccine in persons who refuse to take vaccines. Boiron has collected the evidence-based data for *Oscillococcinum*, which proves that it is both safe and effective. As with all homeopathic remedies, there are no side effects. The FDA has not received any reports of adverse effects. It can be combined with all prescription medicines as well as with the flu vaccine. It is considered safe for elderly persons and pregnant and lactating women. *Oscillococcinum* is considered to be homeopathy's answer to "bird flu" becoming an epidemic in humans.

How should you use it? *Oscillococcinum* comes in tubes. The directions are to dissolve the entire contents of one tube in the mouth. For prevention, give one tube of *Oscillococcinum* every week during flu season, generally from November through March. This is a rationale for elderly people, especially those with heart or respiratory ailments, as well as for young infants. For treatment of flu, give one tube as early as possible after onset, then repeating every 6 hours as needed depending on severity of symptoms. When the patient has improved, you may stop.

Influenzinum

What is it? This is the homeopathic remedy made from influenza virus strains taken from the current year's influenza vaccine. It is used both for prevention by some homeopaths instead of the flu vaccine and for treatment after flu infection. It is certainly safer than the flu vaccine, but whether it is as effective is not known because research has never been done to find out.

When should you use it? The **keynote** symptom for using *Influenzinum* after infection with the flu virus is the patient's conviction that "She (or He) has never been well since coming down with the flu." *Influenzinum* is also used by homeopaths to prevent infection with the influenza virus.

How should you use it? Give one dose of the pellets of *Influenzinum* 200C once a month during the flu season, generally from November through

March to prevent flu infection. If you are treating yourself or a family member who complains of "never been well since," use *Influenzinum* 200C once a week until symptoms are resolved. Then stop.

Colds and Flu Treatment

Aconitum napellus or *Aconite*

See how and when to use *Aconite* under **Prevention of Colds and Flu**. In homeopathy the prevention and treatment of an illness may be administered in the same way.

Oscillococcinum

See how and when to use *Oscillococcinum* under **Prevention of Colds and Flu**. In homeopathy the prevention and treatment of an illness may be administered in the same way.

Ferrum phosphoricum

What is it? This is the homeopathic form of iron phosphate salt found in many tissues of the body. It is often used to help stop bleeding, and for fever, but it also has a place in the treatment of colds and flu.
When should you use it? The **keynote** symptom leading you to use *Ferrum phos* (as it is called for short) is mild symptoms with a slow onset. *Ferrum phos* is most often used for the early or prodromal stage of an illness, that is, with muscle aches and pains, low-grade fever, general not feeling well.
How should you use it? Give *Ferrum phos* 30C pellets or liquid drops every ½-2 hours until more definite symptoms appear which require different homeopathic remedies. Then you may stop *Ferrum phos*. It is possible that if you start *Ferrum phos* at the first signs of an impending cold or flu, you may be able to completely prevent or at least to lessen the later stages.

Belladona

What is it? This is the homeopathic remedy made from the plant, *Atropa belladonna*, a member of the *Solanaceae* botanical family. The common name is *deadly nightshade*. The plant and its berries are very poisonous. The toxic chemical is atropine, which dilates the pupils, hence the name *Belladonna*, or "beautiful lady." The homeopathic remedy is non-toxic and has no side effects. The homeopathic remedy is made from the whole plant.
When should you use it? The **keynote** symptoms leading you to use *Belladonna* for colds and flu are rapid onset of the illness with high fever along with throbbing headache. *Belladonna* is commonly used as a treatment for high fever.
How should you use it? Give *Belladonna* 30C pellets or liquid drops every ½-2 hours, then tapering the frequency quickly as the throbbing headache and high fever decreases.

Gelsemium sempervirens

What is it? This is the poisonous plant whose common name is *yellow jasmine*, a member of the *Loganiaceae* botanical family. The homeopathic remedy is made from the bark.
When should you use it? The **keynote** symptoms leading you to give *Gelsemium* are those colds and flu that come on slowly with fever alternating with chills, weakness, a feeling of heaviness of the limbs and even the eyelids, and a strange lack of thirst.
How should you use it? Give *Gelsemium* 30C pellets or liquid drops every ½-2 hours, then tapering the frequency as the severity of the symptoms decrease.

Pulsatilla nigricans

What is it? This is the plant whose common name is *windflower*, a member of the *Ranunculaceae* botanical family. The whole plant is used for the homeopathic remedy. *Pulsatilla* is most commonly used as a constitutional remedy for girls and women who tend to be timid, yielding, and sympathetic, with a desire to please.
When should you use it? The **keynote** symptom

leading you to use *Pulsatilla* in men or women is yellow or yellow-green mucus discharge in large amounts occurring during colds, flu, coughs, eye infections, and sinus infections. *Pulsatilla* is especially indicated for those persons who feel warm all the time and who are thirstless.

How should you use it? Give *Pulsatilla* 30C pellets or liquid drops every ½-2 hours, rapidly decreasing the frequency when the mucus is decreased or becomes clear.

Allium cepa

What is it? This is the plant whose common name is *red onion*, a member of the *Liliaceae* botanical family. The whole plant is used to make the homeopathic remedy. If you have ever cut an onion and suffered your eyes stinging and watering with your nose dripping, then you instinctively know which symptoms the onion as the homeopathic remedy can cure.

When should you use it? The **keynote** symptoms leading you to use *Allium* are the profuse, stinging, watery eye discharge with profuse, watery, nasal discharge. This may be accompanied by sneezing and a tickle in the throat, which are also symptoms of allergy.

How should you use it? Give *Allium* 30C in pellets or liquid drops every ½-2 hours, decreasing in frequency as the watery discharges start to improve, stopping when the mucus membranes of the eyes and nose are no longer so inflamed.

Arsenicum album

What is it? This is the homeopathic remedy made from the chemical compound arsenic oxide which is highly poisonous if not given in homeopathic dilution. *Arsenicum album* is often used as a constitutional remedy and for asthma, as well as for burns.

When should you use it? The **keynote** symptoms leading you to choose *Arsenicum album* are great chilliness with excessive thirst for cold drinks (from which she takes frequent small sips), and burning, watery mucus discharges from the nose and eyes. There is often great anxiety with weakness and restlessness and there may be fear of death.

How should you use it? Give *Arsenicum album* 30C every ½-2 hours until the anxiety and restlessness have improved. Then you may decrease the frequency, stopping when the watery mucus discharges are no longer dominant.

Nux vomica

What is it? This is a poisonous plant, *Nux vomica*, common name *Poison nut*, a member of the *Loganiaceae* botanical family. The poisonous seeds are used to produce the gentle homeopathic remedy. The plant's poison is strychnine. *Nux vomica* is often used as a constitutional remedy, especially for angry, frustrated men who are workaholics ("Type A" personality) and over-indulge in alcohol, nicotine, and caffeine.

When should you use it? The **keynote** symptoms for the use of *Nux vomica* are when there is nausea, vomiting, and diarrhea with respiratory symptoms of the flu, especially if the nose is blocked at night, but runs during the day. A person needing *Nux vomica* may be excessively chilly, complaining, irritable, and impatient. *Nux vomica* is also used to treat asthma.

How should you use it? Give *Nux vomica* 30C every ½-2 hours until the abdominal symptoms of the flu have decreased. Then you may decrease the frequency, and stop when the patient has improved.

Baptisia

What is it? This plant is *Baptisia tinctoria*, commonly called *Wild indigo*, a member of the *Leguminosae* botanical family. The plant root is used to make the homeopathic remedy.

When should you use it? The **keynote** symptoms leading you to use *Baptisia* are rapid, sudden onset with feeling bruised all over and aching, heavy limbs. The patient may be drowsy and tends to fall asleep while talking. There may be vomiting and diarrhea as well. The sick person tends to be very thirsty.

How should you use it? Give *Baptisia* 30C every ½-2 hours quickly decreasing the frequency as soon as the bruised feeling diminishes.

Eupatorium perfoliatum

What is it? This is the plant commonly called *Boneset*, a member of the *Compositae* botanical family. The whole plant in flower is used to make the homeopathic remedy. The common name comes from its use as an herbal remedy to treat a form of influenza called *Break-Bone Fever*.

When should you use it? The **keynote** symptom leading you to choose *Eupatorium* is the severe muscle aches and pains with bone pain, to the point of feeling that one's bones are broken. The symptoms come on suddenly. There may be high fever with shaking chills along with exhaustion.

How should you use it? Give *Eupatorium* 30C every ½-2 hours quickly decreasing the frequency as soon as the bruised feeling diminishes.

Umcka ColdCare

What is it? *Umcka ColdCare* is a combination homeopathic remedy manufactured by Nature's Way. It is a low potency (1X) homeopathic solution of *Pelargonium sidoides*. *Umcka ColdCare* is one of Europe's leading homeopathic remedies for colds.

When should you use it? The **keynote** symptoms leading you to use *Umcka ColdCare* are nasal congestion, cough, and sore throat. *Umcka ColdCare* lessens the duration and severity of upper respiratory tract symptoms associated with the common cold.

How should you use it? *Umcka ColdCare* comes in drops for ages 12 and over and in alcohol-free drops (with vegetable glycerin instead) for ages 6 and over. It also comes in menthol syrup for ages 12 and over and in cherry syrup for ages 6 and over. Drops are more concentrated than the syrup and can be mixed with juice or water whereas the syrup can be used to soothe a cough or sore throat. Read the directions on the bottle and take as directed.

Echinacea Compound

What is it? *Echinacea Compound* is a combination homeopathic remedy manufactured by Weleda. It consists of: *Lachesis, Echinacea, Equisetum, Vespa,*

Apis, Thuja and *Baptisia*, in very low potencies, in an alcohol solution.

When should you use it? The **keynote** symptoms leading you to use *Echinacea Compound* are sore throat, congestion, and other symptoms of the common cold. If taken early enough in the sequence of common cold symptoms, *Echinacea Compound* can prevent a cold from taking its hold upon you. If you miss the opportunity to prevent the viral infection, you should begin *Echinacea Compound* as soon thereafter as possible.

How should you use it? For adults take 7-10 drops 4 times daily. For children 2-7, take 1 drop per year of age 4 times daily. *Echinacea Compound* functions best when used at the very first inkling that you have a cold coming on.

After Colds and Flu

Gelsemium sempervirens

What is it? This is the poisonous plant whose common name is *yellow jasmine*, a member of the *Loganiaceae* botanical family. The homeopathic remedy is made from the bark.

When should you use it? The **keynote** symptoms leading you to give *Gelsemium* are those colds and flu that come on slowly with fever alternating with chills, weakness, a feeling of heaviness of the limbs and even the eyelids, and a strange lack of thirst. In the weeks to months after a particularly bad cold or flu, *Gelsemium* is also appropriate to give whenever there is physical and emotional weakness long after the flu and you would say, "She has not been well since."

How should you use it? Give *Gelsemium* 30C pellets or liquid drops every ½-2 hours, then tapering the frequency as the severity of the symptoms decrease. For treatment when you believe, "She has not been well since," give *Gelsemium* 200C once a week for four weeks.

Kali phosphoricum

What is it? This is potassium phosphate, a chemical reaction of potassium carbonate and phosphoric acid.

When should you use it? The **keynote** symptom for using *Kali phos*, as it is called, is when someone complains of exhaustion and depression after having had the flu. It is also used one of the homeopathic remedies often prescribed for chronic fatigue syndrome.

How should you use it? Give *Kali phos* 30C pellets or liquid drops every ½-2 hours, then tapering the frequency as the severity of the symptoms decrease

Coughs

Bryonia alba

What is it? The common name for this plant is *wild hops*, a member of the *Cucurbitaceae* botanical family. The homeopathic remedy is prepared from the root of the plant before it flowers. *Bryonia* is useful to treat persons with muscle or bone injuries.

When should you use it? The **keynote** symptoms for use of the homeopathic remedy *Bryonia* are colds and flu when the sick person has a striking reluctance to move. The cold or flu comes on slowly, without much bothersome mucus discharge from the nose but with a dry, painful, bothersome cough starting up whenever the patient moves, so that the patient resists moving.

How should you use it? Give *Bryonia* 30C every ½-2 hours at first, then decreasing the frequency as soon as the cough has improved and the patient no longer resists moving.

Pulsatilla

What is it? This is the plant whose common name is *windflower*, a member of the *Ranunculaceae* botanical family. The whole plant is used for the homeopathic remedy. *Pulsatilla* is most commonly used as a constitutional remedy for girls and women who tend to be timid, yielding, and sympathetic, with a desire to please.

When should you use it? The **keynote** symptoms for using *Pulsatilla* for cough are coughs that interfere with sleep, with thick yellow or greenish-yellow mucus in the morning but dry at night. There may be gagging and choking from mucus. The person needing Pulsatilla will likely have little to no thirst even though having a dry mouth. She will likely feel hot and be made worse from warmth.

How should you use it? Give *Pulsatilla* 30C pellets or liquid drops every ½-2 hours, rapidly decreasing the frequency when the mucus is decreased or becomes clear.

Aconitum napellus

What is it? This homeopathic remedy, called in short *Aconite*, is made from the plant commonly called *monkshood* or *wolfsbane*, a member of the *Ranunculaceae* botanical family. The whole plant just before flowering is used to make the remedy. The plant is highly toxic so the homeopathic remedy is never used below the 3X potency.

When should you use it? The **keynote** symptom for using *Aconite* for cough is a dry cough coming on after exposure to cold. You may try *Aconite* for cough after exposure to any other extreme environmental condition, often a cold, dry wind (such as becoming ill after the air-conditioning of an airplane). The cough is constant and may be sound croupy. When awakening at night, the sick person has many fears and anxieties. The person needing *Aconite* may be thirsty for ice-cold water.

How should you use it? Use *Aconite* 30C every ½-2 hours depending on the severity of the cough. You may always use *Aconite* along with other homeopathic remedies. You may decrease the frequency of administration of *Aconite* and stop it when the patient has improved.

Spongia tosta

What is it? The homeopathic remedy is made from the fresh sea sponge which is roasted.

When should you use it? The **keynote** symptoms leading you to choose *Spongia* are dry, spasmodic cough, often with a sense of suffocation, which is worse before midnight. *Spongia* is useful in croup, asthma, and laryngitis. Sometimes the cough is described as "barking" because it sounds like a bark of a dog.

How should you use it? Give *Spongia* 30C every ½-2 hours at first, decreasing the frequency as soon as the spasms of cough have improved.

Drosera rotundifolia

What is it? This is the plant *Drosera rotundifolia* whose common name is *Sundew*, a member of the *Droseraceae* botanical family. The *Drosera* plant eats insects so it is called insectivorous. The homeopathic remedy is made from the whole plant in flower.

When should you use it? The **keynote** symptoms leading you to choose *Drosera* are strong spasmodic or barking coughs, beginning as a tickling in the throat. The cough is worse after midnight and can be severe. *Drosera* is useful in croup, asthma, bronchitis, and whooping cough.

How should you use it? Give *Drosera* 30C every ½-2 hours at first, decreasing the frequency as soon as the spasms of cough have improved.

Rumex crispus

What is it? The common name for the plant *Rumex crispus* is *Yellow Dock*, a member of the *Polygonaceae* botanical family. The homeopathic remedy *Rumex* is made from the fresh root of the plant.

When should you use it? The **keynote** symptoms leading you to choose *Rumex* are tickling dry cough especially after 11 p.m. and after exposure to cold air, even moving from one room to a cooler one.

How should you use it? Give *Rumex* 30C every ½-2 hours at first, decreasing the frequency as soon as the tickling cough has improved.

Kali bichromicum

What is it? The homeopathic remedy *Kali bich* as it is called is made from the chemical compound potassium dichromate.

When should you use it? The **keynote** symptoms leading you to choose *Kali bich* are strong cough producing a small amount of yellow or white stringy, sticky mucus. *Kali bich* is useful for colds with cough, sinus infections, chronic ear infections that come with fluid in the middle ear, and postnasal drip.

How should you use it? Give *Kali bich* 30C every ½-2 hours at first, decreasing the frequency as soon as the strong cough with mucus production has improved.

Chestal

What is it? This is a combination remedy made by Boiron, a leading homeopathic pharmaceutical supply house. The homeopathic active ingredients are: *Bryonia alba, Coccus cacti, Drosera rotundifolia, Ipecacuanha, Pulsatilla, Rumex crispus, Spongia tosta* and *Sticta pulmonaria*.

When should you use it? The combination remedy *Chestal* is generally helpful for many types of cough (dry, phlegmy, croupy, irritative) that occur with viral illnesses of the upper respiratory tract as well as with allergies. It may also be useful for coughs due to bronchitis (in the lower respiratory tract). The only disadvantage to its use is that it contains honey. Honey is contraindicated for children under the age of about nine months because of the possibility of it containing *Botulinum* spores, which could cause the disease called botulism.

How should you use it? Give 1-2 teaspoons (depending on age) as often as every 2 hours as needed to ease cough. *Chestal* is not recommended for infants under the age of nine months.

Sore Throats and Laryngitis

Throat Infections in General

When throat infections are due to the bacteria called Group A beta-hemolytic *Streptococcus*, antibiotic therapy is indicated because if untreated, this germ can cause rheumatic fever. Rheumatic fever may manifest itself as a life-threatening heart ailment and may last a lifetime. When a throat culture or a Rapid Strep test is negative, it shows that the throat infection is due to any number of viruses and no antibiotic therapy is needed. If you or your family member has a sore throat and you suspect a throat infection, you must pay strict attention to the **Guidelines for Consulting Your Health Care Provider** at the end of this chapter in order to know when a throat culture is necessary to find out whether the sore throat is caused by a bacteria or a virus.

Aconitum napellus

What is it? This homeopathic remedy, called in short *Aconite*, is made from the plant commonly called *monkshood* or *wolfsbane*, a member of the *Ranunculaceae* botanical family. The whole plant just before flowering is used to make the remedy. The plant is highly toxic so the homeopathic remedy is never used below the 3X potency.

When should you use it? You will find that *Aconite* has pride of place in both the prevention and treatment of many forms of upper respiratory infections. The **keynote** symptoms leading you to choose *Aconite* to prevent sore throats are dry, scratchy throat after exposure to cold weather or cold from air conditioning. *Aconite* is suitable to prevent sore throat and hoarseness (laryngitis) after the following environmental conditions: cold and dry winds; cold and wet weather; extremely hot weather. Take *Aconite* as soon as possible after the exposure. Giving *Aconite* right after the exposure without waiting for symptoms to develop may completely prevent the illness from developing. The **keynote** symptoms for using *Aconite* to treat sore throat are a raw burning throat that comes on suddenly.

How should you use it? It is possible that just one dose of *Aconite* 30C will prevent the illness if given early enough just after the exposure or just at the first feeling of dry, scratchy throat.

For treatment, you may use *Aconite* 30C every $\frac{1}{2}$-2 hours depending on the severity of the sore throat. You may always use *Aconite* along with other homeopathic remedies. You may decrease the frequency of administration of *Aconite* and stop it when the patient has either averted the sore throat or has improved.

Hepar sulphuris calcareum

What is it? This homeopathic remedy (called *Hepar sulph* for short) is made from heating sulphur with calcium carbonate from oyster shells.

When should you use it? The **keynote** symptoms leading you to choose *Hepar sulph* are sore throat with infection of the tonsils (tonsillitis) with pus. This remedy helps to expel pus from the body. *Hepar sulph* is also useful to treat earache and sinusitis. The patient needing *Hepar sulph* is usually very sensitive to pain and cold air. Touching the affected part is very painful.

How should you use it? Give *Hepar sulph* 30C every $\frac{1}{2}$-2 hours until the tonsil infection has improved. Then use *Hepar sulph* 200C once daily until the pus is gone.

Mercurius solubilis

What is it? The homeopathic remedy, commonly called *quicksilver*, is made from the action of nitric acid and ammonia on the chemical element mercury.

When should you use it? It is the main homeopathic remedy for infections of the mouth, teeth, and gums, including mouth and gum ulcers and sinusitis. The **keynote** symptoms pointing to the use of *Merc sol*, as it is called in short, in persons with throat infection or tonsillitis are burning, smelly, offensive secretions (sweat, pus) accompanied by excessive salivation (and the saliva burns when swallowed), bad breath, and a metallic taste in the mouth.

How should you use it? Give *Merc sol* 30C every $\frac{1}{2}$-2 hours until the throat infection and bad breath has improved. Then use *Merc sol* 200C once daily until the infection is gone.

Phosphorus

What is it? The chemical element *Phosphorus* is a mineral that is present in every living cell in the form of genetic material (DNA and RNA) as well as many other chemical compounds. It is made into the homeopathic remedy that is a frequently prescribed polychrest or constitutional remedy.

When should you use it? The **keynote** symptoms pointing to the use of *Phosphorus* are colds, sore throats, and hoarseness accompanied by nosebleeds and phlegm with a salty taste. *Phosphorus* is often used for recurrent chest inflammations like asthma as well as respiratory infections such as bronchitis and pneumonia. People who need *Phosphorus* love any touch to the body and love massages. In fact, stroking the body while they suffer from upper respiratory complaints may actually make them improve. *Phosphorus* needing patients feel better from company and desire sympathy.

How should you use it? Give *Phosphorus* 30C every ½-2 hours until the nosebleed associated with cold, sore throat, or hoarseness has improved. You may then give *Phosphorus* 200C once daily for a few days until the patient has recovered whereupon you would stop.

Dulcamara

What is it? The plant *Solanum dulcamara*, common names *Woody nightshade* and *Bittersweet*, is a member of the *Solanaceae* botanical family. The homeopathic remedy *Dulcamara* is made from the stems and leaves before the plant flowers. The berries of the plant are poisonous.

When should you use it? The **keynote** symptoms pointing to use of *Dulcamara* is sore throat with hoarseness after any of these exposures: cold, damp weather, becoming soaked, or being chilled after overheating and sweating. *Dulcamara* is often used to treat asthma.

How should you use it? Give *Dulcamara* 30C every ½-2 hours after exposure causing sore throat with hoarseness. Decrease the frequency as soon as the sore throat and the hoarseness have improved.

Causticum

What is it? The homeopathic remedy is a chemical compound prepared from calcium hydroxide (lime) and potassium bisulphate.

When should you use it? The **keynote** symptoms leading you towards using *Causticum* are loss of voice, hoarseness and laryngitis, from almost any cause, often with cough. People who need *Causticum* tend to be excessively empathetic and acutely feel the suffering of others. *Causticum* is also useful to treat burns.

How should you use it? Give *Causticum* 30C every ½-2 hours after exposure causing loss of voice or hoarseness. Decrease the frequency as soon as the symptoms have improved.

Erpace

What is it? *Erpace* is a lip balm made by Dolisos, a leading homeopathic pharmaceutical supply house. The homeopathic ingredient is *Lappa major* and the essential oils of *Chamomilla*, *Oregano* and *Marjoram* are included for petroleum-free moisturization and aroma.

When should you use it? *Erpace* is very effective for cold sores and fever sores that are often accompanied by sore throat and colds.

How should you use it? *Erpace* is most effective if the roller ball is applied to the area of the lip as soon as itching and burning is detected. Do not wait for the cold sore to become apparent. *Erpace* applied early enough may completely prevent the cold sore from forming. Apply the roller ball over the sensitive area every 1-3 times daily, decreasing the frequency when the lip sensitivity decreases.

Echina-Spray

What is it? *Echina-Spray* is a sore throat spray that is directed by a flip-up nozzle into the back of the throat. It is produced by Boericke & Tafel, a leading homeopathic pharmaceutical supply house. The ingredients are: *Echinacea angustifolia*, *Salvia officinalis* and *Sambucus nigra*, in an alcohol base which is sweetened with xylitol. Since the active ingredients are each present in mother tincture potency, *Echina-Spray* is technically an herbal remedy rather than a homeopathic remedy.

When should you use it? The **keynote** symptoms for which you would use Echina-Spray are sore throat, hoarseness and pain on swallowing. *Echina-Spray* can be used to relieve sore throat pain even if you are taking antibiotics.

How should you use it? Spray *Echina-Spray* 2-4 times directly into the back of the throat, repeating every 1-4 hours as needed, depending on severity, not exceeding 8 times in 24 hours. Children 2-12 years should use 1-2 sprays into the throat.

Ear Infections

Belladonna

What is it? This is the homeopathic remedy made from the poisonous plant, *Atropa belladonna*, common name *deadly nightshade*, a member of the *Solanaceae* botanical family.

When should you use it? The **keynote** symptoms leading you to choose *Belladonna* for ear infection are throbbing pain type of earache in an ear that has turned bright red, accompanied by high fever.

How should you use it? Give *Belladonna* 30C pellets or liquid drops every ½-2 hours, then tapering the frequency quickly as the throbbing earache improves.

Hepar sulphuris calcareum

What is it? This homeopathic remedy (called *Hepar sulph* for short) is made from heating sulphur with calcium carbonate from oyster shells.

When should you use it? The **keynote** symptoms leading you to choose *Hepar sulph* are severe earache pain in an ear that is very sensitive to touch. This, together with *Merc sol*, are homeopathy's "antibiotics" for ear infections.

How should you use it? Give *Hepar sulph* 30C every ½-2 hours until the earache has improved. Then use *Hepar sulph* 200C once daily until the earache is gone.

Mercurius solubilis

What is it? The homeopathic remedy, commonly called *quicksilver*, is made from the action of nitric acid and ammonia on the chemical element mercury.

When should you use it? The **keynote** symptoms leading you to choose *Merc sol* for earache are those ear infections that progress to rupture of the eardrum with smelly pus leaking out of the ear.

How should you use it? Give *Merc sol* 30C every ½-2 hours until the ear infection has improved. Then use *Merc sol* 200C once daily until the infection is gone.

Earache

What is it? The combination remedy, *Earache*, made by Dolisos is a good choice for something to have on hand at all times for children who are prone to ear infections. It contains the following homeopathic remedies in low potency: *Arsenicum album*, *Belladonna*, *Capsicum annuum*, *Chamomilla* and *Ferrum phosphoricum*.

When should you use it? The **keynote** symptoms pointing you to choose *Earache* are any and all signs that you or your family member is having ear pain, such as holding the ear, inclining the ear towards the shoulder, redness of the ear or ear lobe. *Earache* may be used as an ear infection preventive even when simple undue irritability or fever in a child with a cold exists.

How should you use it? Give 5-20 drops of *Earache* depending on age every 1-2 hours until the earache pain has decreased. Then decrease the frequency and continue with once or twice daily in order to prevent ear infection. If the earache becomes an ear infection, you may combine with one or more of the single homeopathic remedies described above.

Eye Infections

Euphrasia officinales

What is it? This is the homeopathic remedy made from the plant *Euphrasia officinalis*, common name *Eyebright*, a member of the *Rhinanthaceae* botanical family.

When should you use it? The **keynote** symptoms pointing towards use of *Euphrasia* for eye infections (conjunctivitis) are profuse tearing (lachrymation), swollen eyelids, and sensitivity to light (photosensitivity) with a burning feeling in the eyes. *Euphrasia* is also used to improve vision and for allergy symptoms when the eye is involved.

How should you use it? Give *Euphrasia* 30C every ½-2 hours until the tearing and burning are decreased. Then decrease the frequency to once or twice a day until the infection is gone.

Apis mellifica

What is it? This is an animal homeopathic remedy made from the whole *honeybee*.

When should you use it? The **keynote** symptoms leading you to consider using *Apis* are burning, stinging pains along with swelling (edema) of the eyelid and itch. The pains are made better from applying cold compresses. *Apis* is often used for allergic conjunctivitis.

How should you use it? Give *Apis* 30C every ½-2 hours until there is relief from the burning and stinging eye pain. Then continue once or twice a day until the infection is gone.

Staphysagria

What is it? The homeopathic remedy comes from the seeds of the plant *Delphinium staphysagria*, common name *stavesacre*, a member of the *Ranunculaceae* botanical family.

When should you use it? The **keynote** symptoms leading you to choose *Staphysagria* are lacerating eye pains and itching at the eye margins with the development of styes. *Staphysagria* is also used to treat a laceration.

How should you use it? Give *Staphysagria* 30C every ½-2 hours until the pains have subsided. Then continue once or twice a day until the stye is gone.

Sinus Infections

Kali bichromicum

What is it? The homeopathic remedy *Kali bich* as it is called is made from the chemical compound potassium dichromate.

When should you use it? The **keynote** symptoms leading you to choose *Kali bich* are sinus infections with yellow or white stringy or sticky mucus from the nose.

How should you use it? Give *Kali bich* 30C every ½-2 hours at first, decreasing the frequency as soon as the mucus discharge has decreased. Then continue once or twice daily until the sinus infection is gone.

Pulsatilla

What is it? This is the plant *Pulsatilla nigricans*, whose common name is *windflower*, a member of the *Ranunculaceae* botanical family.

When should you use it? The **keynote** symptoms leading you to use *Pulsatilla* to treat sinus infections are yellow or yellow-green mucus discharge in large amounts from the nose. *Pulsatilla* is especially indicated for those persons who feel warm to hot all the time and who are thirstless. The typical person needing Pulsatilla is needy emotionally, sensitive, timid and weepy.

How should you use it? Give *Pulsatilla* 30C every ½-2 hours, decreasing the frequency when the mucus is decreased or becomes clear. Then continue once or twice daily until the sinus infection is gone.

Hepar sulphuris calcareum

What is it? *Hepar sulph* is made from heating sulphur with calcium carbonate from oyster shells.

When should you use it? The **keynote** symptoms leading you to choose *Hepar sulph* are severe sinus pain when the facial bones are very sensitive to touch in a patient who is chilly and irritable.

How should you use it? Give *Hepar sulph* 30C every ½-2 hours until the sinus pain has improved. Then use *Hepar sulph* 200C once daily until the sinus infection is gone.

Mercurius solubilis

What is it? The homeopathic remedy, commonly called *quicksilver*, is made from the action of nitric acid and ammonia on the chemical element mercury.

When should you use it? The **keynote** symptoms leading you to choose *Merc sol* for sinus infection are when there is thick, smelly white or yellow mucus leaking out of the nose.

How should you use it? Give *Merc sol* 30C every ½-2 hours until the sinus infection has improved. Then use *Merc sol* 200C once daily until the sinus infection is gone.

Sinus Relief

What is it? This combination remedy by King Bio (in their *SafeCareRx* line of products) comes as a spray for the mouth. It contains the following homeopathic remedies in a pure water base: *Apis mellifica, Baptisia tinctoria, Colocynthis, Hepar sulphuris calcareum, Histaminum, Hydrastis canadensis, Ignatia amara, Kali bichromicum, Lemna minor, Mercurius vivus, Pulsatilla, Rhus toxicodendron, Sabadilla* and *Thuja occidentalis.* Each ingredient comes in a broad spectrum of low to high potencies.

When should you use it? The **keynote** symptoms pointing towards the use of *Sinus Relief* are recurrent sinus infections. This may be effective in reducing the frequency of recurrences. The recurrent bouts may completely disappear.

How should you use it? As soon as you suspect that a sinus infection is beginning, spray *Sinus Relief* 3 times onto or under the tongue 2-4 times a day until sinus pain is relieved. Then continue with once or twice daily until the sinus infection is gone.

Guidelines for Consulting Your Health Care Provider

You should consult your health care provider if:
- the patient doesn't look right or act right (trust your instincts!)
- the patient is getting worse instead of better over the course of the illness
- the patient has a sustained high fever (103°F [39.5°C] to 104°F [40°C])
- the patient is complaining of ear or throat pain or chest pains with coughing that you are unable to control
- the patient has difficulty swallowing saliva or severe pain on swallowing with sore throat and needs a throat culture
- there are conditions suggestive of Streptococcus throat infections and the patient needs a throat culture or a rapid *Strep* test: sudden onset of sore throat with fever more than 102°F (39°C), usually in a person 5-15 years of age, with possible headache, vomiting, abdominal pain, and large painful lymph nodes in the neck but usually not accompanied by cold symptoms
- the patient is uninterested in eating or drinking or playing
- the patient has not had a wet diaper or urinated in the past 12 hours
- the patient has had more than 2 days of vomiting or diarrhea
- the patient is having trouble breathing or complaining of chest pains or there is mental confusion or lethargy or irritability

Note: Do not discontinue taking any pharmaceutical medication that has been prescribed by your health care provider unless you or your family member is under the supervision of a physician.

Remember: The elderly, the very young, and people with chronic diseases tend to have more difficulty coping with even uncomplicated viral upper respiratory infections. The commonest chronic ailments are cardiovascular disease (congestive heart failure and hypertension), stroke, diabetes, arthritis, cancer, and emotional disorders. Please watch out especially for people with any ailment of the endocrine glands, like disorders of the pancreas (diabetes mellitus), thyroid, adrenals, or any metabolic disorder, like hypoglycemia (low blood sugar), ketoacidosis (acidic pH in the blood), hypo- or hypercalcemia (low or high blood calcium), hypo-or hyperkalemia (low or high blood potassium).

Note: *Zicam nasal gels* is a homeopathic preparation of *zinc gluconate* (*zincum gluconicum*) in very low potency in a liquid nasal gel. The FDA has begun to investigate *Zicam nasal gels* (including *Zicam Cold Remedy* and *Zicam Allergic Relief*) for reports that they may cause ansomia, the loss of the sense of smell. At this point, until more information becomes available, I do not recommend the use of any of the *Zicam nasal gels* family of cold and allergy remedies. For more information on Zicam products, visit www.Zicam.com or call 1-877-942-2626. *Cold-Eeze* is a brand of zinc lozenges containing 13.3mg of *zinc gluconate glycine* in each lozenger. This is not a homeopathic remedy. *Cold-Eeze* may shorten the duration of colds. *Airborne* is a vitamin—mineral—herbal effervescent tablet preparation that may be effective in preventing viral infections of the upper respiratory tract if taken at the onset of the very first symptom. But the amount of Vitamin A in *Airborne* is too high to be considered safe for repeated dosages. So, if you do take it, use only 1 or 2 over the course of 1 week and do not give them to children. *Emer'gen-C* is another such preparation, skipping Vitamin A all together and offering 1000mg of Vitamin C in every fizzy tablet.

Recommendations for Homeopathic Remedies

Colds and Flu
<u>Prevention</u>
Aconite 30C—in pellets and liquid drops
Oscillococcinum—in unit-dose pellets
Influenzinum 200C—in pellets
<u>Treatment</u>
Aconite 30C—in pellets and liquid drops
Belladonna 30C—pellets and liquid drops
Gelsemium 30C and 200C—pellets and liquid drops
Ferrum phos 30C—pellets and liquid drops
Pulsatilla 30C—pellets and liquid drops
Allium 30C—in pellets and liquid drops
Arsenicum album 30C—in pellets and liquid drops
Nux vomica 30C—in pellets and liquid drops
Baptisia 30C—in pellets and liquid drops
Eupatorium perfoliatum 30C—in pellets and liquid drops
Zicam Cold Remedy—liquid nasal gel, nasal swabs (adult size and kids size)
<u>After Colds and Flu</u>
Gelsemium 30C and 200C—pellets and liquid drops
Kali phosphoricum 30C and 200C—pellets and liquid drops

Coughs
Bryonia 30C—in pellets and liquid drops
Pulsatilla 30C—in pellets and liquid drops
Aconitum napellus 30C—in pellets and liquid drops
Spongia tosta 30C—in pellets and liquid drops
Drosera rotundifolia 30C—in pellets and liquid drops
Rumex crispus 30C—in pellets and liquid drops
Kali bichromicum 30C—in pellets and liquid drops

Sore Throats and Laryngitis
Aconitum napellus 30C—in pellets and liquid drops
Hepar sulphuris calcareum 30C and 200C—in pellets and liquid drops
Mercurius solubilis 30C and 200C—in pellets and liquid drops
Phosphorus 30C and 200C—in pellets and liquid drops
Dulcamara 30C—in pellets and liquid drops
Erpace by Dolisos—lip balm
Echina-Spray by Boericke & Tafel—sore throat spray

Ear Infections

Belladonna 30C—in pellets and liquid drops
Hepar sulphuris calcareum 30C and 200C—in pellets and liquid drops
Mercurius solubilis 30C and 200C—in pellets and liquid drops
Earache combination remedy made by Dolisos—liquid drops

Eye Infections

Euphrasia officinales 30C—in pellets and liquid drops
Apis mellifica 30C—in pellets and liquid drops
Staphysagria 30C—in pellets and liquid drops

Sinus Infections

Kali bichromicum 30C—in pellets and liquid drops
Pulsatilla 30C—in pellets and liquid drops
Hepar sulphuris calcareum 30C and 200C—in pellets and liquid drops
Mercurius solubilis 30C and 200C—in pellets and liquid drops
Sinus Relief—a combination remedy by King Bio in oral spray

Guidelines for Administration of Homeopathic Remedies

Once you have chosen the homeopathic remedy and the potency that is likely to help you or your family member, you should try to give as few repetitions of the remedy as you can. You start off repeating it more frequently in a severe, acute situation, quickly decreasing the frequency once improvement has begun, stopping the remedy as soon as the problem has resolved.

> **Note:** For more information on *how often* to give the homeopathic remedy please see **Potency and Frequency**, in **Chapter 2: Basic Homeopathy**. For information on *how much* of the homeopathic remedy to give and the importance of a *"clean tongue,"* please see **How to take homeopathic remedies** in the same chapter.

Lower potency remedies, such as 30C and below, are used to treat acute ailments. They are usually repeated often, every ½-2 or ½-4 hours. You should notice improvement in symptoms after just one to perhaps a few repetitions. If you do not see improvement, it is wise to stop the remedy and try a different one, guiding yourself by the **keynote** symptoms. You may use different single remedies together or you may try a combination remedy. And you may use homeopathic remedies together with pharmaceutical prescription and non-prescription drugs without any effect of interference.

General guidelines to treat serious, chronic, relapsing ailments include using single remedies at potencies of 200C. These are generally administered once weekly to once monthly, but they may be used once or twice daily at first if the condition warrants it, quickly decreasing the frequency as you see improvement. Do not continue giving the remedy if it becomes apparent that it is not working. You may always stop one remedy and choose to administer another remedy on the basis of the **keynote** symptoms of the new remedy. In addition, you may administer more than one remedy at a time.

Putting It All Together

People with infections of the eyes, ears, nose, and throat generally require all the vitamins and minerals necessary to repair and replenish tissues (please refer to **Chapter 23: Vitamins and Minerals**), as well as a general antioxidant supplement (please refer to **Chapter 24: Antioxidant Phytochemicals**). Increased doses of *Vitamin C* may be especially useful to repair tissues during and after upper respiratory infections.

In addition, it is a good idea to consider giving the sick person's homeopathic constitutional remedy (please refer to **Chapter 9: Homeopathic Remedies for Constitutional Problems in Infants, Children, and Adolescents** or to **Chapter 18: Homeopathic Constitutional Remedie**s if you are dealing with an adult).

Depending on the chronicity of the infection episodes, you may want to consider learning about nutritional supplements to augment the immune system, especially *medicinal mushrooms* (please refer to **Chapter 27: Nutritional Supplements to**

Prevent Cancer and Augment Your Immune System).

If you are dealing with chronic, recurrent infections (for example, recurrent sinus infections), you may want to investigate certain herbal remedies (please refer to **Chapter 20: Herbs You Need to Know**) such as *Echinacea, Goldenseal, Astragalus* and *Garlic*.

Note: *Sambucus nigra* or *Black Elderberry* extract, specifically a product called *Sambucol* by Nature's Way, is another potent herbal remedy that has been proven to shorten the length of an illness with the flu virus and other upper respiratory viruses.

Chapter 6

Homeopathic Remedies for Allergies and Asthma

Allergies and Asthma in General

Ailment/Disorder/Symptom	Homeopathic Remedy
Asthma and wheezing and cough in chilly, anxious people	*Arsenicum album*
Asthma, wheezing and cough, feeling of suffocation	*Spongia tosta*
Asthma, lower respiratory tract infections, bronchitis and pneumonia	*Phosphorus*
Burning, stinging pains in throat, itchy eyes	*Apis mellifica*
Asthma with wheezing and white-coated tongue	*Antimonium tartaricum*
Tingling and fullness at the root of the nose	*Gelsemium sempervirens*
Allergies with post-nasal drip with thick, stringy mucus	*Kali bichromicum*
Allergies with post-nasal drip with yellow-green mucus	*Pulsatilla*
Allergies with profuse, clear mucus from nose or throat with sneezing	*Nux vomica*
Allergies with runny nose alternating with stuffy nose	*Natrum muriaticum*
Allergies with shortness of breath and nausea	*Ipecac*
Allergies with violently strong or spasmodic coughs	*Drosera rotundifolia*
Asthma and allergies with wheezy coughs with profuse, yellow mucus	*Dulcamara*
Allergies with profuse watery discharges from eyes and nose	*Allium cepa*
Allergies with tingling, itching of soft palate with sneezing	*Sabadilla*
Allergic, itchy, red skin rashes with burning and blistering	*Rhus toxicodendron*
Allergic, itchy, red skin rashes with burning, worse with water	*Sulphur*
Allergic red skin rashes with violent itching and scratching	*Psorinum*
Allergies with severe itching of the soft palate	*Wyethia*
Eye irritations from any and all reasons	*Optique 1*
Allergies with runny nose, sneezing, itchy, watery eyes, congestion	*Allergy Relief Tree Pollen*
Allergies with runny nose, sneezing, itchy, watery eyes, congestion	*Allergy Relief Pollen and Hay Fever*
Sinus pressure and headache, congestion	*Sinus and Allergy Relief*
Hay fever and other respiratory allergies	*Allergies and Hay Fever*
Asthma symptoms	*Asthma Clear*
Allergic skin rashes, eczema, contact dermatitis	*Psoriaflora Cream*

Guidelines for Consulting Your Health Care Provider
Putting It All Together

Allergies and Asthma in General

There is a continuum of allergic reactions in the human body that extends from mild skin itching and hives to sneezing and itchy eyes to coughing and asthma to laryngeal spasms and anaphylactic life-threatening reactions. This chapter will help you with self-care for the lesser allergic reactions and asthma. If you or a family member has a history of allergic reactions accompanied by laryngeal spasms or anaphylaxis, then you should not attempt self-care for allergic reactions, but rather you must use the proper prescription medicines from your health care provider (such as injectable epinephrine). These medications must be available in case of exposure to the offending allergen at all times. Only then you may augment your treatment with a constitutional homeopathic remedy as prescribed by your professional homeopath.

Allergies and asthma are manifestations of a strongly functioning immune system. Homeopathic remedies are well suited to treating allergies and asthma because they act as immunoregulators or modulators. This means that homeopathic remedies will energize a sluggish immune system or dampen an overly enthusiastic immune system, depending on the need.

Homeopathic remedies may be combined with prescription medicines from your health care provider. The only prescription medicine that seems to impede the work of homeopathic remedies is steroids. This can occur when any one of the popular forms of steroids is used, including cremes and ointments for eczema, inhaled steroids in inhalers or nebulizers for asthma, or prednisone tablets or liquid prescribed for many allergic reactions including hives. When a patient is using steroids it is important not to discontinue them abruptly because that can cause one of several different kinds of life-threatening reactions. Instead, I recommend that you first begin taking homeopathic remedies and when you notice that they have eased the allergy or asthma, then the time has come to taper the steroid medicines. But, you must work with your health care provider or your homeopath to taper the steroids appropriately so as not to incur any dangerous medical complications.

Homeopathic remedies for allergies and asthma should be taken along with common-sense precautions. When the offending allergen is known, I recommend that you try to limit the exposure to that chemical compound. Common *allergens* include ragweed pollen, trees, grasses, dust, molds, dog and cat dander, certain foods and food additives, and certain medicines, especially aspirin and antibiotics. If your goal is to decrease the severity and frequency of allergic reactions or asthmatic attacks, then I suggest you try some of the homeopathic remedies listed below according to their **keynote** symptoms.

However, if your goal is to be able to undergo exposure to a known allergen without having an allergic or asthmatic episode, then you are seeking a cure. In this case, I recommend that you engage the services of a professional homeopath because it is likely that a constitutional remedy will be required. Self-prescription of a constitutional remedy is possible, but finding the correct constitutional remedy and its proper administration usually takes formal training in homeopathy.

Besides allergens, some people have triggers that can cause an allergic reaction or an asthmatic episode because they act as irritants in the breathing tubes. Common triggers include cigarette or cigar smoke, viral upper respiratory infections (colds), exercise (called exercise-induced asthma), and cold air. It is a good idea to steer clear of known triggers as well until the homeopathic remedies take effect. After homeopathic treatment, it is sometimes possible to be exposed to known triggers without developing the allergic or asthmatic reaction.

The numbers of children and adults with asthma is growing every year in the U.S.A. Asthma causes approximately 5,000 deaths every year along with about 500,000 hospitalizations. There is no doubt but that asthma can be a serious disease. The best approach to a serious, chronic, recurrent disease is prevention. Homeopathy is uniquely suited to helping you prevent asthmatic attacks.

As with any and all medical conditions, when dealing with allergic and asthmatic reactions you must pay strict attention to the **Guidelines for Consulting Your Health Care Provider** at the end of this chapter. You may want to refer to the last section **Putting It All Together** for ideas on how to integrate the essential natural alternatives, homeopathy, herbal remedies, and nutritional supplements.

Arsenicum album

What is it? This is the homeopathic remedy made from the chemical compound arsenic oxide which is highly poisonous if not given in homeopathic dilution. *Arsenicum album* is one of homeopathy's often-used polychrests or constitutional remedies. *Arsenicum album* is also useful to treat emotional disorders.

When should you use it? The **keynote** symptoms leading you to choose *Arsenicum album* are wheezing with cough in a chilly person along with great anxiety and restlessness. The patient may express a sense of impending doom or fear of death. The asthma is worse after midnight. The patient is thirsty but prefers to drink small sips of cold water. *Arsenicum album* is also a treatment for allergies when there is a burning feeling in the nose and eyes with watery nasal discharge along with incessant sneezing, throbbing headache, and thirst for small sips of water.

How should you use it? Give *Arsenicum album* 30C every ½-2 hours until the asthma or the sneezing is improved. Then continue with *Arsenicum album* 200C once a week until the asthma or hay fever is gone. For some people, continuing with Arsenicum album 200C once a week may prevent recurrences.

> **Note:** *Arsenicum iodatum* may be used instead of *Arsenicum album* when the nasal discharge is particularly burning or corrosive with especially violent tingling and sneezing. *Arsenicum iodatum* is also helpful for the wheezing of asthma when it comes after violent symptoms of hay fever. Use the same directions.

Spongia tosta

What is it? The homeopathic remedy is made from the fresh *sea sponge* which is roasted.

When should you use it? The **keynote** symptoms leading you to choose *Spongia* are dry, spasmodic, wheezing cough, often with a sense of suffocation, and the need to throw the head backwards. The cough sound deep in the chest. The asthmatic episode may have been triggered by a viral upper respiratory infection.

How should you use it? Give *Spongia* 30C every ½-2 hours at first, decreasing the frequency as soon as the allergic or asthmatic symptoms have improved.

Phosphorus

What is it? The chemical element *Phosphorus* is a mineral that is present is every living cell in the form of genetic material (DNA and RNA) as well as many other compounds. It is made into a homeopathic remedy that is an often-prescribed polychrest or constitutional remedy.

When should you use it? The **keynote** symptoms pointing to the use of *Phosphorus* are asthmatic coughs (especially recurrent asthma) in a person who loves massages and loves to be touched. In fact, stroking the body while they are in the midst of an asthmatic coughing episode may actually make them improve. *Phosphorus* needing patients feel better from company and desire sympathy. *Phosphorus* is often used for recurrent chest inflammations like asthma as well as respiratory infections such as bronchitis and pneumonia.

How should you use it? Give *Phosphorus* 30C every ½-2 hours until the asthmatic cough has improved. You may then give *Phosphorus* 200C once daily for a few days until the patient has recovered.

Apis mellifica

What is it? This is a homeopathic remedy from the animal kingdom, made from the whole, crushed *honeybee*.

When should you use it? The **keynote** symptoms leading you to consider using *Apis* for allergic reactions are burning, prickly, stinging pains in the throat along with itchy eyes and swelling of the eyelids. *Apis* treats bee, wasp, and hornet stings.

How should you use it? Give *Apis* 30C every ½-2 hours, decreasing the frequency as soon as the allergic reaction has improved. For insect stings, give *Apis* as soon as possible after the sting.

Antimonium tartaricum

What is it? The homeopathic remedy is made from the oxide of antimony and potassium tartrate. It was once used as an agent to cause vomiting (emetic) in conventional medicine. Its common name is tartar emetic.

When should you use it? The **keynote** symptoms leading to the use of *Antimonium tartaricum* are wheezing in very young and very old people who may not be able to expectorate mucus even though there is a mucus-laden cough. The tongue is thickly coated white. There is little or no thirst. There may be flaring of the nostrils and gasping for air.

How should you use it? Give *Antimonium tartaricum* 30C every ½-2 hours until the asthma is improved. Then continue with *Antimonium tartaricum* 200C once a week until the asthma is gone. For some people, continuing with *Antimonium tartaricum* 200C once a week may prevent recurrences.

Gelsemium sempervirens

What is it? This is the plant whose common name is *yellow jasmine*, a member of the *Loganiaceae* botanical family.

When should you use it? The **keynote** symptoms leading you to give *Gelsemium* are those allergic reactions which come with tingling and fullness at the root of the nose, with thirstlessness, heavy eyelids, and a heavy, dull, lethargic feeling throughout.

How should you use it? Give *Gelsemium* 30C every ½-2 hours, decreasing the frequency as soon as the allergic reaction has improved.

Kali bichromicum

What is it? The homeopathic remedy *Kali bich* (as it is called) is made from the chemical compound potassium dichromate.

When should you use it? The **keynote** symptoms leading you to choose *Kali bich* for allergic reactions causing postnasal drip are thick yellow or white stringy, sticky mucus from the nose or throat. *Kali bich* is useful for sinus infections that come as a result of allergies.

How should you use it? Give *Kali bich* 30C every ½-2 hours at first, decreasing the frequency as soon as the symptoms are improved.

> **Note:** *Kali iodatum* may be useful for especially violent sneezing attacks along with thick mucus similar to that of *Kali bich*. Use the same directions.

Pulsatilla

What is it? This is the plant *Pulsatilla nigricans*, whose common name is *windflower*, a member of the *Ranunculaceae* botanical family.

When should you use it? The **keynote** symptoms leading you to use *Pulsatilla* to treat postnasal drip or sinus infections as a result of allergies are yellow or yellow-green mucus discharge in large amounts from the nose or throat. *Pulsatilla* is especially indicated for those persons who feel warm to hot all the time and who do not feel thirsty. The typical person (usually female) for whom *Pulsatilla* will likely help is emotionally needy, sensitive to insult, timid and an easy-crier. *Pulsatilla* people easily share details of their intimate lives.

How should you use it? Give *Pulsatilla* 30C every ½-2 hours, decreasing the frequency when the allergic reaction is improved. You may continue with *Pulsatilla* 200C once daily and then once weekly during the allergy season to forestall further allergic reactions.

Nux vomica

What is it? This is a poisonous plant, *Nux vomica*, containing strychnine, common name *Poison nut*, a member of the *Loganiaceae* botanical family. *Nux vomica* is often used as a constitutional remedy, especially for angry, frustrated men who are workaholics ("Type A" personality), who over-indulge in alcohol, nicotine, and caffeine. They may manifest a concrete intellectualism while being emotionally superficial although they may display a volatile temper.

When should you use it? The **keynote** symptoms for the use of *Nux vomica* is when during the day there is profuse clear runny nasal discharge along with much sneezing, but during the night there is a blocked, stuffy nose. A person needing *Nux vomica* may be excessively chilly, complaining, irritable, and impatient.

How should you use it? Give *Nux vomica* 30C every ½-2 hours, decreasing the frequency when the excessive sneezing and nasal discharge have improved. You may continue with *Nux vomica* 200C once daily and then once weekly during the allergy season to forestall further allergic reactions.

Natrum muriaticum

What is it? This is the polychrest *Natrum muriaticum*, a homeopathic remedy made from common table salt. Its use is mostly as a constitutional remedy, but it can be used for many specific ailments as well, such as allergic reactions.

When should you use it? The **keynote** symptoms indicating *Natrum muriaticum* are stuffy nose alternating with runny nose along with sneezing and headache in a person who either craves or is averse to salt and salty foods. The nasal mucus can look like egg whites. She may manifest the symptoms of depression which can be severe. She usually has had many occasions for grief in her life, with disappointed love being prominent.

How should you use it? Give *Natrum muriaticum* 30C every ½-2 hours, decreasing the frequency when the nasal symptoms have improved. You may continue with *Natrum muriaticum* 200C once daily and then once weekly during the allergy season to forestall further allergic reactions.

Ipecac

What is it? The homeopathic remedy *Ipecac* is made from the root of the plant *Cephaelis ipecacuanha*, a member of the *Rubiaceae* botanical family. *Ipecac* is used in Western medicine to induce vomiting to eliminate toxic substances that have been ingested into the body. It makes sense, following the **Law of Similars** that the homeopathic remedy *Ipecac* would be used to treat nausea and vomiting. Homeopathic *Ipecac* is used to treat asthmatic symptoms as well.

When should you use it? The **keynote** symptoms directing you to use *Ipecac* are shortness of breath with feelings of choking and suffocation, along with nausea and a cough that does not bring up mucus. *Ipecac* is also indicated when the asthmatic cough leads to a nosebleed with bright red blood.

How should you use it? Give *Ipecac* 30C every ½-2 hours, decreasing the frequency when the asthmatic symptoms have improved.

Drosera rotundifolia

What is it? This is the insect-eating plant *Drosera rotundifolia* whose common name is *Sundew*, a member of the *Droseraceae* botanical family.

When should you use it? The **keynote** symptoms leading you to choose *Drosera* are violently strong, spasmodic coughs, worse after midnight. *Drosera* is often chosen to treat whooping cough as well as other strong coughs that seem to come from deep down in the chest.

How should you use it? Give *Drosera* 30C every ½-2 hours at first, decreasing the frequency as soon as the allergic or asthmatic symptoms have improved.

Dulcamara

What is it? This is the plant *Solanum dulcamara*, common names *Woody nightshade* and *Bittersweet*, a member of the *Solanaceae* botanical family.

When should you use it? The **keynote** symptoms for which you would consider using *Dulcamara* are for asthmatic, wheezy coughs with profuse thick, yellow mucus that result from exposure to cold and damp or cold and wet weather conditions.

How should you use it? Give *Dulcamara* 30C every ½-2 hours at first, decreasing the frequency as soon as the allergic or asthmatic symptoms have improved.

Allium cepa

What is it? This is the plant *Allium cepa*, common name *red onion*, a member of the *Liliaceae* botanical family. The fresh bulb is used to make the homeopathic remedy.

When should you use it? The **keynote** symptoms urging you to use *Allium cepa* are profuse tearing from reddened eyes with profuse mucus discharge from the nose and frequent, violent sneezing, such as that found with hay fever and other allergic reactions. The nostrils and upper lip may turn red and raw from the nasal mucus which can be burning.

How should you use it? Give *Allium cepa* 30C every ½-2 hours at first, decreasing the frequency as soon as the allergic symptoms have improved.

Sabadilla

What is it? This plant has many Latin names, among them *Veratrum sabadilla* and *Sabadilla officinarum*. It is a member of the *Liliaceae* botanical family. The seeds are used to make the homeopathic remedy.

When should you use it? The **keynote** symptoms leading you to try *Sabadilla* are tingling, tickling, or itching of the soft palate with paroxysms of sneezing and watery eyes.

How should you use it? Give *Sabadilla* 30C every ½-2 hours at first, decreasing the frequency as soon as the allergic symptoms have improved.

Rhus toxicodendron

What is it? The botanical name for this plant is *Rhus toxicodendron* (usually abbreviated as *Rhus tox*), common name *poison ivy*, a member of the *Anacardiaceae* botanical family.

When should you use it? The **keynote** symptoms leading you to use *Rhus tox* for skin problems are itchy, red, scaly skin with burning pains and blisters. *Rhus tox* is often called for in treating eczema, poison ivy, and other itchy skin conditions such as contact dermatitis. There are three other **keynote** symptoms that may help you to choose *Rhus tox*. The first is the red-tipped tongue. You may try *Rhus tox* whenever you notice that the triangular tip of the tongue is reddened. The second is the person's extreme sensitivity to cold and damp, making the problem worse. The third is very hot water makes the skin rash feel less itchy.

How should you use it? *Rhus tox* works best in the 200C potency, even for acute conditions. Give *Rhus tox* 200C once daily (or more frequently if needed) until the itchiness has decreased. Then continue with *Rhus tox* 200C once weekly until the problem is

gone. If you wish to prevent poison ivy, oak, or sumac you may give *Rhus tox* 200C a few hours before a possible exposure, but it is also advisable to wear long sleeves, long pants, and gardening gloves.

Note: When treating a break-out of poison ivy, oak, or sumac, you may wish to use topical *Zanfel Poison Ivy, Oak and Sumac Wash*, a Western medicine skin preparation, actually a kind of soap, that washes away the toxic *urushiol* oil from the skin. It is safe and effective. It is safe for use during pregnancy. Detailed instructions are on the tube. *Zanfel* can be used together with *Rhus tox*, or any other homeopathic remedy. For more information about *Zanfel* call 1-800-401-4002 or visit www.zanfel.com.

Sulphur

What is it? The mineral element *Sulphur*, common name *brimstone*, is present in every cell of the human body. *Sulphur* is a polychrest constitutional remedy exerting its main effects on the skin.

When should you use it? The **keynote** symptoms pointing towards the use of *Sulphur* are red, dry, flaky, burning, itchy skin rashes that are worse after any immersion in water and wearing wool. *Sulphur* is often used to treat allergic eczema. Constitutionally, people who need *Sulphur* may resemble the "absent-minded professor" in that they tend to be disheveled with sloppy personal habits, and talk at great length about obscure concepts and abstractions.

How should you use it? Give *Sulphur* 30C every ½-2 hours, decreasing the frequency when the allergic eczema has improved. You may continue with *Sulphur* 200C once daily and then once weekly during the allergic eczema season to forestall further outbreaks.

Note: *Sulphur* is often useful to treat eczema and other allergy-based skin rashes. You may be able to alleviate the itching of these ailments by using topical *Castor Oil* (from the *Castor Oil* plant, *Ricinus communis*). You may use topical

Castor Oil together with homeopathic *Sulphur*.

Psorinum

What is it? This homeopathic remedy is made form the complex biological material of a *scabies* vesicle (sore). The main effects of *Psorinum* are on the skin. **When should you use it**? The **keynote** symptoms leading you towards consideration of *Psorinum* are when the skin rashes are red with violent itching tending towards raw, bleeding sores, especially in people who always feel cold (with great sensitivity to cold and cold air). Paradoxically, their allergic eczema is made worse from being heated, such as covering the part. People who need *Psorinum* show a great sensitivity to the environment making *Psorinum* a hay fever and asthma remedy as well. *Psorinum* should be considered when asthma occurs years later after having had eczema.
How should you use it? Give *Psorinum* 30C every ½-2 hours, decreasing the frequency when the allergic eczema or asthma has improved. You may continue with *Psorinum* 200C once daily and then once weekly during the allergic eczema or asthma season to forestall further outbreaks.

Wyethia

What is it? *Wyethia* is the homeopathic remedy made from the root of the plant *Wyethia helenoides*, common name *Poison weed*, a member of the *Compositae* botanical family.
When should you use it? The **keynote** symptoms leading you towards using *Wyethia* are severe itching of the soft palate along with dryness of the nose and mouth. Trying to relieve the itching by tongue clucking does not help.
How should you use it? Give *Wyethia* 30C every ½-2 hours, decreasing the frequency when the itching of the soft palate has improved. You may continue with *Wyethia* 200C once daily and then once weekly to forestall further outbreaks.

Optique 1

What is it? This is a combination remedy manufactured by Boiron. These eye drops come in single-use doses that you apply directly into the eye. This combination remedy contains the following homeopathic remedies in low potencies: *Cineraria maritima, Euphrasia officinalis, Calendula officinalis, Kali muriaticum, Calcarea fluorica, Magnesia carbonica* and *Silicea*.
When should you use it? It is recommended for treatment of eye irritations (red, dry, itchy, burning, or tired eyes) resulting from eye fatigue or allergic reactions to airborne allergens.
How should you use it? Apply the contents of one single-use dose of *Optique 1* into the eye via the applicator tip. This may be repeated 2-6 times daily, or as often as you require. This preparation is safe for persons with glaucoma. For persons with contact lenses, it is probably better to remove them before applying the drops.

Allergy Relief Tree Pollen

What is it? This is a homeopathic combination remedy manufactured by bioAllers. It contains *Adrenalinum (Adrenaline), Allium cepa (Red onion), Arsenicum iodatum (Arsenic iodide), Euphrasia officinalis (Eyebright), Sabadilla officinarum (Cevadilla), Sanguinaria canadensis (Blood root), Acer negundo (Box elder), Acer rubrum (Maple), Ailanthus altissima (Tree of Heaven), Alnus rhombifolia (Alder), Betula nigra (Birch), Carya tomentosa (Hickory), Fraxinus americana (Ash), Histaminum (Histamine), Juniperus virginiana (Cedar), Ligustrum (Privet), Liquidamber styraciflua (Sweet gum), Morus alba (Mulberry), Pinus strobus (Pine), Populus deltoids (Cottonwood), Quercus rubra (Oak), Salix nigra (Willow)* and *Ulmus parvifolia (Elm)* in 6X-12X potencies, in purified water and alcohol.
When should you use it? *Allergy Relief Tree Pollen* is recommended for use when runny nose, sneezing, itchy and watery eyes, congestion, sinus pressure, and headache symptoms are due to allergy to tree pollen.
How should you use it? Take 15 drops (for children 2-12 take 3-5 drops) under the tongue every 3-4 hours until symptoms are relieved. Then continue with 15 drops (for children 2-12 take 3-5 drops) 3

times daily. You may continue to take it once daily throughout the tree pollen allergy seasons as this may decrease your reactivity to these allergens. For those people with asthmatic symptoms to tree pollen, take 1-5 drops once daily, increasing gradually until the full dosage.

Allergy Relief Pollen and Hay Fever

What is it? This is a homeopathic combination remedy manufactured by bioAllers. It contains *Adrenalinum (Adrenaline), Allium cepa (Red onion), Arsenicum iodatum (Arsenic iodide), Euphrasia officinalis (Eyebright), Sabadilla officinarum (Cevadilla), Silicea (Silica), Ambrosia artemisiaefolia (Ragweed), Artemisia vulgaris (Mugwort), Bellis perennis (Daisy), Brassica napus (Mustard), Chenopodium anthelminticum (Wormseed), Histaminum (Histamine), Lonicera periclymenum (Honeysuckle), Medicago sativa (Alfalfa), Phleum pratense (Timothy grass), Rumex crispus (Yellow dock), Solidago virgaurea (Goldenrod), Taraxacum officinale (Dandelion), Trifolium repens (White clover), Xanthium strumarium* and *(Cocklebur)* in 6X-12X potencies, in purified water and alcohol.

When should you use it? *Allergy Relief Pollen and Hay Fever* is recommended for use when runny nose, sneezing, itchy and watery eyes, congestion, sinus pressure, and headache symptoms are due to hay fever allergies.

How should you use it? Take 15 drops (for children 2-12 take 3-5 drops) under the tongue every 3-4 hours until symptoms are relieved. Then continue with 15 drops (for children 2-12 take 3-5 drops) 3 times daily. You may continue to take it once daily throughout the hay fever allergy season as this may decrease your reactivity to these allergens. For those people with asthmatic symptoms to tree pollen, take 1-5 drops once daily, increasing gradually until the full dosage.

Sinus and Allergy Relief

What is it? This is a homeopathic combination remedy manufactured by bioAllers. It is administered as a nasal spray rather than as oral drops. It contains *Adrenalinum (Adrenaline), Allium cepa (Red onion),*

Ambrosia artemisiaefolia (Ragweed), Echinacea angustifolia (Echinacea), Gelsemium sempervirens, Sanguinaria canadensis (Blood root), Sticta pulmonaria and *Kali iodatum (Potassium iodide)* in 6X-12X potencies, in purified water along with other inactive ingredients.

When should you use it? *Sinus and Allergy Relief* is used for relief of sinus pressure, sinus headache, congestion, runny nose, dry nasal passages, and sneezing, when these symptoms are due to allergy to inhaled allergens.

How should you use it? For adults and children 12 years and over, insert nozzle into nostril and depress pump, breathing through nose while spraying twice into each nostril every 4 hours. You may repeat more frequently than every 4 hours during the acute phase. When you have some relief of symptoms, decrease the frequency. You may want to use this nasal spray once daily during the allergy season to prevent sinus infection.

Allergies and Hay Fever

What is it? This combination remedy manufactured by King Bio (in their *SafeCareRx* line of products) is used as a spray into the mouth. The combination remedy contains the following homeopathic remedies in low potencies in a pure water base: *Allium cepa, Ambrosia artemisiaefolia, Arsenicum album, Arundo muritanica, Arum triphyllum, Euphrasia officinalis, Sabadilla, Naphthalinum, Natrum muriaticum* and *Wyethia helenioides*. Each ingredient comes in a broad spectrum of low to high potencies.

When should you use it? It is recommended for treatment of hay fever and other allergic symptoms such as nasal congestion, runny nose, hoarseness, cough, sore throat, and itchy, watery eyes.

How should you use it? Spray *Allergies and Hay Fever* onto or under the tongue, 2-3 sprays, every 2-4 hours until the allergic symptoms improve. Then use once daily for prevention during the allergic season.

Asthma Clear

What is it? This combination remedy manufactured by King Bio is used as a spray into the mouth.

When should you use it? It is recommended for treatment of asthmatic symptoms such as, shortness of breath, wheezing, and a feeling of tightness in the chest. The combination remedy contains the following homeopathic remedies in low potencies in a pure water base: *Adrenalinum, Antimonium tartaricum, Aralia racemosa, Arsenicum album, Eriodictyon californicum, Eucalyptus globulus, Grindelia robusta, Ipecacuanha, Lobelia inflata, Natrum sulphuricum* and *Quebracho.*

How should you use it? Spray *Asthma Clear* onto or under the tongue, 2-3 sprays, every 2-4 hours until the asthmatic symptoms improve. Then use once daily for asthma prevention during the allergic season.

Florasone Cream

What is it? This homeopathic cream is made by the pharmaceutical manufacturers Boericke & Tafel. The active ingredient is the plant *Cardiospermum halicacabum*, common name *Balloon-vine*, a member of the *Sapindaceae* botanical family, in very low potency.

When should you use it? The **keynote** symptoms for the use of *Florasone Cream* use are allergic rashes of the skin, such as itchy, scaling, red eczema or hives. It is sometimes dubbed the "homeopathic cortisone," but of course it does not act like steroids and has no side effects.

How should you use it? You may apply *Florasone Cream* to the rash 3-4 times daily, stopping when the rash has improved. You do not have to be concerned with over-usage. If the skin rash you believe to be eczema, an allergic rash, is being treated with *Florasone Cream* and does not respond within 2 weeks, then it is possible that the rash may actually be psoriasis (of unknown cause). If that is the case, I then recommend trying *Psoriaflora Cream* (please see below) as well as consultation with both your homeopath health care provider and dermatologist.

Psoriaflora Cream

What is it? This homeopathic cream is made by the pharmaceutical manufacturers Boericke & Tafel. The active ingredient is *Berberis aquifolium*, common

name *Mountain Grape,* a member of the *Berberidaceae* botanical family.

When should you use it? The **keynote** symptoms for the use of *Psoriaflora Cream* are areas of dry skin with itching and silvery white or gray flakes or scales. *Psoriaflora Cream* is included in this section because eczema and psoriasis may look very similar.

How should you use it? Apply *Psoriaflora Cream* 1-4 times daily to the affected area. *Psoriaflora Cream* is indicated for adults and children over the age of 2 years. I recommend that you try *Florasone Cream* first. If the skin rash you are treating does not respond to Florasone Cream, I recommend that you try *Psoriaflora Cream.* If the rash responds, it is likely that you are dealing with psoriasis. If this is the case, I strongly recommend that you consult with both your homeopath health care provider and dermatologist to help you care for psoriasis. There may be severe complications accompanying psoriasis which will require diagnosis and perhaps treatment from your homeopath health care provider or dermatologist.

Guidelines for Consulting Your Health Care Provider

You should consult your health care provider if:
- the patient doesn't look right or act right (trust your instincts!)
- the patient is getting worse instead of better over the course of the illness
- the patient's asthma symptoms (usually cough with wheeze along with a feeling of tightness in the chest) are increasing in severity
- the patient has a sustained high fever (103°F [39.5°C] to 104°F [40°C])
- the patient is having trouble breathing or complaining of chest pains or there is mental confusion or lethargy or irritability
- the patient is having trouble breathing: making grunting sounds, working hard to breathe every breath, breathing much more quickly than before the episode, not able to eat or drink because breathing takes all his energy, turning blue at the lips or fingernails

• the patient's rash is thought to be eczema but does not respond to treatment for eczema, but rather, does respond to treatment for psoriasis.

Remember: Severe allergic reactions like laryngeal spasms or anaphylaxis must be treated with prescription medicines from your health care provider.

Remember: If you want to discontinue steroid prescription medicines, I recommend that you first begin taking homeopathic remedies and when you notice that it has eased the allergy or asthma, then the time has come to taper the steroid medicines. But, you must work with your health care provider or your homeopath to taper the steroids appropriately so as not to incur any dangerous medical complications.

Note: Do not discontinue taking any pharmaceutical medication that has been prescribed by your health care provider unless you or your family member is under the supervision of a physician.

Note: The herbal remedy *Urtica dioica* (*Stinging Nettle*) may be helpful to treat hay fever symptoms during the allergy season. The dose is 400-600mg capsules twice daily of the freeze-dried herb. Children over the age of six take one capsule once daily.

Note: *Butterbur* (*Petasites hybridus*) is an herbal remedy that may be helpful to treat hay fever as well as the migraine headaches that often accompany seasonal allergies. *Butterbur*, in some studies, has been shown to be as effective as the prescription medications *Allegra* and *Zyrtec* in treating seasonal allergies. *Petadolex* is the brand that has been used in medical research. The dosage is 50mg 2-3 times daily. Children over the age of 6 may take 50mg once daily. You should not take *Butterbur* if you are pregnant or breastfeeding. The herbal remedy *Rosmarinic acid* derived from *Rosemary leaf* (*Rosmarinus officinalis*), is sometimes coupled together with *Butterbur* to help with allergies.

Note: With increasing concerns about mosquito-borne West Nile virus, it's important to have an effective and safe mosquito repellent. DEET used to be the only one and many people never liked its chemical smell. Now we have 2 new ones with similar repellent abilities against mosquitoes and safety profiles: *Picaridin* (*Cutter Advanced*) and *Oil of Lemon Eucalyptus* (*Off! Botanicals* and *Repel Lemon Eucalyptus*). But remember that only a Deet-based insect repellant protects against ticks as well as mosquitoes.

Note: *Zicam nasal gels* is a homeopathic preparation of *zinc gluconate* (*zincum gluconicum*) in very low potency in a liquid nasal gel. The FDA has begun to investigate *Zicam nasal gels* (including *Zicam Cold Remedy* and *Zicam Allergic Relief*) for reports that they may cause ansomia, the loss of the sense of smell. At this point, until more information becomes available, I do not recommend the use of any of the *Zicam nasal gels* family of cold and allergy remedies. For more information on *Zicam* products, visit www.Zicam.com or call 1-877-942-2626.

Recommended Internet Sites for More Information on Allergies and Asthma

Internet web address	Name of Organization
www.aaaai.org 1-800-822-2762	The American Academy of Allergy, Asthma, and Immunology
www.aanma.org	The Allergy and Asthma Network—Mothers of Asthmatics Inc.
www.aafa.org	The Asthma and Allergy Foundation of America
www.lungusa.org/asthma 1-800-LUNG USA	The American Lung Association

Recommendations for Homeopathic Remedies

Arsenicum album 30C and 200C—in pellets and liquid drops

Spongia tosta 30C—in pellets and liquid drops

Phosphorus 30C and 200C—in pellets and liquid drops

Apis mellifica 30C—in pellets and liquid drops

Gelsemium sempervirens 30C—in pellets and liquid drops

Kali bichromicum 30C—in pellets and liquid drops

Pulsatilla 30C and 200C—in pellets and liquid drops

Nux vomica 30C and 200C—in pellets and liquid drops

Natrum muriaticum 30C and 200C—in pellets and liquid drops

Ipecac 30C—in pellets and liquid drops

Drosera rotundifolia 30C—in pellets and liquid drops

Dulcamara 30C —in pellets and liquid drops

Allium cepa 30C—in pellets and liquid drops

Sabadilla 30C—in pellets and liquid drops

Rhus toxicodendron 200C—in pellets and liquid drops

Sulphur 30C and 200C —in pellets and liquid drops

Psorinum 30C and 200C—in pellets and liquid drops

Optique 1, combination remedy by Boiron—eye drops in single-use doses

Allergies and Hay Fever—combination remedy by King Bio—oral spray

Asthma Clear—combination remedy by King Bio—oral spray

Florasone Cream—manufactured by Boericke & Tafel

Psoriaflora Cream—manufactured by Boericke & Tafel

Guidelines for Administration of Homeopathic Remedies

Once you have chosen the homeopathic remedy and the potency that is likely to help you or your family member, you should try to give as few repetitions of the remedy as you can. You start off repeating it more frequently in a severe, acute situation, quickly decreasing the frequency once improvement has begun, stopping the remedy as soon as the problem has resolved.

> **Note:** For more information on *how often* to give the homeopathic remedy please see **Potency and Frequency**, in **Chapter 2: Basic Homeopathy**. For information on *how much* of the homeopathic remedy to give and the importance of a "clean tongue," please see **How to take homeopathic remedies** in the same chapter.

Lower potency remedies, such as 30C and below, are used to treat acute ailments. They are usually repeated often, every ½-2 or ½-4 hours. You should notice improvement in symptoms after just one to perhaps a few repetitions. If you do not see improvement, it is wise to stop the remedy and try a different one, guiding yourself by the **keynote** symptoms. You may use different single remedies together or you may try a combination remedy. And you may use homeopathic remedies together with pharmaceutical prescription and non-prescription drugs without any effect of interference.

General guidelines to treat serious, chronic, relapsing ailments include using single remedies at potencies of 200C. These are generally administered once weekly to once monthly, but they may be used once or twice daily at first if the condition warrants it, quickly decreasing the frequency as you see improvement. Do not continue giving the remedy if it becomes apparent that it is not working. You may always stop one remedy and choose to administer another remedy on the basis of the **keynote** symptoms of the new remedy. In addition, you may administer more than one remedy at a time.

Putting It All Together

Asthma and allergies are considered to be ailments with underlying inflammation at their center cores. Coping with chronic, recurrent inflammation is best done utilizing a multilevel attack incorporating all the essential natural alternatives, homeopathy, herbal remedies, and nutritional supplements.

People with allergies and asthma generally suffer from recurrent symptoms which can either be chronic or acute in nature. These people require all the vitamins and minerals necessary to repair and replenish tissues (please refer to **Chapter 23: Vitamins and Minerals**) as well as a general antioxidant supplement (please refer to **Chapter 24: Antioxidant Phytochemicals**).

In addition, it is a good idea to consider giving the sick person's homeopathic constitutional remedy (please refer to **Chapter 9: Homeopathic Remedies for Constitutional Problems in Infants, Children, and Adolescents** or to **Chapter 18: Homeopathic Constitutional Remedies** if you are dealing with an adult).

Depending on the chronicity of the allergic or asthmatic episodes, you may want to consider learning about nutritional supplements to augment the immune system, especially *medicinal mushrooms* (please refer to **Chapter 27: Nutritional Supplements to Prevent Cancer and Augment Your Immune System**).

If you are dealing with chronic, recurrent bouts of inflammation, you may want to investigate certain herbal remedies such as *Echinacea*, *Goldenseal*, *Astragalus* and *Garlic* (please refer to **Chapter 20: Herbs You Need to Know**) as well as *omega-3 fatty acids* (please refer to **Chapter 31: Oils and Fats**). In addition, it is a good idea to incorporate *probiotics* (please refer to **Chapter 30: Prebiotics and Probiotics**) into your daily supplements because your may find your allergies and asthma to be sensitive to enhanced gastrointestinal health.

Chapter 7

Homeopathic Remedies for Infections

Infections in General

Ailment/Disorder/Symptom	Homeopathic Remedy
Chronic infections with profuse, thick, yellow, or greenish pus	*Silicea*
Burning, smelly, offensive secretions (sweat, pus)	*Mercurius solubilis*
Infections with pus; touching the infected part is extremely painful	*Hepar sulphuris calcareum*
Infected skin wounds	*Calendula*
Profuse amounts of yellow-green mucus or pus	*Pulsatilla*
Lower respiratory tract infections (bronchitis, pneumonia)	*Phosphorus*
Breast inflammations and infections	*Phytolacca*

Guidelines for Consulting Your Health Care Provider
Putting It All Together

Infections in General

The person who is looking into homeopathic treatment for infections generally wishes to prevent the chronic, relapsing infection to which he or she has become prone, such as recurrent sinus infections or chronic ear infections. On the other hand, that person may require homeopathic treatment for an acute recurrence of his or her usual chronic, relapsing infection.

For best results in prevention of chronic, recurring infections the patient's constitutional remedy should be determined and administered. This is possible for you to do, but it is sometimes difficult to find the appropriate homeopathic constitutional remedy. Finding the proper constitutional remedy will likely require the services of your homeopath.

Another instance in which homeopathic remedies may be appropriate to use against infections is when a sick person requires treatment of an acute infection that does not tend to recur, such as an abscess or boil, or a tooth infection.

Whatever the situation, homeopathy is well suited to the prevention and treatment of chronic and acute infections, including those that come with pus, without the use of antibiotics. A good way to approach the problem is to try homeopathic remedies first and then if you feel you are not making progress you should consider using antibiotics. Antibiotics may be used along with homeopathic remedies without diluting the effect of the antibiotics. Although it is theoretically possible that antibiotics would interfere with the action of your homeopathic remedies, in my clinical experience this does not occur.

It is important to have a diagnosis from your health care provider when an infection is present because some infections, such as meningitis and bone infections, are serious and may be life threatening. Serious and life-threatening infections require the use of antibiotics, although you may achieve a swifter cure using homeopathic remedies at the same time.

When throat infections are due to the bacteria called *Group A beta-hemolytic Streptococcus*, antibiotic therapy is indicated because if untreated, this germ can cause rheumatic fever. Rheumatic fever may manifest itself as a life-threatening heart ailment and may last a lifetime. When a throat culture or a Rapid Strep test is negative, it means that the throat infection is due to any number of viruses and no antibiotic therapy is needed. However, this is a situation when the use of homeopathic remedies is urgently required.

It is good common sense to use the old standbys to treat infections, such as soaking with warm water or elevating the part, along with homeopathic remedies.

The homeopathic remedies should be chosen according to their **keynote** symptoms.

Please refer to **Chapter 4: Homeopathic Remedies for Fever** if fever is a prominent part of the infection process. Homeopathic treatment of fever may be combined with homeopathic treatment of infections.

As with any and all medical conditions, when dealing with infections you must pay strict attention to the **Guidelines for Consulting Your Health Care Provider** at the end of this chapter. You may want to refer to the last section **Putting It All Together** for ideas on how to integrate the essential natural alternatives, homeopathy, herbal remedies, and nutritional supplements.

Silicea

What is it? The common name for the homeopathic chemical mineral remedy *Silicea* is *silica* or *quartz* or *flint*. *Silicea* (alternative spellings are *Silicia* and *Silica*) is the mineral constituent of quartz rock, which when it breaks down forms sand. *Silicea* is also a component of both soil and the human body. *Silicea* is a constitutional remedy most often used for young children.

When should you use it? The **keynote** symptoms pointing you towards the use of *Silicea* are chronic infections with profuse thick yellow or greenish pus that have weakened the immune system and have produced generalized weakness and fatigue. Homeopathic *Silicea* is used to expel pus from deep places in the body such as abscesses, boils, and foreign bodies (including splinters). *Silicea* is indicated for the treatment of infections of the lymph glands when they have become swollen and hard. *Silicea* is also useful to treat pustular infections that tend to leave scars, such as facial acne. People who need *Silicea* often feel cold, are sensitive to cold weather, and tend to have cold, clammy, sweaty feet and hands.

How should you use it? Give *Silicea* 30C 2-4 times daily before the pus is expelled. Then use *Silicea* 200C once or twice daily when the infection has responded. Then continue with once weekly until there are no further signs of infection.

Mercurius solubilis

What is it? The homeopathic remedy, commonly called *quicksilver*, is made from the action of nitric acid and ammonia on the chemical element mercury. Mercury was once used to treat syphilis and other infections because it possesses anti-inflammatory, antibacterial, and antifungal properties. However, mercury vapors are toxic to the nervous, respiratory, and kidney systems. Ingested mercury may also be toxic. Fish is the major source of mercury toxicity.

> **Note:** For more information on mercury in seafood, please see **Chapter 31: Fat and Oils**.

Some of the signs of mercury poisoning are tightness in the chest, paroxysmal coughing, shortness of breath, sore throat with chills and fever, and a metallic taste in the mouth. Understanding what happens in a case of mercury poisoning allows us to understand what can be cured when mercury is used as a homeopathic remedy. *Merc sol* as the homeopathic remedy is called, is used to treat infections of the mouth, teeth, and gums, including mouth and gum ulcers, and sinusitis.

When should you use it? The **keynote** symptoms pointing to the use of *Merc sol* are burning, smelly, offensive secretions (sweat, pus) accompanied by excessive salivation (and the saliva burns when swallowed), bad breath, and a metallic taste in the mouth. The person needing *Merc sol* would likely be hurried and nervous.

How should you use it? Give *Merc sol* 30C every ½-2 hours until the infection has improved. Then use *Merc sol* 200C once daily until the infection is gone.

Hepar sulphuris calcareum

What is it? This homeopathic remedy (called *Hepar sulph* for short) is made from heating sulphur with calcium carbonate from oyster shells.

When should you use it? The **keynote** symptoms leading you to choose *Hepar sulph* are infections with pus while touching the infected part is extremely painful. *Hepar sulph* helps to expel pus from the body. The patient needing *Hepar sulph* is irritable out of proportion to the illness and is usually very sensitive to pain and cold air. The sweat and other secretions smell sour. Some infections for which *Hepar sulph* may be particularly helpful are: gingivitis, mouth ulcers, tonsillitis, ear infections, sinusitis, lymphadenitis (lymph gland inflammations), boils, abscesses, folliculitis (infections around the hair root), as well as other skin infections such as acne.

How should you use it? Give *Hepar sulph* 30C every ½-2 hours until the infection has improved. Then use *Hepar sulph* 200C once daily until the infection and pus are gone.

Calendula

What is it? This is the plant *Calendula officinalis*, common name *marigold*, a member of the *Compositae* botanical family. The leaves and orange flowers are used to prepare the tincture of Calendula and from that, the herbal ointments and creams are made, as well as the homeopathic remedy. When *Calendula* is used as a topical herbal remedy for the skin, it does not go through the dilutions and succussions that are necessary to make the oral homeopathic remedy.

When should you use it? The **keynote** symptoms indicating use of *Calendula* are skin wounds (abrasions, lacerations) that have become infected with pus accompanied by complaints of severe pain that may be out of proportion to the injury.

How should you use it? Give *Calendula* 30C every ½-2 hours until the infection has improved. Then use *Calendula* 200C once daily until the infection and pus are gone. *Calendula* as the oral homeopathic remedy may be given together with *Calendula* as the herbal remedy, applied topically to the skin as creams, ointments, and tinctures.

Pulsatilla

What is it? This is the plant, *Pulsatilla nigricans*, whose common name is *windflower*, a member of the *Ranunculaceae* botanical family.

When should you use it? The **keynote** symptoms leading you to use *Pulsatilla* to treat infections are yellow or yellow-green mucus or pus discharges in large amounts from the infected part. *Pulsatilla* is commonly used for infections of the sinuses, swollen glands with upper respiratory infections, and vaginitis. *Pulsatilla* is especially indicated for those persons who feel warm to hot all the time and who are thirstless. The typical person needing *Pulsatilla* is needy emotionally, sensitive, childlike, moody, timid and weepy.

How should you use it? Give *Pulsatilla* 30C every ½-2 hours until the infection has improved. Then use *Pulsatilla* 200C once daily until the infection and greenish drainage are gone.

Phosphorus

What is it? The chemical element *Phosphorus* is a mineral that is present in every living cell in the form of genetic material (DNA and RNA) as well as many other compounds. It is made into a homeopathic remedy that is an often-prescribed polychrest or constitutional remedy.

When should you use it? The **keynote** symptoms pointing to the use of *Phosphorus* are lower respiratory tract infections (such as bronchitis and pneumonia) in a person who loves massages and loves to be touched. Patients needing *Phosphorus* feel better from company and desire sympathy. Patients who require *Phosphorus* for respiratory tract infections often have a history of recurrent pneumonias. They may be clairvoyant and be sensitive to thunderstorms and lightening. *Phosphorus* is also useful in asthmatic conditions.

How should you use it? Give *Phosphorus* 30C every ½-2 hours until the infection has improved. Then use *Phosphorus* 200C once daily until the infection has gone.

Phytolacca

What is it? This is the plant *Phytolacca decandra*, common name *Pokeroot*, a member of the *Phytolaccaceae* family.

When should you use it? The homeopathic remedy *Phytolacca* has a special affinity for breast inflammations, including infections (mastitis), benign nodules, and malignant cancers. The **keynote** symptoms pointing to the use of *Phytolacca* are a breast that has a purplish caste and is swollen and hard. The pains in the breast may feel like electric shocks. The nipples may be fissured and very painful when the infant suckles.

How should you use it? Give *Phytolacca* 30C every ½-2 hours until the infection has improved. Then use *Phytolacca* 200C once daily until the infection has gone. *Phytolacca* is indicated just after delivery to prevent breast inflammations in the woman who intends to nurse her baby.

Guidelines for Consulting Your Health Care Provider

You should consult your health care provider if:
- the patient doesn't look right or act right (trust your instincts!)
- the patient is getting worse instead of better over the course of the illness
- the patient has a sustained high fever (103°F [39.5°C] to 104°F [40°C])
- the patient is having trouble breathing or complaining of chest pains or there is mental confusion or lethargy or irritability
- the infection appears to be spreading over a greater area
- the infection has become very painful to the touch
- there appears to be a red line (indicating lymphatic spread of the infection) leading from the infection towards the body's center, for example, there is a red line from a pus-filled abscess on a finger leading towards the upper arm
- the infection is interfering with function of that part, such as a pus-filled abscess in the armpit has impeded the movement of the entire arm

Remember: There are some infections that are life- threatening such as meningitis, certain abdominal infections, and certain fast spreading bacterial infections that can kill quickly. It is important that you are comfortable knowing what infection you are dealing with. If you have any questions about the nature of the infection, you must consult with your health care provider.

Note: Do not discontinue taking any pharmaceutical medication that has been prescribed by your health care provider unless you or your family member is under the supervision of a physician.

Remember: The elderly, the very young, and people with chronic diseases tend to have more difficulty coping with even uncomplicated infections. The commonest chronic ailments are cardiovascular disease (congestive heart failure and hypertension), stroke, diabetes, arthritis, cancer, and emotional disorders. Please watch out especially for people with any ailment of the endocrine glands, like disorders of the pancreas (diabetes mellitus), thyroid, adrenals, or any metabolic disorder, like hypoglycemia (low blood sugar), ketoacidosis (acidic pH in the blood), hypo- or hypercalcemia (low or high blood calcium), hypo-or hyperkalemia (low or high blood potassium).

Note: *Colloidal silver* products are sometimes used by patients to treat infections as an alternative to antibiotics. *Colloidal silver* is not a homeopathic remedy. *Colloidal silver* consists of tiny silver particles in a liquid to be taken by mouth or sprayed topically on the skin. *Colloidal silver* products are not recommended because unregulated use may result in the irreversible build up of silver in your body (silver poisoning, called argyria). People with argyria have a bluish-gray discoloration of their skin, nails, gums, and deep tissues. Silver may damage your kidneys and cause seizures.

Recommendations for Homeopathic Remedies
Silicea 30C and 200C—in pellets and liquid drops
Mercurius solubilis 30C and 200C—in pellets and liquid drops
Hepar sulphuris calcareum 30C and 200C—in pellets and liquid drops
Calendula 30C and 200C—in pellets and liquid drops
Pulsatilla 30C and 200C—in pellets and liquid drops
Phosphorus 30C and 200C—in pellets and liquid drops
Phytolacca 30C and 200C—in pellets and liquid drops

Guidelines for Administration of Homeopathic Remedies
Once you have chosen the homeopathic remedy and the potency that is likely to help you or your family member, you should try to give as few repetitions of the remedy as you can. You start off repeating it more frequently in a severe, acute situation, quickly decreasing the frequency once improvement has begun, stopping the remedy as soon as the problem has resolved.

> **Note:** For more information on *how often* to give the homeopathic remedy please see **Potency and Frequency**, in **Chapter 2: Basic Homeopathy**. For information on *how much* of the homeopathic remedy to give and the importance of a "*clean tongue*," please see **How to take homeopathic remedies** in the same chapter.

Lower potency remedies, such as 30C and below, are used to treat acute ailments. They are usually repeated often, every $\frac{1}{2}$-2 or $\frac{1}{2}$-4 hours. You should notice improvement in symptoms after just one to perhaps a few repetitions. If you do not see improvement, it is wise to stop the remedy and try a different one, guiding yourself by the **keynote** symptoms. You may use different single remedies together or you may try a combination remedy. And you may use homeopathic remedies together with pharmaceutical prescription and non-prescription drugs without any effect of interference.

General guidelines to treat serious, chronic, relapsing ailments include using single remedies at potencies of 200C. These are generally administered once weekly to once monthly, but they may be used once or twice daily at first if the condition warrants it, quickly decreasing the frequency as you see improvement. Do not continue giving the remedy if it becomes apparent that it is not working. You may always stop one remedy and choose to administer another remedy on the basis of the **keynote** symptoms of the new remedy. In addition, you may administer more than one remedy at a time.

Putting It All Together

Infections may be either chronic or acute in nature. Some infections are recurrent. Most of the time infections are considered to be ailments with underlying inflammation at their center cores. Coping with chronic, recurrent inflammation is best done utilizing a multilevel attack incorporating all the essential natural alternatives, homeopathy, herbal remedies, and nutritional supplements.

Depending on the chronicity of the fever episodes with the infections, you may decide to incorporate certain homeopathic remedies from **Chapter 4: Homeopathic Remedies for Fever.** Depending on the source of the infection, it may be a good idea to read **Chapter 5: Homeopathic Remedies for Upper Respiratory Infections:** **Colds, Flu, Coughs, Sore Throats, Laryngitis, Ear Infections, Eye Infections, Sinus Infections;** **Chapter 11: Homeopathy for Digestive Tract Ailments** and **Chapter 12: Homeopathy for Urinary Tract Ailments.**

People with infections require all the vitamins and minerals necessary to repair and replenish tissues (please refer to **Chapter 23: Vitamins and Minerals**) as well as a general antioxidant supplement (please refer to **Chapter 24: Antioxidant Phytochemicals**).

For people with chronic, recurrent infections, it is a good idea to consider giving the homeopathic constitutional remedy (please refer to **Chapter 9: Homeopathic Remedies for Constitutional Problems in Infants, Children, and Adolescents** or to **Chapter 18: Homeopathic Constitutional Remedies** if you are dealing with an adult).

Depending on the chronicity of the infection episodes, you may want to consider learning about nutritional supplements to augment the immune system, especially *medicinal mushrooms* (please refer to **Chapter 27: Nutritional Supplements to Prevent Cancer and Augment Your Immune System**).

If you are dealing with chronic, recurrent bouts of infection and inflammation, you may want to investigate certain herbal remedies such as *Echinacea, Goldenseal, Astragalus* and *Garlic* (please refer to **Chapter 20: Herbs You Need to Know**) as well as *omega-3 fatty acids* (please refer to **Chapter 31: Oils and Fats**). In addition, it is a good idea to incorporate *probiotics* (please refer to **Chapter 30: Prebiotics and Probiotics**) into your daily supplements because your may find your infections to be sensitive to enhanced gastrointestinal health.

Chapter 8

Homeopathic Remedies for Emotional Problems

Emotional Problems in General

Ailment/Disorder/Symptom	Homeopathic Remedy
Denying that anything is wrong, saying, "Leave me alone, I'm okay."	*Arnica montana*
Fear and anxiety with sudden onset, panic attacks, shock, fright, loss	*Aconitum napellus*
Grief after loss, bereavement, severed relationship	*Ignatia amara*
Panic attacks	*Argentum nitricum*
Great anxieties and fears, fear of death	*Arsenicum album*
Deep grief reactions, depression	*Natrum muriaticum*
Dramatic, hysterical grief reactions	*Pulsatilla*
Great fears, "something bad will happen"	*Calcarea carbonica*
Constant worrying, insomnia	*Cocculus indicus*
Despairing depression, may express suicidal ideas	*Aurum metallicum*
Emotional shock from getting bad news	*Gelsemium*
Depression from empty nest syndrome, indifference and apathy	*Sepia*
Depression in over-empathetic people	*Causticum*
Suppressed emotions, suppressed anger, indignation	*Staphysagria*
Depression with anguished weeping	*Veratrum album*
Depression and anxiety in menopausal women	*Lachesis*
Depression resulting from head injury	*Natrum sulphuricum*
Depression after influenza	*Kali phosphoricum*
Feelings of being out-of-control, stress, helplessness	*911 Stress Control*
Stress and anxiety	*Rescue Remedy*

Guidelines for Consulting Your Health Care Provider
Putting It All Together

Emotional Problems in General

Today, emotional problems have become so prevalent in our society that we find ourselves in the midst of an epidemic. Western medicine patients in this epidemic are treated with psychiatric medications and psychological counseling. Conventional wisdom is that the emotional ailment will likely be chronic and recurrent and treatment may be life long. Homeopathic wisdom is that it is possible to **treat** emotional disorders and then to **prevent** their recurrence.

A basic tenet of homeopathic philosophy is that the mind and body are interconnected and that both directly influence each other. Homeopaths do not treat physical complaints without paying attention to the emotional, intellectual (or mental), sexual, and spiritual parts of that person. Homeopathy is a holistic medical science.

Homeopathic remedies are uniquely suited to **treating** many emotional problems, such as: grief and loss, depression, seasonal affective disorder, bipolar disorder, anxiety disorders, panic attacks, eating disorders, phobias, stress, substance abuse, alcoholism, schizophrenia, obsessive compulsive disorder, anger and rage, certain personality disorders, and post-traumatic stress disorder. Sometimes homeopathic remedies are utilized along with psychological counseling.

Since there is no interaction between psychiatric medications and homeopathic remedies, it is possible to use both at the same time, and many people do that. The appropriate homeopathic remedy may strengthen and deepen the action of psychiatric medications, making them more effective. However, many people begin homeopathic remedies for emotional disorders in the hopes that they will be able to taper and then discontinue their prescription medicines.

For best results in **preventing** chronic, recurring emotional disorders the patient's constitutional remedy should be determined and administered. This is possible for you to do, but it is sometimes difficult for an untrained person to find the appropriate constitutional remedy. Finding the proper constitutional remedy will likely require the services of your homeopath.

Stress-related ailments may be the commonest form of emotional distress in our society. Chronic stress gives rise to complications such as depression, insomnia, headaches, substance abuse, alcoholism, eating disorders, obesity, cancer, cardiovascular disease, high blood pressure (hypertension), and stroke. Homeopathy is a healthy first choice for both stress prevention and treatment.

Emotional problems come in many forms and a layperson may find them hard to diagnose. A psychiatrist and your homeopath as well as other health care providers are trained in making emotional diagnoses by fitting the patient's symptoms to those listed in the *Diagnostic and Statistical Manual of Mental Disorders*. If you have trouble deciding whether you or a person in your family has a certain emotional problem, you must consult with your health care provider.

Some emotional disorders can be life-threatening, for example, some people with depression try to commit suicide and a certain percentage succeed, even though they may be taking psychiatric medications, or even homeopathic remedies, for that matter. Some persons with certain forms of emotional disorders such as schizophrenia may be dangerous to themselves and to others. It is important that you do not exceed your limitations in dealing with the self-care of emotional problems. It is hard to make a mistake with homeopathy. The biggest mistake you are likely to make would be to use homeopathy exclusively while not consulting with your health care provider for potentially serious emotional disorders.

As with any and all medical conditions, when dealing with emotional problems you must pay strict attention to the **Guidelines for Consulting Your Health Care Provider** at the end of this chapter. You may want to refer to the last section **Putting It All Together** for ideas on how to integrate the essential natural alternatives, homeopathy, herbal remedies, and nutritional supplements.

Arnica montana

What is it? This is the plant *Arnica montana*, common name *Leopard's bane*, a member of the *Compositae* botanical family. *Arnica* helps injured people to cope, physically and emotionally, with the physiological stress of the injury.

When should you use it? The **keynote** symptom

leading you to use *Arnica* is that the injured person denies that anything is wrong, saying, "Leave me alone, I'm okay." This kind of reaction tends to happen during the shock following loss of a dear one and the accompanying bereavement period. Another instance when you would give *Arnica* is when an injured person awakens suddenly in the middle of the night from dreaming of an accident, whether recent or long past. This is one of the prominent symptoms of post-traumatic stress disorder. You should consider using *Arnica* whenever PTSD occurs, even long after the accident itself.

How should you use it? Administer *Arnica* 30C every ½-2 hours, as needed at first, then decreasing to 3-4 times daily, then once or twice daily.

Aconitum napellus

What is it? This homeopathic remedy, called in short *Aconite*, is made from the plant commonly called *monkshood* or *wolfsbane*, a member of the *Ranunculaceae* botanical family.

When should you use it? *Aconite* is the homeopathic substitute for *Valium*, because of its calming effect on anxiety. The **keynote** symptoms leading you to use *Aconite* are fear or anxiety and restless agitation with a sudden onset. *Aconite* is useful for treating the emotional shock or fright after a traumatic injury. It is often used along with *Arnica* to control the pain and shock from trauma and to speed the healing process. *Aconite* is used to treat panic attacks, fear of death during labor, and fear of dying when sick. Fear, anxiety, pains and restlessness are worse after midnight. *Aconite* is also useful during bereavement to ease the emotional shock of death of a loved one. *Aconite* treats the emotional shock and numbness that sets in after a particularly traumatic injury.

How should you use it? Administer *Aconite* 30C every ½-2 hours, as needed at first, then decreasing to 3-4 times daily as the fear and anxiety improves, and stopping when the condition is under control. *Aconite* is often administered along with *Arnica*. They complement each other well in their actions on the emotional and physical parts of the self. Remember you may give *Aconite* and *Arnica* along with another remedy chosen by its **keynote** symptoms.

Ignatia amara

What is it? This is the plant *Ignatia amara*, common name *St. Ignatius's bean*, a member of the *Loganiaceae* botanical family. The homeopathic remedy is made from the seeds of the plant. *Ignatia amara* is poisonous as it contains strychnine, as does *Nux vomica*, so the homeopathic remedy is never given in potency less than 3X.

When should you use it? The **keynote** symptoms leading you to consider the use of *Ignatia* are grief after loss: bereavement through death or great loss through the severing of a love relationship. Persons in need of *Ignatia* display obvious depression but their expressions of grief are suppressed. Their depression is accompanied by features of hysteria, such as: inappropriate laughing, dramatic sighing, much crying, extreme mood swings, self-pity, insomnia, and an inability to express emotions appropriately. *Ignatia* is often prescribed as an acute constitutional remedy for persons (female gender, mostly) who are emotionally fragile especially in response to the depression seen after disillusioned romance or disappointed love or betrayal in love.

How should you use it? Give *Ignatia* 30C 3-4 times daily depending on severity of symptoms until the patient is able to express emotions of grief and anger. Then give *Ignatia* 200C once daily until the mood swings are less violent. Then continue with *Ignatia* 200C once weekly until the bereavement reactions have subsided.

Argentum nitricum

What is it? This is the soluble chemical compound *Silver nitrate*.

When should you use it? The **keynote** symptoms leading you towards trying *Argentum nitricum* are panic attacks with palpitations in the chest, sweating, hyperventilation, along with restlessness. There may be associated claustrophobia, fear of heights, impulsiveness, and a hurried manner in walking, speaking, and eating. *Argentum nitricum* is also a constitutional remedy suiting some actors and actresses because of their over-active imaginations, quick thinking abilities, and rapid talking and gesturing. *Argentum nitricum* is also used to control anticipatory anxiety, such as stage fright.

How should you use it? Give *Argentum nitricum* 30C every ½-2 hours at first, then decreasing the frequency to 1-2 times daily as the panic attack subsides. In treating long-standing phobias, give *Argentum nitricum* 200C once daily until the panic phase associated with the action has diminished. Then continue with *Argentum nitricum* 200C once weekly until the phobic situation is no longer associated with panic reaction symptoms.

Arsenicum album

What is it? This is the homeopathic remedy made from the chemical compound *arsenic oxide* which is highly poisonous if not given in homeopathic dilution. *Arsenicum album* is one of homeopathy's often-used polychrests or constitutional remedies. *Arsenicum album* is often used to treat asthma.

When should you use it? The **keynote** symptoms leading you to consider the use of *Arsenicum album* are great restlessness, fears of one's own health and dying, fear of one's own physical and financial security in a very insecure world, in a person who is chilly, restless, and anxious. Fears are worse after midnight. Additionally, *Arsenicum album* is often useful to treat depression with anxiety and guilt. The person needing *Arsenicum album* is often a perfectionist, fastidious in habits and dress. He or she is likely to feel chilly most of the time and suffer from burning type of pains.

How should you use it? Give *Arsenicum album* 30C 3-4 times daily depending on severity of symptoms until the patient's fears and anxieties are under control. Then give *Arsenicum album* 200C once daily and then once weekly until the fears and insecurities are gone.

Natrum muriaticum

What is it? This is the polychrest *Natrum muriaticum*, a homeopathic remedy made from common table salt. *Natrum muriaticum* is a polychrest, used mostly as a constitutional remedy, however it is also used to treat emotional disorders.

When should you use it? The **keynote** symptoms leading you towards the use of *Natrum muriaticum* are deep-seated grief reactions, including depres-

sion, after the loss of a loved one, or after several cumulative losses. *Natrum muriaticum* is indicated for sensitive but private people who suffer with great sadness but who have difficulty crying. When they do cry, although never with gusto, they tend to cry alone, and the crying does not make them feel better. People needing *Natrum muriaticum* desire to be alone even when they are acutely depressed and they feel worse if someone tries to console them. *Natrum muriaticum* people tend to suffer deeply and may express an existential personal belief system.

How should you use it? Give *Natrum muriaticum* 30C 3-4 times daily depending on severity of symptoms until the patient's depression has lessened. Then give *Natrum muriaticum* 200C once daily and then once weekly until the emotional problem has resolved.

Pulsatilla

What is it? This is the plant *Pulsatilla nigricans*, whose common name is *windflower*, a member of the *Ranunculaceae* botanical family.

When should you use it? The **keynote** symptoms leading you to consider the use of *Pulsatilla* are grief reactions with dramatic weeping and expressions of emotion. *Pulsatilla* is indicated for people, usually women and girls, who are affectionate, compassionate, empathetic, and hypersensitive to their own or others' sufferings. Crying (and they can cry with great gusto) gives them relief from their grief. Depressed people who are likely to benefit from *Pulsatilla* express a need for company almost all the time.

How should you use it? Give *Pulsatilla* 30C 3-4 times daily depending on severity of symptoms until the acute grief reaction has lessened. Then give *Pulsatilla* 200C once daily and then once weekly until the emotional problem has resolved.

Calcarea carbonica

What is it? This is the chemical mineral compound *calcium carbonate* which is obtained from oyster shells. *Calcarea carbonica* is a polychrest constitutional remedy and is also an important homeopathic remedy for infants, children, and adolescents. The homeopathic action of *Calcarea carbonica* is exerted primarily on bones and teeth, especially for problems due to delayed and imperfect development.

When should you use it? The **keynote** symptoms leading you towards choosing *Calcarea carbonica* are much anxiety from fears, especially fear that "something bad will happen" in persons who are obese, clumsy, and easily constipated, fatigued, and frightened. Persons needing *Calcarea carbonica* may be depressed and appear slow-witted.

How should you use it? Give *Calcarea carbonica* 30C 3-4 times daily depending on severity of symptoms until the anxiety or depression has lessened. Then give *Calcarea carbonica* 200C once daily and then once weekly until the emotional problem has resolved.

Cocculus indicus

What is it? This is the plant *Cocculus indicus*, common name *Levant nut*, or *Fish berry*, a member of the *Menispermaceae* botanical family. The poisonous seeds are used to make the homeopathic remedy. The poison is *picrotoxine*. The homeopathic remedy is non-toxic.

When should you use it? The main use of homeopathic *Cocculus* is to treat motion sickness with its attendant nausea and vertigo. The **keynote** symptoms of using *Cocculus* for emotional problems are an empty, hollow feeling with an almost constant worrying about loved ones causing a loss of sleep. The insomnia may cause the daytime personality to be dominated by irritability and anger.

How should you use it? Give *Cocculus* 30C 1-2 times daily depending on severity of symptoms until the worrying and resultant insomnia have decreased. Then continue with *Cocculus* 200C once daily and then once weekly until the emotional problem has resolved.

Aurum metallicum

What is it? This is the element *gold*, one of the metals in the periodic table of chemicals.

When should you use it? The **keynote** symptoms leading you to consider using *Aurum metallicum* are deep, dark, despairing depression with expressions of suicidal ideas (suicidal ideation) in gloomy persons who are apt to explode with anger, then using meditation and prayer to control themselves.

> **Note:** If someone you are caring for has suicidal thoughts it is imperative that you seek consultation with your health care provider in conjunction with giving *Aurum metallicum*. The **Guidelines for Consulting Your Health Care Provider for Emotional Problems** at the end of this chapter stresses this point.

The depression is likely to be worse in the winter months making *Aurum metallicum* a remedy for seasonal affective disorder (SAD). A person needing *Aurum metallicum* feels better when listening to music, which is often sad and gloomy.

How should you use it? Give *Aurum metallicum* 30C 3-4 times daily depending on severity of symptoms until the depression has decreased. Then give *Aurum metallicum* 200C once daily and then once weekly until the emotional problem has resolved. *Aurum metallicum* may be used together when necessary with prescription psychiatric medications.

Gelsemium

What is it? This is the poisonous plant whose common name is *yellow jasmine*, a member of the *Loganiaceae* botanical family.

When should you use it? The **keynote** symptoms leading you towards using *Gelsemium* are trembling from shock or surprise from getting bad news that leads to intellectual (or mental) dullness with confusion. The person needing *Gelsemium* complains of heaviness in the limbs and body along with thirstlessness. *Gelsemium* is also used for anticipatory anxiety (such as going for a medical test) in a person who can be paralyzed from fears. *Gelsemium* may be used for jet lag when all parts of the body feel tired and heavy.

How should you use it? Give *Gelsemium* 30C 3-4 times daily depending on severity of symptoms until the shock from bad news has decreased. Then give *Gelsemium* 200C once daily and then once weekly until the emotional problem has resolved.

Sepia

What is it? The homeopathic remedy *Sepia* is made from the black ink sac of *Sepia officinalis*, the *cuttlefish*, a species of mollusk.

When should you use it? The **keynote** symptoms for using *Sepia* are those of the empty nest syndrome, usually but not exclusively present in the female gender, or depression (worse in the winter, so used for seasonal affective disorder [SAD]) with indifference and apathy towards one's own children and husband. *Sepia* is the treatment of choice for the physically and emotionally exhausted or worn out housewife who has been a workaholic until now.

How should you use it? Give *Sepia* 30C 3-4 times daily depending on severity of symptoms until the empty nest syndrome or the physical and emotional exhaustion symptoms have decreased. Then give *Sepia* 200C once daily and then once weekly until the emotional problem has resolved.

Causticum

What is it? This is the chemical *potassium hydrate* which is prepared as a homeopathic remedy by the action of *potassium bisulphate* and water on lime.

When should you use it? The **keynote** symptoms suggesting the use of *Causticum* are depression in over-sympathetic or over-empathetic persons who suffer to an exaggerated degree when others suffer. These persons tend to become active in organizations whose goals are to alleviate injustice in the world. Persons needing *Causticum* tend to worry that "something bad will happen."

How should you use it? Give *Causticum* 30C 3-4 times daily depending on severity of symptoms until the obsessive worries or depression have decreased. Then give *Causticum* 200C once daily and then once weekly until the emotional problem has resolved.

Staphysagria

What is it? This is the plant *Delphinium staphysagria*, common name *stavesacre*, a member of the *Ranunculaceae* botanical family.

When should you use it? The **keynote** symptoms indicating the use of *Staphysagria* are anger and indignation (taking offense easily) with wounded pride, with much of the anger being suppressed. All of this commonly leads to clinical depression. This scenario is exacerbated after a loss. The person needing *Staphysagria* feels resentful after experiencing humiliating insults, betrayal, and bullying, yet he or she generally suppresses strong emotions.

How should you use it? Give *Staphysagria* 30C 3-4 times daily depending on severity of symptoms until the suppressed anger and indignation or depression have decreased. Then give *Staphysagria* 200C once daily and then once weekly until the emotional problem has resolved.

Veratrum album

What is it? This is the poisonous plant *Veratrum album*, common name *White Hellebore*, a member of the *Liliaceae* botanical family. The root before flowering is used to make the homeopathic remedy, which is non-toxic.

When should you use it? The **keynote** symptoms indicating the use of *Veratrum album* are depression with anguished weeping after loss or disappointed love in people who feel better when they are busy. They tend to turn to prayer as a coping mechanism. The most common use for *Veratrum album* is for severe gastrointestinal infections, such as cholera, accompanied by copious amounts of diarrhea and violent vomiting with icy cold hands and a cold, sinking feeling in the whole body.

How should you use it? Give *Veratrum album* 30C 3-4 times daily depending on severity of symptoms until the depression and weeping have decreased. Then give *Veratrum album* 200C once daily and then once weekly until the emotional problem has resolved.

Lachesis

What is it? This is *Trigonocephalus lachesis*, common name *Surukuku snake* or the *Bushmaster snake*. The homeopathic remedy is made from the venom of the snake. It is non-toxic.

When should you use it? The **keynote** symptoms

indicating the use of *Lachesis* are depression and anxiety with accompanying insomnia during the menopause with intolerance of wearing constricting clothing. The woman needing *Lachesis* may exhibit traits of jealousy, suspiciousness, loquacity and maliciousness. *Lachesis* is most commonly used for menopausal symptoms.
How should you use it? Give *Lachesis* 30C 3-4 times daily depending on severity of symptoms until the depression and anxiety have decreased. Then give *Lachesis* 200C once daily and then once weekly until the emotional problem has resolved.

Natrum sulphuricum

What is it? This is the non-metallic chemical compound *sodium sulphate*, a naturally occurring salt in the body.
When should you use it? The **keynote** symptom leading you to use *Natrum sulphuricum* (or *Natrum sulph* as it is usually called) is depression resulting from head injury.
How should you use it? Give *Natrum sulph* 30C 3-4 times daily depending on severity of symptoms until the depression has decreased. Then give *Natrum sulph* 200C once daily and then once weekly until the emotional problem has resolved.

Kali phosphoricum

What is it? This is the chemical compound *Potassium phosphate* that is produced by adding phosphoric acid to *potassium carbonate*.
When should you use it? The **keynote** symptom for using *Kali phos*, as it is called, is when someone complains of weakness, exhaustion and depression after having had the flu. It is also used one of the homeopathic remedies often prescribed for chronic fatigue syndrome and the depression that accompanies it. People needing *Kali phos* may develop physical ailments as a result of emotional stress and overwork.
How should you use it? Give *Kali phos* 30C 3-4 times daily depending on severity of symptoms until the depression has decreased. Then give *Kali phos* 200C once daily and then once weekly until the emotional problem has resolved.

911 Stress Control

What is it? This is a combination remedy made by King Bio (in their *SafeCareRx* line of products), a leading homeopathic pharmaceutical supply house. It is composed of the following ingredients in a pure water base: *Aconitum napellus, Apis mellifica, Arnica montana, Arsenicum album, Belladonna, Bellis perennis, Bryonia alba, Calendula officinalis, Chamomilla, Cistus canadensis, Clematis erecta, Ferrum phosphoricum, Histaminum, Hypericum perforatum, Ignatia amara, Impatients glandulifera, Ornithogaium umbellatum, Passiflora incarnata, Phosphorus, Prunus cerasifera, Rhus toxicodendron, Sulphur, Symphytum officinalis* and *Veratrum album*. Each ingredient comes in a broad spectrum of low to high potencies.
When should you use it? The **keynote** symptoms for the use of *911 Stress Control* are feelings of out-of-control stress and helplessness, oftentimes occurring after a traumatic event. It is also useful for post-traumatic stress disorder.
How should you use it? Spray *911 Stress Control* 2-3 times onto or under the tongue 3-4 times daily depending on severity of symptoms until anxieties are diminished. Then continue with once daily until the perceived threats to self-harm are gone.

Rescue Remedy

What is it? This is a combination *Bach Flower Remedy* that is strictly speaking, not homeopathic. *Rescue Remedy* is a combination of five flower essences.
When should you use it? It is very useful for the **keynote** symptoms of stress and anxiety. Whenever you or one of your family members is confronted with a sudden, unexpected threat to emotional health, whether from an accident or any other cause, it is worthwhile to give a few doses of *Rescue Remedy* to restore calm and a sense of well being. Think of *Rescue Remedy* as a preventive whenever you or a family member may be encountering a frightening or worrying situation, such as doctors' appointments.
How should you use it? Give *Rescue Remedy* as the liquid drops, 4 drops or as the spray, 2 sprays every $\frac{1}{2}$-1 hour for as long as the oppressive feelings of stress and anxiety persist. Decrease the frequency of

administration depending on depending on severity of symptoms and control of the symptoms. To prevent anxiety, give *Rescue Remedy* 4 drops or 2 sprays twice daily the day before the anxiety-producing event, and then every 2 hours on the day of the event.

Guidelines for Consulting Your Health Care Provider

You should consult your health care provider if:
• the patient doesn't look right or act right (trust your instincts!)
• the patient is getting worse instead of better over the course of the illness
• the patient is having trouble breathing or complaining of chest pains or there is mental confusion or lethargy or irritability
• the patient expresses a wish to die, commit suicide, "end it all"
• the patient is having sustained difficulties with "survival" functions, such as sleeping, eating, anger, anxiety
• the patient has developed new symptoms, such as obsessions with germs or cleanliness along with compulsive hand washing or cleaning
• the patient has developed new phobias or the old phobias have intensified
• the patient has developed hallucinations and/or delusions
• the patient wishes to discontinue his/her Western medications and requires directions for tapering along with ongoing supervision from a health care provider

> **Remember:** Homeopathic remedies may be used in conjunction with Western psychiatric prescription medicines.

> **Note:** Do not discontinue taking any pharmaceutical medication that has been prescribed by your health care provider unless you or your family member is under the supervision of a physician.

Recommendations for Homeopathic Remedies
Arnica montana 30C—in pellets and liquid drops
Aconitum napellus 30C—in pellets and liquid drops
Ignatia amara 30C and 200C—in pellets and liquid drops
Argentum nitricum 30C and 200C—in pellets and liquid drops
Arsenicum album 30C and 200C—in pellets and liquid drops
Natrum muriaticum 30C and 200C—in pellets and liquid drops
Pulsatilla 30C and 200C—in pellets and liquid drops
Calcarea carbonica 30C and 200C—in pellets and liquid drops
Cocculus indicus 30C and 200C—in pellets and liquid drops
Aurum metallicum 30C and 200C—in pellets and liquid drops
Gelsemium 30C and 200C—in pellets and liquid drops
Sepia 30C and 200C—in pellets and liquid drops
Causticum 30C and 200C—in pellets and liquid drops
Staphysagria 30C and 200C—in pellets and liquid drops
Veratrum album 30C and 200C—in pellets and liquid drops
Lachesis 30C and 200C—in pellets and liquid drops
Natrum sulphuricum 30C and 200C—in pellets and liquid drops
Kali phosphoricum 30C and 200C—in pellets and liquid drops
911 Stress Control—spray combination remedy by King Bio
Rescue Remedy—in liquid drops and spray

Guidelines for Administration of Homeopathic Remedies
Once you have chosen the homeopathic remedy and the potency that is likely to help you or your family member, you should try to give as few repetitions of the remedy as you can. You start off repeating it more frequently in a severe, acute situation, quickly decreasing the frequency once improvement has begun, stopping the remedy as soon as the problem has resolved.

Note: For more information on *how often* to give the homeopathic remedy please see **Potency and Frequency**, in **Chapter 2: Basic Homeopathy**. For information on *how much* of the homeopathic remedy to give and the importance of a "*clean tongue*," please see **How to take homeopathic remedies** in the same chapter.

Lower potency remedies, such as 30C and below, are used to treat acute ailments. They are usually repeated often, every ½-2 or ½-4 hours. You should notice improvement in symptoms after just one to perhaps a few repetitions. If you do not see improvement, it is wise to stop the remedy and try a different one, guiding yourself by the **keynote** symptoms. You may use different single remedies together or you may try a combination remedy. And you may use homeopathic remedies together with pharmaceutical prescription and non-prescription drugs without any effect of interference.

General guidelines to treat serious, chronic, relapsing ailments include using single remedies at potencies of 200C. These are generally administered once weekly to once monthly, but they may be used once or twice daily at first if the condition warrants it, quickly decreasing the frequency as you see improvement. Do not continue giving the remedy if it becomes apparent that it is not working. You may always stop one remedy and choose to administer another remedy on the basis of the **keynote** symptoms of the new remedy. In addition, you may administer more than one remedy at a time.

Putting It All Together

Coping with chronic, recurrent emotional problems is best done utilizing a multi-pronged approach incorporating all the essential natural alternatives, homeopathy, herbal remedies, and nutritional supplements.

Depending on the chronicity of the emotional problems, you may decide to incorporate certain homeopathic remedies from **Chapter 16: Homeopathy for Neurologic Disorders** and **Chapter 15: Homeopathy for Eating Disorders and Weight Control**. Depending on the age of the patient, it may be a good idea to read **Chapter 13: Homeopathy for Elderly Persons**.

For people with chronic, recurrent emotional ailments, it is a good idea to consider giving the homeopathic constitutional remedy (please refer to **Chapter 9: Homeopathic Remedies for Constitutional Problems in Infants, Children, and Adolescents** or to **Chapter 18: Homeopathic Constitutional Remedies** if you are dealing with an adult).

People with emotional ailments require all the vitamins and minerals necessary to repair and replenish tissues (please refer to **Chapter 23: Vitamins and Minerals**) as well as a general antioxidant supplement (please refer to **Chapter 24: Antioxidant Phytochemicals**).

You may want to investigate certain herbal remedies such as *Valerian* and *St. John's Wort* (please refer to **Chapter 20: Herbs You Need to Know**) as well as *omega-3 fatty acids* (please refer to **Chapter 31: Oils and Fats**). In addition, it is a good idea to incorporate *probiotics* (please refer to **Chapter 30: Prebiotics and Probiotics**) into your daily supplements because your may find your emotional problems to be sensitive to enhanced gastrointestinal health.

You may wish to investigate additional nutritional supplements for specific neurologic ailments in **Chapter 29: Nutritional Supplements for Neurologic Disorders**.

Chapter 9

Homeopathic Remedies for Constitutional Problems in Infants, Children, and Adolescents

Constitutional Problems in Infants, Children and Adolescents in General

Ailment/Disorder/Symptom	Homeopathic Remedy
Inferiority, lack of self-confidence, memory difficulties	*Anacardium*
Fears, anxieties, and worries	*Arsenicum album*
Delayed development, shyness	*Baryta carbonica*
Placidity, clumsiness, obesity, flabbiness, lethargy	*Calcarea carbonica*
Rigid thinking, over-empathetic	*Causticum*
Fidgety, impulsivity, thinness	*Iodum*
Domineering, bossiness, controlling	*Lycopodium*
Hyperactivity, self-centeredness	*Medorrhinum*
Pervasive sense of sadness	*Natrum muriaticum*
Creativity, excitability, optimism, easily frightened	*Phosphorus*
Shyness, timidity, insecurity, submissiveness	*Pulsatilla*
Lack of physical stamina	*Silicea*
Suppression of anger leading to rage	*Staphysagria*
Nightmares, night terrors, impulsivity, post-traumatic stress disorder	*Stramonium*
Domineering, selfishness	*Sulphur*
Complications from immunization	*Thuja*
Hyperactivity, impulsivity, difficulties with concentration	*Tuberculinum*
Hyperactivity, restlessness	*Zincum metallicum*
Teething, colic, restlessness, irritability	*Viburcol*
Common ailments in children	*Children's Kit*

Guidelines for Consulting Your Health Care Provider
Putting It All Together

Constitutional Problems in Infants, Children and Adolescents in General

Every child is different. This is true up to a point. We know there are similarities between children as well. It is sometimes possible to categorize children by considering both their differences and similarities into groupings according to their personality traits, temperament, likes and dislikes, abilities, and tendencies. Constitutional homeopathic remedies for infants and children may be determined according to these groupings. The important thing is to appreciate what stands out about your child and try to fit those things to the **keynote** symptoms for the homeopathic remedy.

This chapter will help you to determine your child's *constitutional homeopathic remedy* so that you may treat such common childhood problems as:

aggressive behavior, anxiety, biting or hitting, bossiness, complaining or whining, concentration or focus problems, cruelty to animals, delayed developmental milestones such as slow progress in talking or walking, depression, difficulties adjusting to change or learning new tasks, disorganization, distractibility, clinginess, excitability, fearfulness, hyperactivity, hypersensitivity to insults or criticism, immaturity, impatience, impulsivity, indecisiveness, jealousy, learning difficulties, lying, obstinacy or defiant behavior, obsessive behavior, memory problems, messiness or sloppiness, moodiness, poor self-confidence, poor self-esteem, post-traumatic stress disorder after abuse or violence, restlessness, school failure, perfectionism, school phobia, shyness, sibling rivalry, stealing, substance abuse, temper tantrums, tics, timidity, weepiness, wildness, as well as many other problems.

Determining and using your child's constitutional remedy may help your child in many other ways. It may help with preventing a chronic reoccurring medical condition such as asthma, eczema, or recurrent otitis media. It may help your child cope with new situations in a different, healthier way. And you may expect it to help in ways that might surprise you.

Determining your infant's or child's *constitutional homeopathic remedy* may be possible for you to do, but it is sometimes difficult for an untrained person to find the appropriate *constitutional homeopathic remedy*. Finding the proper *constitutional homeopathic remedy* may require the services of a homeopath. In addition, if you find you have achieved only partial results after administering the *constitutional homeopathic remedy* that you have prescribed, I recommend that you consult with your homeopath.

Once you or your homeopath determines the constitutional remedy for your infant or child, you may start reading about the remedy and the constitutional type either on the internet or by choosing a book from the **Homeopathic Educational Services** catalogue, or from the other sources listed in the **Appendix**.

As with any and all medical conditions, when dealing with constitutional problems of infants and children you must pay strict attention to the **Guidelines for Consulting Your Health Care Provider** at the end of this chapter. You may want to refer to the last section **Putting It All Together** for ideas on how to integrate the essential natural alternatives, homeopathy, herbal remedies, and nutritional supplements.

Anacardium

What is it? This is the plant *Anacardium orientale*, common name *Marking nut tree*, a member of the *Anacardiaceae* botanical family.

When should you use it? The **keynote** symptoms telling you to try using *Anacardium* are when the child manifests difficulties with memory, a marked lack of self-confidence and an exaggerated sense of inferiority. These children tend to show cruelty to animals and to use curse words. *Anacardium* is a remedy that is useful for children who have suffered abuse. Some people who need *Anacardium* describe the strange sensation to feeling a band around the body or any part of the body.

How should you use it? Begin *Anacardium* 200C once or twice weekly, depending on the severity of the situation or condition, and then quickly decrease the repetitions of the remedy once you notice improvement, stopping the remedy as soon as the problem has resolved. If the problem is not improved within 1-3 months, I recommend consultation with your homeopath.

Arsenicum album

What is it? This is the homeopathic remedy made from the chemical compound *arsenic oxide* which is highly poisonous if not given in homeopathic dilution. *Arsenicum album* is often used as a constitutional remedy for adults and for asthma as well as for burns.

When should you use it? The **keynote** symptoms leading you to choose *Arsenicum album* are many fears, anxieties, and worries in a child who is easily frightened, restless, and chilly. The anxieties tend to be about one's own health, often accompanied by a prominent fear of death. Children needing *Arsenicum album* tend to be well-organized, fastidious, neat, and perfectionistic.

How should you use it? Begin *Arsenicum album* 200C once or twice weekly, depending on the severity of the situation or condition, and then quickly decrease the repetitions of the remedy once you notice improvement, stopping the remedy as soon as the problem has resolved. If the problem is not improved within 1-3 months, I recommend consultation with your homeopath.

Baryta carbonica

What is it? This is the poisonous mineral compound *barium carbonate*, which is used in imaging procedures (barium enemas and barium swallows) because it is opaque to x-rays (shows up white) and is very, very slowly absorbed by the body. But the homeopathic remedy is non-toxic.

When should you use it? The **keynote** symptoms telling you when to choose *Baryta carbonica* are when there is slow development of all types, physical, emotional, and mental (or intellectual) with short stature and excessive shyness. This remedy is for infants and children who are developmentally delayed, late in talking and walking. Youngsters needing *Baryta carbonica* tend to be afraid of strangers and are so averse to change in routine or structure that they may react violently.

How should you use it? Begin *Baryta carbonica* 200C once or twice weekly, depending on the severity of the situation or condition, and then quickly decrease the repetitions of the remedy once you notice improvement, stopping the remedy as soon as the problem has resolved. If the problem is not improved within 1-3 months, I recommend consultation with your homeopath.

Calcarea carbonica

What is it? This is the chemical mineral compound *calcium carbonate* which is obtained from oyster shells. *Calcarea carbonica* is a polychrest constitutional remedy and is also an important homeopathic remedy for emotional ailments. The homeopathic action of *Calcarea carbonica* is exerted primarily on bones and teeth, especially for problems due to delayed and imperfect development.

When should you use it? The **keynote** symptoms leading you toward choosing *Calcarea carbonica* are low levels of mental and physical energy in an infant or child who is placid, clumsy, fat, flabby, chilly, and lethargic. The infant needing *Calcarea carbonica* tends to have a large head and sweats easily about the head. These are serious children who tend to learn slowly but they are not mentally retarded. They need to work hard to learn. They may have delayed dentition (teething) and problems with tissues that rely on calcium metabolism such as bone, hair, and nails. This is a good remedy to try in a child who is tending towards obesity.

How should you use it? Begin *Calcarea carbonica* 200C once or twice weekly, depending on the severity of the situation or condition, and then quickly decrease the repetitions of the remedy once you notice improvement, stopping the remedy as soon as the problem has resolved. If the problem is not improved within 1-3 months, I recommend consultation with your homeopath.

Causticum

What is it? The homeopathic remedy is a chemical compound prepared from *calcium hydroxide* (lime) and *potassium bisulphate*.

When should you use it? The **keynote** symptoms leading you towards using *Causticum* are timid children who are rigid in their thinking and who cry when other children are hurt. They may have an exaggerated sense of empathy.

How should you use it? Begin *Causticum* 200C once or twice weekly, depending on the severity of the situation or condition, and then quickly decrease the repetitions of the remedy once you notice improvement, stopping the remedy as soon as the problem has resolved. If the problem is not improved within 1-3 months, I recommend consultation with your homeopath.

Iodum

What is it? This is the chemical element *iodine*. Homeopathic *Iodum* is usually used to treat the symptoms of an overactive thyroid gland.

When should you use it? The **keynote** symptoms pointing you towards trying *Iodum* are impulsive children who are constantly restless and fidgeting. Children who may need *Iodum* tend to be thin although they are always hungry and eat a fair amount, but they do not gain weight. They are warm or even hot when others are not. They tend to be excessively talkative and disorganized.

How should you use it? Begin *Iodum* 200C once or twice weekly, depending on the severity of the situation or condition, and then quickly decrease the repetitions of the remedy once you notice improvement, stopping the remedy as soon as the problem has resolved. If the problem is not improved within 1-3 months, I recommend consultation with your homeopath.

Lycopodium

What is it? This plant is the primitive moss, *Lycopodium clavatum*, common name *Club moss*, a member of the *Lycopodiaceae* botanical family. The spores of the moss are used to produce the homeopathic remedy.

When should you use it? The **keynote** symptoms helping you to choose *Lycopodium* are children who are domineering, bossy, controlling, and tyrannical at home but not outside the home because they fear public humiliation. Children needing *Lycopodium* tend to be indecisive and preoccupied with their looks. This is a good remedy to try when a prepubertal girl has become obsessed with her hair, clothing, and jewelry. This type of child may have dyslexia with mistakes in reading and writing and this may lead to procrastination in doing his or her schoolwork.

How should you use it? Begin *Lycopodium* 200C once or twice weekly, depending on the severity of the situation or condition, and then quickly decrease the repetitions of the remedy once you notice improvement, stopping the remedy as soon as the problem has resolved. If the problem is not improved within 1-3 months, I recommend consultation with your homeopath.

Medorrhinum

What is it? This homeopathic remedy is made from the complex biological material of gonorrheal discharge. The homeopathic remedy is non-toxic.

When should you use it? The **keynote** symptoms leading you to consider *Medorrhinum* are hyperactivity to the point of wildness in children who have been ill from birth, usually with a serious illness. Children who may need *Medorrhinum* tend to be self-centered, selfish, and engage in sibling rivalry. They may grow up to experiment early with smoking, drugs, and sex. They may have temper tantrums as young children, then throwing things and striking out at adults or anyone who reprimands them as a preschooler, then go on to display much fighting in school. The child who needs *Medorrhinum* has a strange need for punishment, egging the parent on with bad behavior and lying until he or she is finally punished, thereby ending a cycle, which then tends to start up again. The *Medorrhinum* child may show poor attention span with deficiencies in concentration.

How should you use it? Begin *Medorrhinum* 200C once or twice weekly, depending on the severity of the situation or condition, and then quickly decrease the repetitions of the remedy once you notice improvement, stopping the remedy as soon as the problem has resolved. If the problem is not improved within 1-3 months, I recommend consultation with your homeopath.

Natrum muriaticum

What is it? This is the polychrest *Natrum muriaticum*, a homeopathic remedy made from common table salt. Its use is mostly as an adult constitutional remedy, but it can be used as a child's constitutional remedy as well.

When should you use it? The **keynote** symptoms indicating *Natrum muriaticum* are profound emotions, often manifesting as a pervasive sense of sadness, in an intelligent, perfectionistic child who prefers to be left alone rather than be comforted by the mother. They also prefer their own company to the company of others. Children who may need *Natrum muriaticum* tend to develop depression after medical illnesses. They may become obsessively concerned with cleanliness. They may have either a special craving or aversion to salt and salty foods.

How should you use it? Begin *Natrum muriaticum* 200C once or twice weekly, depending on the severity of the situation or condition, and then quickly decrease the repetitions of the remedy once you notice improvement, stopping the remedy as soon as the problem has resolved. If the problem is not improved within 1-3 months, I recommend consultation with your homeopath.

Phosphorus

What is it? The chemical element *Phosphorus* is a mineral that is present in every living cell in the form of genetic material (DNA and RNA) as well as many other compounds. It is made into a homeopathic remedy that is an often-prescribed polychrest or adult constitutional remedy.

When should you use it? The **keynote** symptoms pointing to the use of *Phosphorus* are very bright, creative, excitable, impressionable, expressive, optimistic, good-hearted children who are very easily frightened. Children needing *Phosphorus* tend to

grow tall quickly, looking thin and gangly as a result. These children do not like to be left alone. They crave affection and they return affection, something that is rare in the homeopathic *Materia Medica*. Their fears and illnesses tend to be better when they are rubbed, stroked, or massaged. They are hypersensitive to pain. They are afraid of thunderstorms and lightening. Preadolescents tend to have strong opinions which are expounded upon passionately. They may have cravings for chocolate.

How should you use it? Begin *Phosphorus* 200C once or twice weekly, depending on the severity of the situation or condition, and then quickly decrease the repetitions of the remedy once you notice improvement, stopping the remedy as soon as the problem has resolved. If the problem is not improved within 1-3 months, I recommend consultation with your homeopath.

Pulsatilla

What is it? This is the plant *Pulsatilla nigricans*, whose common name is *windflower*, a member of the *Ranunculaceae* botanical family.

When should you use it? The **keynote** symptoms leading you to consider the use of *Pulsatilla* are shy, timid, clingy, insecure, submissive, weepy children (usually but not always girls) who crave affection, sympathy, and consolation, but are not as responsive in returning affection as is a child who needs *Phosphorus*. Their fear of being left alone is what makes them seem affectionate. Children needing *Pulsatilla* are jealous of affection shown to others and they can be selfish and possessive. They are warm or even hot when others are not. These children are followers rather than leaders and they tend to dress (and to be dressed) in a childish manner.

How should you use it? Begin *Pulsatilla* 200C once or twice weekly, depending on the severity of the situation or condition, and then quickly decrease the repetitions of the remedy once you notice improvement, stopping the remedy as soon as the problem has resolved. If the problem is not improved within 1-3 months, I recommend consultation with your homeopath.

Silicea

What is it? The common name for the homeopathic chemical mineral remedy *Silicea* is *silica* or *quartz* or *flint*. *Silicea* (alternative spellings are *Silicia* and *Silica*) is the mineral constituent of quartz rock, which when it breaks down forms sand. *Silicea* is also a component of both soil and the human body.

When should you use it? The **keynote** symptoms pointing you towards the use of *Silicea* are bright children who lack physical stamina. You may think of them as delicate children, usually with pale skin and thin hair. They tend to feel cold and to sweat easily, especially on the hands and feet, and their perspiration may have a sour odor, even in young infants and children. Children who may benefit from *Silicea* show poor self-esteem and a lack of self-confidence. They are cautious children who lack courage and are afraid of failure. They avoid challenges and confrontation by developing headaches. They have difficulties coping with the normal changes that are part of life's ups and downs. *Silicea* is often used to treat deep infections with pus.

How should you use it? Begin *Silicea* 200C once or twice weekly, depending on the severity of the situation or condition, and then quickly decrease the repetitions of the remedy once you notice improvement, stopping the remedy as soon as the problem has resolved. If the problem is not improved within 1-3 months, I recommend consultation with your homeopath.

Staphysagria

What is it? The botanical name of this remedy is *Delphinium staphysagria*, common name *stavesacre* or *larkspur*, a member of the *Ranunculaceae* botanical family. The seeds are extremely poisonous. The homeopathic remedy is non-poisonous and non-toxic.

When should you use it? The **keynote** symptoms leading you to consider using *Staphysagria* are deep rage, often not expressed directly, in children who are hypersensitive to humiliation, insults, and perceived insults. They react to criticism whether justified or not with wounded pride, causing at first a suppression of anger, but then they erupt in great anger. They may throw things or hit and bite other children.

How should you use it? Begin *Staphysagria* 200C once or twice weekly, depending on the severity of the situation or condition, and then quickly decrease the repetitions of the remedy once you notice improvement, stopping the remedy as soon as the problem has resolved. If the problem is not improved within 1-3 months, I recommend consultation with your homeopath.

Stramonium

What is it? This is the plant *Datura stramonium*, common name *Thorn apple* or *Stinkweed*, a member of the *Solanaceae* botanical family. The seeds are poisonous, causing hallucinations when ingested. The seeds of the plant are used to make the homeopathic remedy which is non-toxic.

When should you use it? The **keynote** symptoms leading you to use *Stramonium* are nightmares and night terrors (often causing the child to scream out) in an impulsive child who has many fears (especially of the dark, but also of death and evil). The nightmares and night terrors are likely to begin after the child has had a frightening experience such as abuse of any nature or any traumatic experience, such as occurs with post-traumatic stress disorder. The child may be suddenly interested in praying and do so with exaggerated devotion. There may be facial or body tics, stammering or stuttering, muscle spasms, grimacing, rage, wildness, violent outbursts with throwing things, kicking and biting, hallucinations, delusions, or even convulsions. These symptoms have an aspect of violence attached to them and they tend to be worse when the child is in the dark or is left alone.

How should you use it? Begin *Stramonium* 200C once or twice weekly, depending on the severity of the situation or condition, and then quickly decrease the repetitions of the remedy once you notice improvement, stopping the remedy as soon as the problem has resolved. If the problem is not improved within 1-3 months, I recommend consultation with your homeopath.

Sulphur

What is it? The mineral element *Sulphur*, common name *brimstone*, is present in every cell of the human body. *Sulphur* is a polychrest constitutional remedy for adults. *Sulphur* exerts its main effects on the skin.

When should you use it? The **keynote** symptoms pointing towards the use of *Sulphur* are domineering, controlling leadership in an intellectual child who is curious, expressive and smart. Children who may need *Sulphur* want to be the center of attention and are themselves self-centered and selfish. The *Sulphur* child is bright and creative and may be known as "the little professor." They want to understand how the world works and so they may be drawn to engineering or computers, but typically they lack social skills. *Sulphur* needing children may be sloppy in their personal habits, refusing to bathe, dress in clean clothes, or clean up their rooms. They often look like they slept in their clothes. They may suffer from skin problems that come with red, itchy rashes and the skin around their mouth or anus may be red and burning.

How should you use it? Begin *Sulphur* 200C once or twice weekly, depending on the severity of the situation or condition, and then quickly decrease the repetitions of the remedy once you notice improvement, stopping the remedy as soon as the problem has resolved. If the problem is not improved within 1-3 months, I recommend consultation with your homeopath.

> **Note:** *Sulphur* is often useful to treat eczema and other allergy-based skin rashes. You may be able to alleviate the itching of these ailments by using topical *Castor Oil* (from the *Castor Oil* plant, *Ricinus communis*). You may use topical *Castor Oil* together with homeopathic *Sulphur*.

Thuja

What is it? This is the plant *Thuja occidentalis*, common name *Arbor vitae* or *Tree of Life*, a member of the *Coniferae* botanical family. The new green twigs are used to make the homeopathic remedy.

When should you use it? The **keynote** symptoms leading you to choose *Thuja* are fevers and other complications from immunizations or vaccinations in young children as well as teenagers. You may give *Thuja* before immunizations in order to prevent complications and you may give *Thuja* afterwards to treat whatever complications do develop. Together with *Silicea*, *Thuja* is often prescribed to treat warts.

How should you use it? Administer *Thuja* 30C 3 times on the day before the immunizations. Repeat *Thuja* 30C 3 times on the day the immunization is given. Then stop.

> **Note:** To treat warts, you may want to try *Thuja Ointment*, a topical homeopathic remedy manufactured by Boiron. *Thuja Ointment* is for external use only, but not on the face. First soak the wart in warm water for 5 minutes. Then dry the area. Then apply a thin layer of *Thuja Ointment* to the wart and cover with an adhesive bandage (latex-free is best). Do this twice daily for 12 weeks. It is a good idea to get a diagnosis of "wart" from your health care provider before using this ointment so that you don't misidentify what you're treating.

Tuberculinum

What is it? This homeopathic remedy is made from dead tubercular bacteria. The homeopathic remedy has been used to prevent and treat tuberculosis, as well as many other uses.

When should you use it? The **keynote** symptoms pointing towards the use of *Tuberculinum* are hyperactivity, impulsivity, difficulties with concentration, and anger with complete disregard for parental controls. These children seem to be indifferent to the consequences of bad behavior. They are often obstinate and defiant. In order to satisfy this type of child, the parent needs to offer continual change and new experiences, but nevertheless, they become easily dissatisfied with their current activities. They seem not to know what they want. They love to travel. They may manifest self-destructive behaviors such as head banging in infancy or cutting in teen years. Their anger may turn violent towards others with hitting, kicking, and biting. They may manifest cruelty towards animals. Physically, children needing *Tuberculinum* may seem to have inherited a weakness in their immune systems with recurrent respiratory tract illnesses, or they may have midline physical deformities (such as cleft palate, umbilical hernia, or protruding or sunken breastbone). They may grind their teeth at night.

How should you use it? Begin *Tuberculinum* 200C once or twice weekly, depending on the severity of the situation or condition, and then quickly decrease the repetitions of the remedy once you notice improvement, stopping the remedy as soon as the problem has resolved. If the problem is not improved within 1-3 months, I recommend consultation with your homeopath.

Zincum metallicum

What is it? The homeopathic remedy is made from the metal element, *Zinc*.

When should you use it? The **keynote** symptoms leading you towards using *Zincum metallicum* are difficulties learning and remembering new material, in a restless, fidgety, hyperactive child whose legs are always moving. Children needing *Zincum metallicum* may have delayed development. They may manifest extreme exhaustion and weakness.

How should you use it? Begin *Zincum metallicum* 200C once or twice weekly, depending on the severity of the situation or condition, and then quickly decrease the repetitions of the remedy once you notice improvement, stopping the remedy as soon as the problem has resolved. If the problem is not improved within 1-3 months, I recommend consultation with your homeopath.

Viburcol

What is it? This is a combination homeopathic remedy produced by Heel, a homeopathic pharmaceutical supply house. The ingredients are: *Calcarea carbonica, Pulsatilla, Chamomilla, Plantago major, Dulcamara* and *Belladonna* in low potencies, in an alcohol-free saline solution.

When should you use it? The **keynote** symptoms leading you towards using *Viburcol* are restlessness and irritability especially as a result of teething, colic, or minor infections.

How should you use it? *Viburcol* comes in single-dose vials. Twist off the cap of 1 vial and administer the drops onto or under the tongue or directly into the mouth. This may be repeated 2-6 times daily depending on age of the child and severity of the symptoms.

Children's Kit

What is it? This is a kit of 12 different combination homeopathic remedies, indicated for 12 different common ailments in children, manufactured by Washington Homeopathic Products, Inc. The ailments treated are: children's tonic, colic, constipation, coughs and colds, diarrhea, earache, fever, hives, insomnia, motion sickness, teething, and tonsillitis. Each combination remedy contains pellets of appropriate homeopathic remedies in low potencies.

When should you use it? Using this system, you fit the name of the ailment your child is suffering from to the remedy. It is first-line defense against many of the commonest ailments that occur in children.

How should you use it? Depending on the age of the child, dissolve 3-5 pellets in a teaspoon of water and give to your child to drink. Older children will allow 3-5 pellets to dissolve on the tongue. You may repeat every 1-4 hours, as necessary. *Children's Kit* is designed to travel with you for emergencies.

Guidelines for Consulting Your Health Care Providers

You should consult your health care provider if:
- the patient doesn't look right or act right (trust your instincts!)
- the patient is getting worse or developing new symptoms instead of getting better over time (about 1-3 months)
- there is no change in the patient over time (about 1-3 months)
- the patient is having trouble breathing or complaining of chest pains or there is mental confusion or lethargy or irritability

Please refer to **Guidelines for Consulting Your Health Care Provider**: at the end of **Chapter 3: Homeopathic Remedies for Traumatic Injuries**; **Chapter 4: Homeopathic Remedies Fever**; **Chapter 5: Homeopathic Remedies Upper Respiratory Infections: Colds, Flu, Coughs, Sore Throats, Laryngitis, Ear Infections, Eye Infections, Sinus Infections**; **Chapter 6: Homeopathic Remedies for Allergies and Asthma**; **Chapter 7: Homeopathic Remedies for Infections** and **Chapter 8: Homeopathic Remedies for Emotional Problems** because these are the chapters that especially pertain to the non-constitutional problems that often occur in infants and children.

> **Note:** Do not discontinue taking any pharmaceutical medication that has been prescribed by your health care provider unless you or your family member is under the supervision of a physician.

> **Note:** It is very difficult, even for properly trained homeopaths, to treat youngsters with autism spectrum diseases (ASD), so I don't recommend that you attempt this on your own. It is important that you become familiar with the alternatives available for treatment by reading *A Drug-Free Approach to Asperger Syndrome and Autism* by Judyth Reichenberg-Ullman, Robert Ullman, and Ian Leupker. You may order at 800-398-1151 or www.drug freeasperger.com.

Recommendations for Homeopathic Remedies
Anacardium 200C—pellets and liquid drops
Arsenicum album 200C—pellets and liquid drops
Baryta carbonica 200C—pellets and liquid drops
Calcarea carbonica 200C—pellets and liquid drops
Causticum 200C—pellets and liquid drops
Iodum 200C—pellets and liquid drops
Lycopodium 200C—pellets and liquid drops
Medorrhinum 200C—pellets and liquid drops
Natrum muriaticum 200C—pellets and liquid drops
Phosphorus 200C—pellets and liquid drops
Pulsatilla 200C—pellets and liquid drops

Silicea 200C—pellets and liquid drops
Staphysagria 200C—pellets and liquid drops
Stramonium 200C—pellets and liquid drops
Sulphur 200C—pellets and liquid drops
Thuja 30C—pellets and liquid drops
Tuberculinum 200C—pellets and liquid drops
Zincum metallicum 200C—pellets and liquid drops
Viburcol—combination remedy oral drops
Children's Kit—combination remedies, pellets

Guidelines for Administration of Homeopathic Remedies
The recommended potency of the constitutional homeopathic remedy will likely be 200C. I recommend that you start off once or twice weekly, depending on the severity of the situation or condition, and then quickly decrease the repetitions of the remedy once you notice improvement, stopping the remedy as soon as the problem has resolved and good health restored.

Once you have chosen the homeopathic remedy and the potency that is likely to help you or your family member, you should try to give as few repetitions of the remedy as you can. You start off repeating it more frequently in a severe, acute situation, quickly decreasing the frequency once improvement has begun, stopping the remedy as soon as the problem has resolved.

> **Note:** For more information on *how often* to give the homeopathic remedy please see **Potency and Frequency**, in **Chapter 2: Basic Homeopathy**. For information on *how much* of the homeopathic remedy to give and the importance of a "*clean tongue*," please see **How to take homeopathic remedies** in the same chapter.

Lower potency remedies, such as 30C and below, are used to treat acute ailments. They are usually repeated often, every ½-2 or ½-4 hours. You should notice improvement in symptoms after just one to perhaps a few repetitions. If you do not see improvement, it is wise to stop the remedy and try a different one, guiding yourself by the **keynote** symptoms. You may use different single remedies together or you may try a combination remedy. And you may use homeopathic remedies together with pharmaceutical prescription and non-prescription drugs without any effect of interference.

General guidelines to treat serious, chronic, relapsing ailments include using single remedies at potencies of 200C. These are generally administered once weekly to once monthly, but they may be used once or twice daily at first if the condition warrants it, quickly decreasing the frequency as you see improvement. Do not continue giving the remedy if it becomes apparent that it is not working. You may always stop one remedy and choose to administer another remedy on the basis of the **keynote** symptoms of the new remedy. In addition, you may administer more than one remedy at a time.

Putting It All Together

Coping with difficult constitutional problems in infancy, childhood and adolescence is best done utilizing a multi-pronged approach incorporating all the essential natural alternatives, homeopathy, herbal remedies, and nutritional supplements.

Depending on the chronicity of the problems you may decide to incorporate certain homeopathic remedies in **Chapter 16: Homeopathy for Neurologic Disorders** and **Chapter 8: Homeopathic Remedies for Emotional Problems**.

> **Note:** A homeopathic detoxification remedy is the *Detox-Kit*, manufactured by Heel. It consists of 3 components:

Lymphomyosot, Berberis Homaccord and *Nux vomica Homaccord*, each in a 50 ml bottle. *Lymphomyosot* detoxifies the lymphatic system; *Berberis*, the excretory organs, specifically the kidneys, skin, and liver; and *Nux vomica*, the digestive system and liver. Thus, the *Detox-Kit* provides for the elimination of diverse toxins from most sources. The directions for use are to put 30 drops of each of the three solutions into one quart of water and drink it during the day.

People with problems of a constitutional type require all the vitamins and minerals necessary to repair and replenish tissues (please refer to **Chapter 23: Vitamins and Minerals**) as well as a general antioxidant supplement (please refer to **Chapter 24: Antioxidant Phytochemicals**).

You may want to investigate certain herbal remedies such as *Valerian* and *St. John's Wort* (please refer to **Chapter 20: Herbs You Need to Know**) as well as *omega-3 fatty acids* (please refer to **Chapter 31: Oils and Fats**). In addition, it is a good idea to incorporate *probiotics* (please refer to **Chapter 30: Prebiotics and Probiotic**s) into your daily supplements because your may find emotional problems to be sensitive to enhanced gastrointestinal health.

You may wish to investigate additional nutritional supplements for specific neurologic ailments in **Chapter 29: Nutritional Supplements for Neurologic Disorders**.

Chapter 10

Homeopathic Remedies for Disorders of Menstruation, Fertility, Pregnancy, Labor, Childbirth, Lactation, and Menopause

Women's Reproductive Tract Disorders in General

Menstruation:

Ailment/Disorder/Symptom	Homeopathic Remedy
Menstrual pains accompanied by extreme anger	*Chamomilla*
Heavy menstrual bleeding with exhaustion	*China*
Bearing down pains and feeling worn-down	*Sepia*
Bright red menstrual bleeding	*Phosphorus*
Weepiness, sulkiness, and moodiness at the onset of menstruation	*Pulsatilla*
Cramping pains	*Magnesia phosphorica*
Premenstrual syndrome symptoms	*Lachesis*
Swollen, tender breasts before menstruation	*Lac caninum*
Severe abdominal cramping pains on the first day of menstruation	*Colocynthis*
Menstrual cramping associated with back pains	*Cimicifuga racemosa*
General PMS symptoms (pains, bloating, irritability)	*Cyclease PMS*
Menstrual cramps	*Cyclease CRAMP*
Bloating, headaches, tender or swollen breasts, irritability, and mood swings	*PMS Relief*

Infertility:

Ailment/Disorder/Symptom	Homeopathic Remedy
Absence of menstrual cycles after severe emotional shock	*Ignatia*
Infertility from scarring of the Fallopian tubes	*Medorrhinum*
Overwhelming grief and sadness from not conceiving	*Natrum muriaticum*
Indifference to childbearing	*Sepia*

Pregnancy:

Ailment/Disorder/Symptom	Homeopathic Remedy
Constant nausea and vomiting during early pregnancy	*Ipecac*
Nausea and vomiting during pregnancy	*Tabacum*
Nausea and vomiting during pregnancy with exhaustion	*Cocculus indicus*
Nausea with frequent spasms of vomiting	*Nux vomica*
Pressure and pain in the uterus or groin	*Bellis perennis*

Nausea of pregnancy	*Pulsatilla*
Nausea at the sight and smell of food	*Sepia*
Great anxiety about health during pregnancy	*Arsenicum album*
Pregnancy with lower back pains	*Kali carbonicum*

Labor:

Ailment/Disorder/Symptom	Homeopathic Remedy
Physical trauma of labor	*Arnica montana*
Emotional trauma of labor	*Aconitum napellus*
Labor not progressing	*Caulophyllum*
Labor with great crying and screaming	*Coffea*
Labor with ineffective contractions	*Nux vomica*
Prolonged labor with weepiness	*Pulsatilla*
Labor facilitation	*Birth Ease*

Childbirth:

Ailment/Disorder/Symptom	Homeopathic Remedy
Physical trauma of labor	*Arnica montana*
Emotional trauma of labor	*Aconitum napellus*

Lactation:

Ailment/Disorder/Symptom	Homeopathic Remedy
Sudden, violent, throbbing breast inflammation	*Belladonna*
Painful, cracked nipples	*Chamomilla*
Hard nodules of the breast	*Conium*
Breast inflammations and infections (mastitis)	*Phytolacca*

Menopause:

Ailment/Disorder/Symptom	Homeopathic Remedy
Perimenopausal and menopausal symptoms	*Lachesis*
Loss of libido with dry vagina	*Sepia*
Weight gain in menopausal women	*Calcarea carbonica*

Guidelines for Consulting Your Health Care Provider
Putting It All Together

Women's Reproductive Tract Disorders in General

This chapter will help you to choose homeopathic remedies for some of the ailments that women suffer, such as menstrual disorders, infertility, problems during pregnancy, labor, childbirth, and lactation, and ailments that occur during the menopause. Infertility is a condition that can be helped with homeopathy and choosing an appropriate homeopathic remedy from this chapter may help you to conceive. However, it is more likely that solving infertility problems will require that you seek help first from a reproductive endocrinologist to obtain a specific diagnosis and treatment and then secondly from your homeopath. Homeopathic remedies may be given together with prescription medications. If you are trying to conceive it is important that you are already taking prenatal vitamins and 400-800 mcg of folic acid.

This chapter may be helpful to you if you are pregnant and have decided to give birth at a birthing center where homeopathic remedies are commonly used as first-line therapy for easing labor and delivery. It is a good idea to become familiar with the remedies that are likely to be used during labor and delivery.

Sometimes serious menstrual disorders, such as absent or infrequent menses (after the monthly menstrual cycle has been established for more than two years) may indicate an underlying disease that needs attention from a specialist in reproductive endocrinology. You will find that in those cases homeopathy may be combined with prescription medicines for good health effects.

Sometimes other serious diseases may co-exist with reproductive tract disorders, such as eating disorders (anorexia nervosa, bulimia nervosa, binge eating disorder), polycystic ovary syndrome with or without obesity, diabetes mellitus type 2, hypertension, cardiovascular disease, low or high functioning of the thyroid gland, and many other medical disorders. If any of these conditions are present, I strongly recommend that you seek the services of your health care provider and that you read the **Guidelines for Consulting Your Health Care Provider** at the end of this chapter.

Reproductive tract health lends itself to using all three essential natural alternative health care practices, namely, homeopathy, herbal remedies, and nutritional supplements. I recommend that you first master using homeopathy to treat or prevent the ailments that concern you. Homeopathy is the safest of the three alternative health care practices because it has no significant side effects or interactions with prescription medications. Then you should investigate the nutritional supplements specifically for women's health that are used to augment the action of the homeopathic remedies you have chosen. Then I urge you to learn about the use of the appropriate herbal remedies for the women's health issue that concerns you.

You may prefer to use a *combination homeopathic remedy* to treat any of the conditions discussed in this chapter. *Combination remedies* are certainly easier to use than single remedies and are very often effective. Combination remedies will likely include many of the single remedies listed below, but in very low potencies. Using combination remedies is like taking a stab in the dark.

However, many people find that combination remedies do not work well enough so it is important to be able to use single remedies according to their **keynote** symptoms. You may always give a remedy, gauge the reaction, and if necessary, give a different remedy. You may use more than one single remedy at one time. You should have on hand those remedies for treating those **keynote** symptoms that tend to recur in you or members of your family.

As with any and all medical conditions, when dealing with disorders of menstruation, fertility, pregnancy, labor, childbirth, lactation, and menopause you must pay strict attention to the **Guidelines for Consulting Your Health Care Provider** at the end of this chapter. You may want to refer to the last section **Putting It All Together** for ideas on how to integrate the essential natural alternatives, homeopathy, herbal remedies, and nutritional supplements.

Menstruation

Chamomilla

What is it? The homeopathic remedy is made from the plant *Matricaria chamomilla*, common name *Chamomile*, a member of the *Compositae* botanical family. It is a prominent homeopathic remedy for fever and for children with teething problems and colic.

When should you use it? The **keynote** symptoms pointing towards the use of *Chamomilla* are menstrual cramps with extreme pain accompanied by intense anger and irritability. Women needing *Chamomilla* at the time of menstruation may be demanding, quarrelsome, contrary, and temperamental. She may ask for something and then change her mind when she gets it.

How should you use it? Give *Chamomilla* 30C every ½-2 hours, depending on the severity of symptoms, rapidly decreasing the frequency as soon as improvement sets in, then stopping when the symptoms have resolved.

China

What is it? This is the plant *China officinalis*, also called *Cinchona succirubra*, common name *Peruvian bark*, a member of the *Rubiaceae* botanical family.

When should you use it? The **keynote** symptoms leading towards trying *China* are very heavy menstrual bleeding leading to great exhaustion, debilitation, and apathy, with occasional angry outbursts. The menstrual blood may be discharged in dark clots. *China* is often used for extreme loss of body fluids of any nature, such as hemorrhaging, vomiting, or diarrhea.

How should you use it? Give *China* 30C every ½-2 hours, depending on the severity of symptoms, rapidly decreasing the frequency as soon as improvement sets in, then stopping when the symptoms have resolved.

Sepia

What is it? The homeopathic remedy *Sepia* is made from the black ink sac of *Sepia officinalis*, the *cuttlefish*, a species of mollusk.

When should you use it? The **keynote** symptoms pointing towards the use of *Sepia* are feelings of apathy and sadness at the time of the monthly menstruation, accompanied by the feeling that the uterus or another internal organ is falling out of the vagina. *Sepia* is often administered to a woman who has been worn down by taking care of her children and husband while tending to the household chores. A woman needing *Sepia* may complain of backache that is made worse by standing just before the menses begins. There may be long-standing problems with the menstrual cycle, either too frequent or too infrequent, even including absent menses (amenorrhea). *Sepia* is a good remedy to think of when the menstrual cycle has not become normalized after taking birth control pills or after a miscarriage.

How should you use it? Give *Sepia* 30C every 2-4 hours for the apathy and sadness at the time of the menstrual cycle, depending on the severity of symptoms, rapidly decreasing the frequency as soon as improvement sets in, and then stopping when the symptoms have resolved. Give *Sepia* 200C once weekly for normalization of the menstrual cycle, stopping when the cycle has become normal.

Phosphorus

What is it? This is the homeopathic remedy that is made from the non-metallic chemical element *Phosphorus*. It is one of the commonest elements in the human body because it makes up part of ATP (adenosine triphosphate), the chemical that stores our energy. *Phosphorus* is a polychrest constitutional remedy.

When should you use it? The **keynote** symptom for homeopathic *Phosphorus* is profusely bright red vaginal bleeding at the time of menstruation. Homeopathic *Phosphorus* is used to treat bright red bleeding from any site in the body and for this reason it is sometimes called the "homeopathic bandaid." The symptoms of a woman who will benefit from *Phosphorus* at the time of menstruation will likely feel better when parts of her body are stroked, rubbed, or massaged. She will likely be an optimistic, vibrant, extroverted woman. She will have a hypersensitivity to pain and menstrual cramps will be experienced as very painful. She may display some clairvoyant tendencies and have an insight into her nature that is surprising for her age.

How should you use it? Give *Phosphorus* 30C every 2-4 hours, depending on the severity of symptoms, rapidly decreasing the frequency as soon as improvement sets in, then stopping when the symptoms have resolved.

Pulsatilla

What is it? This is the plant *Pulsatilla nigricans*, whose common name is *windflower*, a member of the *Ranunculaceae* botanical family.

When should you use it? The **keynote** symptoms indicating the use of *Pulsatilla* are weepiness, sulkiness, and moodiness at the onset of menstruation along with a strong need for sympathetic company. Her moods can be very changeable. The girl or woman needing *Pulsatilla* will feel better in open air. She will complain of being warm or hot when other people are comfortable. She will likely have a sweet-natured disposition and be non-confrontational in her relationships with family members. She may have a vaginal infection with yellowish-greenish discharge.

How should you use it? Give *Pulsatilla* 30C every 2-4 hours, depending on the severity of symptoms, rapidly decreasing the frequency as soon as improvement sets in, then stopping when the symptoms have resolved.

Magnesia phosphorica

What is it? This is *magnesium phosphate*, a tissue salt present in body cells.

When should you use it? The **keynote** symptoms indicating the use of *Magnesia phosphorica*, abbreviated *Mag phos*, are cramping pains that are colicky or spasmodic in nature (meaning increasing in intensity and then decreasing, in cycles). The pains may cause her to double over. She may find some relief with hot compresses on the lower abdomen or pelvic region, or bathing in hot water. The cramping pains are better once the menstrual flow begins.

How should you use it? Give *Mag phos* 30C every ½-2 hours, depending on the severity of symptoms, rapidly decreasing the frequency as soon as improvement sets in, then stopping when the symptoms have resolved.

Lachesis

What is it? This is *Trigonocephalus lachesis*, common name *Surukuku snake* or the *Bushmaster snake*. The homeopathic remedy is made from the venom of the snake. The remedy is non-toxic.

When should you use it? The **keynote** symptoms pointing you towards using *Lachesis* are PMS (premenstrual syndrome) symptoms such as insomnia, ovarian pain, and sore breasts, which stop when the menstrual flow begins. The person needing *Lachesis* may be talkative, often expressing jealousy and anger.

How should you use it? Give *Lachesis* 30C every 2-4 hours, depending on the severity of symptoms, rapidly decreasing the frequency as soon as improvement sets in, then stopping when the symptoms have resolved.

Lac caninum

What is it? This homeopathic remedy is made from the milk of a female dog, commonly called *Bitch's milk*.

When should you use it? The **keynote** symptoms indicating the use of *Lac caninum* are swollen, tender breasts before menstruation. The symptoms tend to switch back and forth from one breast to the other.

How should you use it? Give *Lac caninum* 30C every 2-4 hours, depending on the severity of symptoms, rapidly decreasing the frequency as soon as improvement sets in, and then stopping when the symptoms have resolved.

Colocynthis

What is it? This is the plant *Citrullus colocynthis*, common name *Bitter apple*, a member of the *Cucurbitaceae* botanical family.

When should you use it? The **keynote** symptoms pointing you towards trying *Colocynthis* are severe abdominal cramping pains on the first day of menstruation that are relieved somewhat when lying down in the knee-chest position and applying hard pressure and on the lower abdomen. The pains may be so intense that they cause her to vomit. The pains are better after a bowel movement. She may express great anger but it may be suppressed.

How should you use it? Give *Colocynthis* 30C every ½-2 hours, depending on the severity of symptoms, rapidly decreasing the frequency as soon as improvement sets in, then stopping when the symptoms have resolved. For women who tend to have dysmenorrhea (severe menstrual pains) recurring every month, I recommend using *Colocynthis* 30C together with *Mag phos* 30C every ½-2 hours on the first day of menstruation. Sometimes only one or two doses are needed.

Cimicifuga racemosa

What is it? This is the plant *Cimicifuga racemosa*, common name *Black cohosh*, a member of the *Ranunculaceae* botanical family. The black root is used to make the homeopathic remedy. It is abbreviated as *Cimic*. *Black cohosh* is a commonly used herbal remedy for menopausal symptoms.

When should you use it? The **keynote** symptoms to help you choose *Cimic* are menstrual cramping associated with back pains, depression with prominent sighing, anxiety, and headaches. She may express the fear that she is going crazy.

How should you use it? Give *Cimic* 30C every ½-2 hours, depending on the severity of symptoms, rapidly decreasing the frequency as soon as improvement sets in, then stopping when the symptoms have resolved.

Cyclease PMS

What is it? This is a combination homeopathic remedy made by Boiron, a homeopathic pharmaceutical supply house. The ingredients are: *Folliculinum* 15C, *Natrum muriaticum* 12C and *Sepia* 12C.

When should you use it? The **keynote** symptoms for which you should consider using this combination remedy are general PMS symptoms such as pain, bloating, and irritability.

How should you use it? The directions are to dissolve 2 tablets in the mouth twice daily. However, this combination remedy could be taken more frequently depending on the severity of the PMS symptoms.

Cyclease CRAMP

What is it? This is a combination homeopathic remedy made by Boiron, a homeopathic pharmaceutical supply house. The ingredients are: *Cimicifuga racemosa*, *Colocynthis* and *Magnesia phosphorica*, all in 6C potency.

When should you use it? The **keynote** symptoms for which you should consider using this combination remedy are menstrual cramps, often associated with muscle aches and pains.

How should you use it? The directions are to dissolve 2 tablets in the mouth every 15 minutes for 3 doses. It may be repeated when necessary depending on the severity of the menstrual cramp symptoms.

PMS Relief

What is it? This is a combination remedy manufactured by King Bio (in their *SafeCareRx* line of products). The ingredients are: *Apis mellifica*, *Chamomilla*, *Cimicifuga racemosa*, *Cyclamen europaeum*, *Helonias dioica*, *Ignatia amara*, *Lac caninum*, *Lycopodium clavatum*, *Natrum muriaticum*, *Nux vomica*, *Platinum metallicum* and *Sepia*, in a pure water base. Each ingredient comes in a broad spectrum of low to high potencies.

When should you use it? The **keynote** symptoms for which you should consider using this combina-

tion remedy are bloating, headaches, tender or swollen breasts, irritability, and mood swings associated with the premenstrual part of your cycle.
How should you use it? Spray 2-3 times onto or under the tongue 1-4 times a day, depending on the severity of the PMS symptoms.

Infertility

Ignatia

What is it? This is the plant *Ignatia amara*, common name *St. Ignatius's bean*, a member of the *Loganiaceae* botanical family.
When should you use it? The **keynote** symptoms indicating the use of *Ignatia* are absence of menstrual cycles (amenorrhea) occurring after a severe emotional shock such as grief, bereavement, or after disappointed love, especially after falling in love with an inappropriate partner. She will display audible sighing. The inability to conceive will cause her great anguish.
How should you use it? Administer *Ignatia* 200C once weekly until conception occurs, then discontinue. It is probably beneficial if the male counterpart of the couple trying to conceive also take his own constitutional remedy at the same time.

Medorrhinum

What is it? This homeopathic remedy is made from the complex biological material of gonorrheal discharge. *Medorrhinum* is a constitutional remedy for infants and children
When should you use it? The **keynote** symptoms leading you to consider *Medorrhinum* are infertility as a result of scarring of the Fallopian tubes from episodes of pelvic inflammatory disease (PID), often but not necessarily due to infections with gonorrhea.
How should you use it? Administer *Medorrhinum* 200C once weekly until conception occurs, then discontinue. It is probably beneficial if the male counterpart of the couple trying to conceive also take his own constitutional remedy at the same time.

Natrum muriaticum

What is it? This is the polychrest *Natrum muriaticum*, a homeopathic remedy made from common table salt. *Natrum muriaticum* is a polychrest constitutional remedy.
When should you use it? The **keynote** symptoms pointing towards the use of *Natrum muriaticum* are overwhelming grief and sadness from not conceiving in a couple without physiologic or anatomic reasons why they have not.
How should you use it? Administer *Natrum muriaticum* 200C once weekly until conception occurs, then discontinue. It is probably beneficial if the male counterpart of the couple trying to conceive also take his own constitutional remedy at the same time.

Sepia

What is it? The homeopathic remedy *Sepia* is made from the black ink sac of *Sepia officinalis*, the *cuttlefish*, a species of mollusk found in the Mediterranean Sea and the Atlantic Ocean.
When should you use it? The **keynote** characteristics guiding you towards using *Sepia* are infertility when childbearing seems to be required out of a sense of duty or responsibility, rather than a yearning to mother a child.
How should you use it? Administer *Sepia* 200C once weekly until conception occurs, then discontinue. It is probably beneficial if the male counterpart of the couple trying to conceive also take his own constitutional remedy at the same time.

Pregnancy

Ipecac

What is it? The homeopathic remedy *Ipecac* is made from the root of the plant *Cephaelis ipecacuanha*, a member of the *Rubiaceae* botanical family.
When should you use it? The **keynote** symptoms helping you to choose *Ipecac* are almost constant nausea and vomiting during early pregnancy

(morning sickness) which are not relieved by vomiting in a women who feels worse when bending over. **How should you use it?** Give *Ipecac* 30C every ½-2 hours, depending on the severity of symptoms, rapidly decreasing the frequency as soon as improvement sets in, then stopping when the symptoms have resolved.

Tabacum

What is it? This is the plant *Nicotiana tabacum*, common name *Tobacco*, a member of the *Solanaceae* botanical family. *Tobacco* when smoked or ingested can cause nausea and vomiting. Therefore, according to the **Law of Similars** when *Tabacum* is prepared as a homeopathic remedy, it can cure those same symptoms.
When should you use it? The **keynote** symptoms leading you to try *Tabacum* are nausea and vomiting while the face is pale and sweaty. The woman feels worse with motion or movement, which is why *Tabacum* is useful for motion sickness as well as for morning sickness.
How should you use it? Give *Tabacum* 30C every ½-2 hours, depending on the severity of symptoms, rapidly decreasing the frequency as soon as improvement sets in, then stopping when the symptoms have resolved.

Cocculus indicus

What is it? This is the plant *Cocculus indicus*, common name *Levant nut*, or *Fish berry*, a member of the *Menispermaceae* botanical family.
When should you use it? The **keynote** symptoms are nausea and vomiting in a woman who feels physically and mentally exhausted, fitting the morning sickness that occurs in the first trimester of pregnancy. *Cocculus* is often used to treat motion sickness because the nausea and vomiting tend to occur while in motion, such as riding in a car, or even while thinking about being in motion.
How should you use it? Give *Cocculus* 30C every ½-2 hours, depending on the severity of symptoms, rapidly decreasing the frequency as soon as improvement sets in, then stopping when the symptoms have resolved.

Nux vomica

What is it? This is a poisonous plant, *Nux vomica*, containing strychnine, common name *Poison nut*, a member of the *Loganiaceae* botanical family. The homeopathic remedy is non-toxic.
When should you use it? The **keynote** symptoms pointing you towards choosing *Nux vomica* are nausea leading to frequent spasms of vomiting, often bringing up close to nothing except some mucus. This often occurs in an irritable, impatient, critical, constipated woman who would ordinarily prefer to drink alcohol, but does not due to her pregnancy.
How should you use it? Give *Nux vomica* 30C every ½-2 hours, depending on the severity of symptoms, rapidly decreasing the frequency as soon as improvement sets in, then stopping when the symptoms have resolved.

Bellis perennis

What is it? This is the plant *Bellis perennis*, common name *Daisy*, a member of the *Compositae* botanical family.
When should you use it? The **keynote** symptoms pointing you towards using *Bellis perennis* are pressure and pain in the uterus or groin as a result of the baby dropping before delivery along with a desire to lie down for relief. *Bellis perennis* is mostly used after childbirth to alleviate the bruising of soft tissues and internal organs.
How should you use it? Give *Bellis perennis* 30C every ½-2 hours, depending on the severity of symptoms, rapidly decreasing the frequency as soon as improvement sets in, then stopping when the symptoms have resolved.

Pulsatilla

What is it? This is the plant *Pulsatilla nigricans*, whose common name is *windflower*, a member of the *Ranunculaceae* botanical family.
When should you use it? The **keynote** symptoms indicating the use of *Pulsatilla* are nausea of pregnancy, worse in the early evening, in a woman who

has a sweet-natured disposition and lacks thirst. She may complain of heartburn.

How should you use it? Give *Pulsatilla* 30C every ½-2 hours, depending on the severity of symptoms, rapidly decreasing the frequency as soon as improvement sets in, then stopping when the symptoms have resolved.

Sepia

What is it? The homeopathic remedy *Sepia* is made from the black ink sac of *Sepia officinalis*, the *cuttlefish*, a species of mollusk.

When should you use it? The **keynote** symptoms leading you to use *Sepia* are nausea at the sight and smell of food, often accompanied by bearing down pains or the feeling that the uterus or another internal organ is falling out of the vagina. The woman needing *Sepia* will likely be gloomy and irritable.

How should you use it? Give *Sepia* 30C every ½-2 hours, depending on the severity of symptoms, rapidly decreasing the frequency as soon as improvement sets in, then stopping when the symptoms have resolved.

Arsenicum album

What is it? This is the homeopathic remedy made from the chemical compound *arsenic oxide* which is highly poisonous if not given in homeopathic dilution. *Arsenicum album* is often used as a constitutional remedy for adults and children as well as for asthma.

When should you use it? The **keynote** symptoms encouraging you to use *Arsenicum album* are great anxiety about her health. At her prenatal visits to her doctor she will emphatically announce that something is wrong. All her pregnancy-related symptoms will be worse around midnight.

How should you use it? Give *Arsenicum album* 30C every ½-2 hours, depending on the severity of symptoms, rapidly decreasing the frequency as soon as improvement sets in, and then stopping when the symptoms have resolved.

Kali carbonicum

What is it? This is the chemical compound *potassium carbonate* found in all plants.

When should you use it? The **keynote** symptoms helping you to decide to use *Kali carbonicum* are lower back pains (with either menstruation or pregnancy) which worsen around 2 a.m. *Kali carbonicum* suits a woman who has a high sense of duty but is closed off emotionally, finding it difficult to get close to anybody, even family members and her husband.

How should you use it? Give *Kali carbonicum* 30C every ½-2 hours, depending on the severity of symptoms, rapidly decreasing the frequency as soon as improvement sets in, and then stopping when the symptoms have resolved.

Labor

Arnica montana

What is it? This the plant *Arnica montana*, common name *Leopard's bane*, a member of the *Compositae* botanical family.

When should you use it? *Arnica* should be taken as soon after labor has begun as is possible in order to help with the healing process on both physical and emotional levels. *Arnica* is homeopathy's painkiller much as acetaminophen or ibuprofen is in Western medicine. The **keynote** symptom leading you to use *Arnica* is that the person in labor denies that anything is wrong, saying, "Leave me alone, I'm okay." However, it is perfectly clear to those around her that her body is undergoing trauma. However, I strongly urge you to consider using *Arnica* for all women in labor, even without the characteristic **keynote** symptom.

How should you use it? Give *Arnica* 30C every ½-2 hours as soon as labor has begun, depending on the severity of the labor pains, rapidly decreasing the frequency as soon as delivery has been accomplished. Then continue with *Arnica* 30C once or twice daily until postpartum aches and pains are improved, and then stop.

Aconitum napellus

What is it? This homeopathic remedy, called in shorthand *Aconite*, is made from the plant commonly called *monkshood* or *wolfsbane*, a member of the *Ranunculaceae* botanical family.

When should you use it? *Aconite* is the homeopathic substitute for *valium*, because of its calming effect on anxiety. The **keynote** symptoms leading you to use *Aconite* are fear and restless agitation with a sudden onset. *Aconite* is useful for treating the emotional shock or fright during or after labor and delivery. It is often used along with *Arnica* to control the pain and shock from labor and delivery and to speed the healing process. *Aconite* is specifically useful to treat the commonly expressed fear of death during labor. Fear, anxiety, pains and restlessness are worse after midnight.

How should you use it? Give *Aconite* 30C every ½-2 hours as soon as labor has begun, depending on the severity of the fears, anxieties, and restlessness, rapidly decreasing the frequency as soon as these are improved. Then continue with *Aconite* 30C once or twice daily for a few days postpartum, and then stop. You may give both *Arnica* and *Aconite* together during labor and delivery for best results.

Caulophyllum

What is it? This is the plant *Caulophyllum thalictroides*, common name *Blue Cohosh*, a member of the *Berberidaceae* botanical family.

When should you use it? The **keynote** symptoms indicating the use of *Caulophyllum* are whenever one needs to accelerate labor, or for a labor that is not progressing properly from any reason.

How should you use it? Give *Caulophyllum* 30C every ½-2 hours to accelerate the labor, rapidly decreasing the frequency when the labor is going well and stopping when delivery has occurred.

Coffea

What is it? This is the plant *Coffea arabica*, common name *coffee*, a member of the *Rubiaceae* botanical family.

When should you use it? The **keynote** symptoms indicating the usefulness of *Coffea* are when labor contractions are accompanied by much crying and screaming with great anxiety in between contractions in a woman whose labor pains are intolerable.

How should you use it? Give *Coffea* 30C every ½-2 hours for the crying and screaming, rapidly decreasing the frequency when the pain is under control, and stopping when delivery has occurred.

Nux vomica

What is it? This is a poisonous plant, *Nux vomica*, containing strychnine, common name *Poison nut*, a member of the *Loganiaceae* botanical family. This homeopathic remedy is non-toxic.

When should you use it? The **keynote** symptoms helping you to choose *Nux vomica* are ineffective contractions in a woman who is hypercritical, angry, and has the urge to urinate or defecate, often with no result.

How should you use it? Give *Nux vomica* 30C every ½-2 hours, depending on the severity of symptoms, rapidly decreasing the frequency as soon as improvement sets in, then stopping when the symptoms have resolved.

Pulsatilla

What is it? This is the plant *Pulsatilla nigricans*, whose common name is *windflower*, a member of the *Ranunculaceae* botanical family.

When should you use it? The **keynote** symptoms leading you to try *Pulsatilla* are prolonged labor in a woman who is weepy and submissive, and who craves company and sympathy.

How should you use it? Give *Pulsatilla* 30C every ½-2 hours, depending on the severity of symptoms, rapidly decreasing the frequency as soon as improvement sets in, then stopping when the symptoms have resolved.

Birth Ease

What is it? This is a combination remedy manufactured by King Bio. The ingredients are: *Aletris farmi-*

nosa, Arnica montana, Apis mellifica, Belladonna, Caulophyllum thalictroides, Chamomilla, Cimicifuga racemosa, Ferrum metallicum, Kali carbonicum, Sabin juniperus, Secale cornutum and *Viburnum opulus*, each in low potency.

When should you use it? The **keynote** symptoms leading you to try *Birth Ease* are an increase in the normal Braxton-Hicks uterine contractions that occur in the last 1-2 months of pregnancy. *Birth Ease* prepares the uterus to contract effectively so that the length of labor will be shortened. Complications of labor are said to be lessened.

How should you use it? Pump 3 sprays of *Birth Ease* onto or under the tongue 3 times daily beginning 1-2 months before expected time of delivery.

Childbirth

Arnica montana and *Aconitum napellus* are the main homeopathic remedies to use during childbirth. Please refer to the sections under **Labor** for when and how to use them. For best results use *Aconite* and *Arnica* together.

Lactation

Belladonna

What is it? This is the homeopathic remedy made from the plant, *Atropa belladonna*, common name *deadly nightshade*, a member of the *Solanaceae* botanical family.

When should you use it? The **keynote** symptoms pointing you towards using *Belladonna* are for a sudden, violent, throbbing breast inflammation with red streaks or red flushing on the skin of a sore breast. There may be a high fever.

How should you use it? Give *Belladonna* 30C every ½-2 hours, depending on the severity of the breast inflammation symptoms, rapidly decreasing the frequency as soon as improvement sets in, then stopping when the symptoms have resolved.

Chamomilla

What is it? The homeopathic remedy is made from the plant *Matricaria chamomilla*, common name *Chamomile*, a member of the *Compositae* botanical family.

When should you use it? The **keynote** symptoms pointing you in the direction of *Chamomilla* are very painful, cracked nipples in a woman who may have low to moderate grade fever (less than 102°F [39°C]) and who may be angry and irritable so that nothing seems to please her.

How should you use it? Give *Chamomilla* 30C every ½-2 hours, depending on the severity of the breast inflammation symptoms, rapidly decreasing the frequency as soon as improvement sets in, then stopping when the symptoms have resolved.

Conium

What is it? This is the plant *Conium maculatum*, common name *Hemlock*, a member of the *Umbelliferae* botanical family. Drinking the poisonous juice of this plant was the method that the Ancient Greeks used to put Socrates to death. The homeopathic remedy is non-toxic.

When should you use it? The **keynote** symptoms indicating the use of *Conium* are hard nodules of the breast in a breastfeeding woman who may be depressed. *Conium* is a remedy that is also used to treat tumors of the breast.

How should you use it? Give *Conium* 30C every ½-2 hours, depending on the severity of the breast nodule symptoms, rapidly decreasing the frequency as soon as improvement sets in, then stopping when the symptoms have resolved.

Phytolacca

What is it? This is the plant *Phytolacca decandra*, common name *Pokeroot*, a member of the *Phytolaccaceae* family.

When should you use it? The homeopathic remedy *Phytolacca* has a special affinity for breast inflammations, including infections (mastitis), benign nodules, and malignant cancers. The **keynote** symptoms pointing to the use of *Phytolacca* are a breast that has a purplish caste and is swollen and hard. The pains in the breast may feel like electric shocks. The nipples may be fissured and very painful when the infant suckles.

How should you use it? Give *Phytolacca* 30C every ½-2 hours until the infection has improved. Then use *Phytolacca* 200C once daily until the infection has gone.

> **Note:** *Weleda Nursing Tea* contains several herbal remedies which help to promote lactation as well as exert a calming effect on both mother and baby.

Menopause

Lachesis

What is it? This is *Trigonocephalus lachesis,* common name *Surukuku snake* or the *Bushmaster snake.* The homeopathic remedy is made from the venom of the snake.

When should you use it? The **keynote** symptoms helping you to choose *Lachesis* are the major symptoms associated with the perimenopausal and menopausal times of the lifecycle: profuse menstrual bleeding, hot flashes, night sweats, insomnia, weight gain, and pounding headaches (especially left-sided). Symptoms tend to occur in a loquacious, suspicious, jealous, excitable, passionate woman who may be afraid of snakes. Her emotional life tends to be intense. All of her symptoms tend to be worse with heat. She tends not to wear anything around her neck. *Lachesis* is the most commonly prescribed homeopathic remedy to alleviate menopausal symptoms.

How should you use it? Give *Lachesis* 200C once weekly until the menopausal symptoms have improved, reducing the frequency to once monthly, stopping when the symptoms have disappeared.

Sepia

What is it? The homeopathic remedy *Sepia* is made form the black ink sac of *Sepia officinalis,* the *cuttlefish,* a species of mollusk.

When should you use it? The **keynote** symptoms pointing towards the use of *Sepia* are dry vaginal lining with loss of libido, accompanied by the feeling that the uterus or another internal organ is falling out of the vagina. There may be an associated dread of sexual intercourse.

How should you use it? Give *Sepia* 200C once weekly until the menopausal symptoms have improved, reducing the frequency to once monthly, stopping when the symptoms have disappeared.

Calcarea carbonica

What is it? This is the chemical mineral compound *calcium carbonate* that is obtained from oyster shells.

When should you use it? The **keynote** symptoms leading you to choose *Calcarea carbonica* are when the most aggravating menopausal symptoms are weight gain and bloating in a chilly woman who fatigues easily. She may express that she is afraid of going insane, or that something bad is going to happen.

How should you use it? Give *Calcarea carbonica* 200C once weekly until the menopausal symptoms have improved, reducing the frequency to once monthly, stopping when the symptoms have disappeared.

Guidelines for Consulting Your Health Care Provider

You should consult your health care provider if:
• the patient doesn't look right or act right (trust your instincts!)
• the patient is getting worse instead of better over the course of the illness
• the patient is having trouble breathing or complaining of chest pains or there is mental confusion or lethargy or irritability

- there are serious menstrual abnormalities such as absent or infrequent menses (after the monthly menstrual cycle has been established for more than two years)
- other serious diseases co-exist with reproductive tract disorders, such as eating disorders (anorexia nervosa, bulimia nervosa, binge eating disorder), polycystic ovary syndrome with or without obesity, diabetes mellitus type 2, hypertension, cardiovascular disease, low or high functioning of the thyroid gland, and many other medical disorders
- you are pregnant and you wish to deliver at a birthing center rather than at a hospital. This requires that you have regular checkups throughout your pregnancy with the health care team at the birthing center
- if you have vaginal bleeding after your monthly menstrual cycles have ceased and you have entered the menopause; this may be a sign of uterine cancer and requires prompt attention

Remember: As soon as a woman becomes sexually active, it is important to visit her gynecologist health care provider in order to get regular checkups including Pap smears (to check for early cervical cancer), internal vaginal examinations (to detect early ovarian cancer), and breast examinations (to rule out possibly cancerous lumps that her mammogram may have missed).

Note: Do not discontinue taking any pharmaceutical medication that has been prescribed by your health care provider unless you or your family member is under the supervision of a physician.

Note: If you want to learn more about your body from a respected source, please read *The New Harvard Guide to Women's Health* by Carlson, Eisenstat, and Ziporyn.

Recommendations for Homeopathic Remedies

Menstruation
Chamomilla 30C—pellets
China 30C—pellets
Sepia 30C and 200C—pellets
Phosphorus 30C—pellets
Pulsatilla 30C—pellets
Magnesia phosphorica 30C—pellets
Lachesis 30C—pellets
Lac caninum 30C—pellets
Colocynthis 30C—pellets
Cimicifuga racemosa 30C—pellets
Cyclease PMS—tablets
Cyclease CRAMP—tablets
PMS Relief—spray

Infertility
Ignatia 200C—pellets
Medorrhinum 200C—pellets
Natrum muriaticum 200C—pellets
Sepia 200C—pellets

Pregnancy
Ipecac 30C—pellets
Tabacum 30C—pellets
Cocculus indicus 30C—pellets
Nux vomica 30C—pellets
Bellis perennis 30C—pellets
Pulsatilla 30C—pellets
Sepia 30C—pellets
Arsenicum album 30C—pellets
Kali carbonicum 30C—pellets

Labor
Arnica montana 30C—pellets
Aconitum napellus 30C—pellets
Caulophyllum 30C—pellets
Coffea 30C—pellets
Nux vomica 30C—pellets
Pulsatilla 30C—pellets
Birth Ease—liquid drops

Childbirth
Arnica montana 30C—pellets
Aconitum napellus 30C—pellets

Lactation
Belladonna 30C—pellets
Chamomilla 30C—pellets
Conium 30C—pellets
Phytolacca 30C and 200C—pellets

Menopause
Lachesis 200C—pellets
Sepia 200C—pellets
Calcarea carbonica 200C—pellets

> **Note:** You may want to try the homeo-pathic personal lubricant formulas for women manufactured by Sensua-organics, such as *Libido Formula* or *Menopause Formula*. The Sensuaorgan-ics topical homeopathic products are available for men as well as for women, and they come in different flavors. Call Sensuaorganics at 1-800-983-1993.

Guidelines for Administration of Homeopathic Remedies
Once you have chosen the homeopathic remedy and the potency that is likely to help you or your family member, you should try to give as few repetitions of the remedy as you can. You start off repeating it more frequently in a severe, acute situation, quickly decreasing the frequency once improvement has begun, stopping the remedy as soon as the problem has resolved.

> **Note:** For more information on *how often* to give the homeopathic remedy please see **Potency and Frequency**, in **Chapter 2: Basic Homeopathy**. For information on *how much* of the homeopathic remedy to give and the importance of a "*clean tongue*," please see **How to take homeo-pathic remedies** in the same chapter.

Lower potency remedies, such as 30C and below, are used to treat acute ailments. They are usually repeated often, every ½-2 or ½-4 hours. You should notice improvement in symptoms after just one to perhaps a few repetitions. If you do not see improvement, it is wise to stop the remedy and try a different one, guiding yourself by the **keynote**

symptoms. You may use different single remedies together or you may try a combination remedy. And you may use homeopathic remedies together with pharmaceutical prescription and non-prescription drugs without any effect of interference.

General guidelines to treat serious, chronic, relapsing ailments include using single remedies at potencies of 200C. These are generally administered once weekly to once monthly, but they may be used once or twice daily at first if the condition warrants it, quickly decreasing the frequency as you see improvement. Do not continue giving the remedy if it becomes apparent that it is not working. You may always stop one remedy and choose to administer another remedy on the basis of the **keynote** symptoms of the new remedy. In addition, you may administer more than one remedy at a time.

Putting It All Together

Coping with disorders of menstruation, fertility, pregnancy, labor, childbirth, lactation, and menopause will sometimes (depending on the ailment) require a multi-pronged approach incorporating all the essential natural alternatives: homeopathy, herbal remedies, and nutritional supplements.

Since disorders of the reproductive tract often require a homeopathic constitutional remedy, it is important to pay attention to **Chapter 18: Homeopathic Constitutional Remedies**.

> **Remember:** Homeopathy is safe for women who are or who may become pregnant and for those who are breastfeeding.

Women with disorders of the reproductive tract require all the vitamins and minerals necessary to repair and replenish tissues (please refer to **Chapter 23: Vitamins and Minerals**, especially *folic acid, iron, calcium* and *magnesium*) as well as a general antioxidant supplement (please refer to **Chapter 24: Antioxidant Phytochemicals**).

You may want to investigate certain herbal remedies for women's health (please refer to **Chapter 21: Herbal Remedies for Women's Health**) as well as *omega-3 fatty acids* (please refer to **Chapter 31: Oils and Fats**). In addition, it is a good idea to incorporate *probiotics* (please refer to **Chapter 30: Prebiotics and Probiotics**) into your daily supplements because your may find your reproductive tract problems to be sensitive to enhanced gastrointestinal health.

Remember: Women who are or who may become pregnant or who are breastfeeding need to ensure that each and every herbal remedy and nutritional supplement is appropriate for those special circumstances before ingesting anything.

Chapter 11

Homeopathy for Digestive Tract Ailments

Digestive Tract Ailments in General

Ailment/Disorder/Symptom	Homeopathic Remedy
Spasmodic abdominal pains and colic	*Chamomilla*
Constipation and straining at stool	*Nux vomica*
Nausea and vomiting	*Ipecac*
Spasmodic abdominal pains, cramps	*Colocynthis*
Flatulence, distention, bloating, and discomfort	*Argentum nitricum*
Diarrhea with burning around the anus	*Sulphur*
Indigestion, flatulence, bloating, distention and discomfort	*Lycopodium*
Violent vomiting and diarrhea	*Veratrum album*
Profuse diarrhea	*Camphor*
Vomiting with metallic taste in mouth	*Cuprum metallicum*
Vomiting and diarrhea with prostration	*China*
Heartburn, indigestion, gassy abdomen	*Carbo vegetalis*
Heartburn, indigestion, gassy abdomen	*Kali carbonicum*
Food poisoning, vomiting and diarrhea with burning pains in the abdomen	*Arsenicum album*
Nausea and indigestion	*Anacardium*
Indigestion with heartburn, bloating, and gas	*Natural Relief Indigestion*
Indigestion with heartburn, bloating, and gas	*Acidil*
Constipation with bloating, distention, abdominal cramping	*Constipation*
Discomfort from hemorrhoids	*Avenoc*
Abdominal gas with bloating, pressure, and pain	*Gasalia*
Indigestion with burning or pressing pain	*Kalium Aceticum Compound*
Pain, burning, itching, bleeding, and oozing at the anal area	*Hemorrhoid Relief*

Guidelines for Consulting Your Health Care Provider
Putting It All Together

Digestive Tract Ailments in General

Some digestive ailments lend themselves to self-care, such as heartburn, diarrhea, and constipation. However, even these ailments can become dangerous to health, so it is always important that you check the **Guidelines for Consulting Your Health Care Provider** at the end of this chapter. Digestive complaints that are accompanied by a slow-down or a cessation of growth in height (in children who are still supposed to be growing) may indicate celiac disease (gluten enteropathy) or one of the inflammatory bowel syndromes, such as Crohn's disease or ulcerative colitis. The proper diagnosis is essential to good health. I recommend that you consult with your primary health care provider or your homeopath.

There is good medical evidence, published in important peer-reviewed medical journals, that the treatment of diarrhea with homeopathy is likely to decrease the number of days sick with diarrhea when compared to any other treatment.

Some digestive ailments lend themselves to treatment with all three essential natural alternatives, namely, homeopathy, herbal remedies, and nutritional supplements. Those digestive problems that will likely require all three essential natural alternatives are: irritable bowel syndrome with chronic abdominal cramps and diarrhea alternating with constipation; chronic constipation; chronic indigestion with or without gastroesophageal reflux (GERD); and chronic enzyme deficiencies leading to abdominal discomfort and diarrhea.

Chronic indigestion with or without gastroesophageal reflux (GERD) is sometimes called "acid indigestion" (a synonym for heartburn). The medical establishment's treatment of the whole issue of "acid indigestion" is based on a false premise. Antacids, Histamine H2-receptor blockers (H2-blockers), and Proton Pump Inhibitors (PPIs) all treat "acid indigestion" as though the cause is *too much acid* in the stomach, whereas the real situation is, in 90% of cases, exactly the opposite, *too little acid* in the stomach. It is a good idea to stay away from those drugs, especially on a chronic basis. If you want to read more about this, I recommend the book, *Why Stomach Acid Is Good for You* by Jonathan Wright and Lane Lenard, published by M. Evans and Company, 2001. A safe and effective way to treat "acid indigestion" is with homeopathy, herbal remedies, and nutritional supplements.

> **Note:** If you want a gentler yet effective antacid, you might try the herbal remedy *deglycyrrhizinated licorice* (*DGL*). It is made from the herb *Glycyrrhiza glabra*. *DGL* exerts a protective coating effect on the lining of the esophagus and stomach. Chew 2 *DGL* tablets before meals. There are no serious side effects. *DGL* is used to treat heartburn, GERD, and peptic ulcers.

> **Note:** Another herbal remedy, *Orange peel* extract, from the plant *Citrus sinensis* may be helpful to treat heartburn and gastroesophageal reflux (GERD). The recommended dose is 1 gram of *Orange peel* extract every other day for 20 days. Buy *Orange peel* extract in capsules that have been standardized to 98.5% *d-limonene*. You may take a capsule if your heartburn returns occasionally after the 20-day period. Do not take *Orange peel* extract if you are pregnant or lactating. But do not use *Orange peel* extract if you have an ulcer. The safety of *Orange peel* extract has not been evaluated in children.

In my experience, disorders of the liver will likely require the prescribing of a *constitutional homeopathic remedy*, as well as certain herbal remedies such as *Milk thistle* and nutritional supplements. Celiac disease (gluten enteropathy) and the inflammatory bowel syndromes, such as Crohn's disease or ulcerative colitis also will likely require a *constitutional homeopathic remedy*. Determining your own or someone else's *constitutional homeopathic remedy* may be possible for you to do, but it is sometimes difficult for an untrained person to find the appropriate constitutional remedy. Finding the proper constitutional remedy may require the services of your homeopath. In addition, if you find you have achieved only partial results after administering the constitutional homeopathic remedy that you have prescribed, I recommend that you consult with your professional homeopath.

If you feel that you need more information on what foods to eat to be healthy yourself and to maintain a healthy home for your family, I urge you to embark on a lifetime of reading about the connections between food and health. You will find that the food-health connection impinges on every system of your body, touching every fiber of your being. You should start by reading the labels on everything you buy at the supermarket. You may be startled at the amount of sugar you have been feeding yourself and your family. You will also want to become educated in order to make informed choices about organic foods, genetically altered foods, pesticides in foods, and food additives.

If you have difficulties digesting food it may be helpful to take a *multi-digestive enzyme* capsule before each meal. This would include digestive enzymes such as amylase to break down starches, lipase to break down fats, and protease to break down proteins. People who lack the enzyme lactase may experience distention of the abdomen with crampy pain, increased gas, and diarrhea after eating dairy products containing the milk sugar lactose. These people can drink *Lactaid milk* or add *Lactaid* to their other dairy meals.

For more information on many different gastrointestinal ailments (including gallbladder disease), I recommend the book, *Healthy Digestion the Natural Way* by D. Lindsey Berkson, published by John Wiley, 2000. If you or your family member suffers from one of the common gastrointestinal ailments, this book will help you to construct a healthy lifestyle to prevent and treat those diseases. You should always include homeopathic remedies in whatever therapies you choose to optimize your health.

Note: Enteric-coated *Peppermint oil* capsules may be beneficial for decreasing the symptoms of irritable bowel syndrome (IBS). *Peppermint oil* is an herbal remedy that acts to relax the intestinal muscles, decreasing spasm and cramping. It is sometimes combined with other herbal remedies, *Rosemary* and *Thyme*, for the treatment of IBS. Always buy enteric-coated *Peppermint oil* so it will act in the small and large intestines rather than be absorbed in the stomach.

Follow the directions on the bottle but take the enteric-coated capsules between meals. Another herbal remedy that may be helpful for IBS is *Clown's mustard* (*Iberis amara*). It may be taken together with enteric-coated *Peppermint oil*.

As with any and all medical conditions, when dealing with digestive tract ailments you must pay strict attention to the **Guidelines for Consulting Your Health Care Provider** at the end of this chapter. You may want to refer to the last section **Putting It All Together** for ideas on how to integrate the essential natural alternatives, homeopathy, herbal remedies, and nutritional supplements.

Chamomilla

What is it? The homeopathic remedy is made from the plant *Matricaria chamomilla*, common name *Chamomile*, a member of the *Compositae* botanical family.

When should you use it? The **keynote** symptoms leading you towards choosing *Chamomilla* are cramping, spasmodic abdominal pains (colic) in irritable infants and children. Nothing satisfies the crying child at this time so he tends to throw away whatever plaything the parent tries to give him. The child cries in a rage, kicking, biting and scratching, until they quiet down while being carried. *Chamomilla* should be given whenever there is anger or rage out of proportion to the situation, for instance, during fever and earache. A peculiar symptom strongly indicating the use of *Chamomilla* is when one cheek is pale and the other is red. *Chamomilla* is also effective in treating indigestion, especially after drinking coffee.

How should you use it? Give *Chamomilla* 30C every ½-4 hours depending on severity of symptoms to relieve colicky pains, quickly decreasing the frequency with improvement. Then give once or twice daily, stopping when the problem has passed.

Note: *Chamomile* is the herbal form of *Matricaria chamomilla*. The herbal tea is used to calm the digestive tract in cases of infant colic, irritable bowel syndrome, indigestion, gas and bloating.

Chamomile acts as an antispasmodic of the intestinal tract. It acts as a mild sedative as well so it is doubly calming. Other herbal remedies helpful for indigestion and colicky pains in infancy are: *Peppermint* (*Mentha piperita*), *Fennel seed* (*Foeniculum vulgare*) and *lemon balm* (*Melissa officinalis*). They are present in *Calma Bebi* herbal tea. *Gripe water* is another remedy worthy to try in cases of infant colic. There are many formulations of *Gripe water* available, but most have *Fennel seed* or *Dill seed oil* or *Ginger* and some have *sodium bicarbonate*.

Nux vomica

What is it? This is a poisonous plant, *Nux vomica*, containing strychnine, common name *Poison nut*, a member of the *Loganiaceae* botanical family. This homeopathic remedy is non-toxic.
When should you use it? The **keynote** symptoms pointing towards the use of *Nux vomica* are constipation with straining at stool with little result. The person needing *Nux vomica* will likely be a workaholic with extreme irritability, anger, and intolerance of others, in large part due to stress from overwork or overindulgence. *Nux vomica* is also indicated for the indigestion associated with smoking cigarettes or drinking too much alcohol or coffee.
How should you use it? Give *Nux vomica* 30C every ½-4 hours depending on severity of symptoms to relieve the constipation or indigestion, quickly decreasing the frequency with improvement. Then give once or twice daily, stopping when the problem has passed. For chronic constipation, you may need to find the person's *constitutional homeopathic remedy*.

Ipecac

What is it? The homeopathic remedy *Ipecac* is made from the root of the plant *Cephaelis ipecacuanha*, a member of the *Rubiaceae* botanical family.
When should you use it? The **keynote** symptoms helping you to choose *Ipecac* are almost constant nausea and vomiting which are not relieved by vomiting, worsening while bending down. Diarrhea and a sweaty, pale face may accompany the nausea and vomiting.
How should you use it? Give *Ipecac* 30C every ½-4 hours depending on severity of symptoms to relieve the nausea and vomiting, quickly decreasing the frequency with improvement. Then give once or twice daily, stopping when the problem has passed.

Colocynthis

What is it? This is the plant *Citrullus colocynthis*, common name *Bitter apple*, a member of the *Cucurbitaceae* botanical family.
When should you use it? The **keynote** symptoms leading you to choose *Colocynthis* are cramping, spasmodic abdominal pains which are relieved when the patient lies down in the knee-chest position.
How should you use it? Give *Colocynthis* 30C every ½-4 hours depending on severity of symptoms to relieve the cramping abdominal pains, quickly decreasing the frequency with improvement. Then give once or twice daily, stopping when the problem has passed.

Argentum nitricum

What is it? This is the soluble chemical compound *Silver nitrate*.
When should you use it? The **keynote** symptoms pointing towards the use of *Argentum nitricum* are severe gassy abdomen (with flatulence, distention, bloating, and discomfort) with or without diarrhea as a result of anticipatory anxiety, such as before an examination or a performance (stage fright).
How should you use it? Give *Argentum nitricum* 30C every ½-4 hours depending on severity of symptoms to relieve the gas and discomfort, quickly decreasing the frequency with improvement, stopping as soon as the gas and discomfort are gone. You may give *Argentum nitricum* 30C every 30 minutes for 3 doses starting 90 minutes before a performance to prevent gassy abdominal symptoms that tend to occur from performance anxiety.

Sulphur

What is it? The mineral element *Sulphur*, common name *brimstone*, is present in every cell of the human body. *Sulphur* is a polychrest constitutional remedy exerting its main effects on the skin.

When should you use it? The **keynote** symptoms indicating *Sulphur* are diarrhea and burning around the anus with an early morning onset, usually around 5 a.m. The symptoms tend to occur in an untidy person with unhygienic personal habits.

How should you use it? Give *Sulphur* 30C every ½-4 hours depending on severity of symptoms to relieve the gas and discomfort, quickly decreasing the frequency with improvement, stopping as soon as the gas and discomfort are gone.

Lycopodium

What is it? This plant is the primitive moss, *Lycopodium clavatum*, common name *Club moss*, a member of the *Lycopodiaceae* botanical family. *Lycopodium* is a major polychrest constitutional remedy.

When should you use it? The **keynote** symptoms directing you to try *Lycopodium* are large amounts of gas in the abdomen, with flatulence, even after eating very small amounts, with bloating, distention, and discomfort. The indigestion symptoms are made worse around 4-8 p.m. The person needing *Lycopodium* tends to be "a little dictator" at home while being conciliatory outside the home. The *Lycopodium* type of person is often considered arrogant but that is a cover for insecurity. *Lycopodium* is useful to treat constipation in elderly people. People needing *Lycopodium* tend to crave sweets.

How should you use it? Give *Lycopodium* 30C every ½-4 hours depending on severity of symptoms to relieve the gas and discomfort, quickly decreasing the frequency with improvement, stopping as soon as the gas and discomfort are gone.

Veratrum album

What is it? This is the poisonous plant *Veratrum album*, common name *White Hellebore*, a member of the *Liliaceae* botanical family. This homeopathic remedy is non-toxic.

When should you use it? The **keynote** symptoms encouraging your use of *Veratrum album* are severe gastrointestinal infections accompanied by copious amounts of diarrhea and violent vomiting leading to prostration with icy cold hands and a cold, sinking feeling in the whole body.

How should you use it? Give *Veratrum album* 30C every ½-4 hours depending on severity of symptoms, quickly decreasing the frequency with improvement, stopping as soon as the diarrhea is under control.

Camphor

What is it? This is the plant *Cinnamonum camphora*, also called *Laurus camphora*, a member of the *Lauraceae* botanical family.

When should you use it? The **keynote** symptoms helping you to choose *Camphor* are copious amounts of diarrhea without much cramping but with an icy coldness of the extremities.

How should you use it? Give *Camphor* 30C every ½-4 hours depending on severity of symptoms, quickly decreasing the frequency with improvement, stopping as soon as the diarrhea is under control and the icy coldness has gone.

Cuprum metallicum

What is it? This is the metal chemical element *Copper*.

When should you use it? The **keynote** symptoms pointing in the direction of using *Cuprum metallicum* are vomiting accompanied by a putrid or metallic taste in the mouth. The vomiting is decreased by drinking cold water.

How should you use it? Give *Cuprum metallicum* 30C every ½-4 hours depending on severity of symptoms, quickly decreasing the frequency with improvement, stopping as soon as the vomiting with metallic taste in the mouth is gone.

China

What is it? This is the plant *China officinalis* (also called *Cinchona succirubra*), common name *Cinchona bark* or *Peruvian bark*, a member of the *Rubiaceae* botanical family. The bark contains quinine. The homeopathic remedy is made from the bark.

When should you use it? The **keynote** symptoms leading you to try *China* are great weakness with prostration from loss of bodily fluids, such as with vomiting and diarrhea from a viral intestinal infection (gastroenteritis).

How should you use it? Give *China* 30C every ½-4 hours depending on severity of symptoms, quickly decreasing the frequency with improvement, stopping as soon as the vomiting and diarrhea is gone.

Carbo vegetalis

What is it? This is the homeopathic remedy made from *charcoal* that is made from partially burned wood.

When should you use it? The **keynote** symptoms pointing towards using *Carbo veg* (as it is called) are heartburn, indigestion, gassy abdomen with flatulence and bloating, and gastroesophageal reflux with a sour taste in the mouth.

How should you use it? Give *Carbo veg* 30C every ½-4 hours depending on severity of symptoms, quickly decreasing the frequency with improvement, stopping as soon as the indigestion symptoms are gone. If you find that the symptoms are relieved by *Carbo veg* but then recur fairly frequently, you should try *Carbo veg* 30C once daily until the recurrences are infrequent.

Kali carbonicum

What is it? This is the chemical compound *potassium carbonate* found in all plants.

When should you use it? The **keynote** symptoms pointing towards using *Kali carb* (as it is called) are abdominal distention, bloating, gas, flatulence, and constipation occurring in a stern person who has an exaggerated sense of duty, and is closed off emotionally.

How should you use it? Give *Kali carb* 30C every ½-4 hours depending on severity of symptoms, quickly decreasing the frequency with improvement, stopping as soon as the constipation and related symptoms are gone.

Arsenicum album

What is it? This is the homeopathic remedy made from the chemical compound *arsenic oxide* which is highly poisonous if not given in homeopathic dilution. *Arsenicum album* is one of homeopathy's often-used polychrests or constitutional remedies.

When should you use it? The **keynote** symptoms directing you towards using *Arsenicum album* are vomiting and diarrhea with burning pains in the abdomen, along with thirst for small but frequent sips of water at a time. *Arsenicum album* is homeopathy's treatment for food poisoning. In fact, *Arsenicum album* is useful to treat intestinal infections (gastroenteritis) from both viral and bacterial causes. *Arsenicum album* can be helpful when there is vomiting and diarrhea from eating fruit that is too ripe or from drinking too much alcohol. The person needing *Arsenicum album* may be anxious about his or her health along with restlessness and chilliness. The symptoms tend to worsen at and after midnight.

> **Note:** *Arsenicum album* is one of the important homeopathic remedies that should be included in your foreign travel medicine kit. You can tailor the other homeopathic remedies that you might need by visiting the *Center for Disease Control* for health information updated every year at www.cdc.gov/travel/yb/index.htm and you may want to join the *International Association for Medical Assistance to Travelers* at www.iamat.org.

How should you use it? Give *Arsenicum album* 30C every ½-4 hours depending on severity of symptoms, quickly decreasing the frequency with improvement, stopping as soon as the vomiting and diarrhea have resolved.

Anacardium

What is it? This is the plant *Anacardium orientale*, common name *Marking nut tree*, a member of the *Anacardiaceae* botanical family.

When should you use it? The **keynote** symptoms helping you to use *Anacardium* are nausea and indigestion with the feeling of a hard plug pressing into the area where the esophagus leads into the stomach (epigastrium) and the feeling of a band around the body or any part of the body. *Anacardium* is often used to treat ulcers in the stomach or duodenum.

How should you use it? Give *Anacardium* 30C every ½-4 hours depending on severity of symptoms, quickly decreasing the frequency with improvement, stopping as soon as the nausea and hard plug feelings have resolved.

Natural Relief Indigestion

What is it? This is a combination remedy produced by Boericke & Tafel, a homeopathic pharmaceutical supply house. *Natural Relief Indigestion* contains the following ingredients in very low potencies: *Arsenicum album, Bismuthum subnitricum, Capsicum annuum, Iris versicolor* and *Robinia pseudoacacia*, in lactose-based tablets which also contain sorbitol.

When should you use it? The **keynote** symptoms leading you to choose *Natural Relief Indigestion* are indigestion with heartburn, bloating, and gas.

How should you use it? Chew or allow to dissolve in the mouth 1-2 tablets of *Natural Relief Indigestion* depending on severity of indigestion every 1-4 hours, but not exceeding 12 tablets in a 24 hour period.

Acidil

What is it? This is a combination remedy produced by Boiron, a homeopathic pharmaceutical supply house. *Acidil* contains the following ingredients in very low potencies: *Abies nigra, Carbo vegetalis, Nux vomica* and *Robinia pseudoacacia*, in a lactose-based tablet.

When should you use it? The **keynote** symptoms leading you to choose *Acidil* are indigestion with heartburn, bloating, and gas.

How should you use it? For acute indigestion, chew or allow dissolving in the mouth 2 tablets and repeating every 15 minutes for 3 more doses, depending on severity. For more chronic use, take 2 tablets 15 minutes before meals.

Constipation

What is it? This is a combination remedy produced by Boericke & Tafel, a homeopathic pharmaceutical supply house. *Constipation* contains the following ingredients in very low potency: *Dioscorea villosa, Nux vomica* and *Natrum muriaticum*, in lactose-based tablets.

When should you use it? The **keynote** symptoms leading you to choose *Constipation* are constipation with associated bloating, distention, and abdominal cramping.

How should you use it? Chew or allow to dissolve in the mouth 1 or 2 tablets depending on severity. This may be repeated 1-4 times daily. Infants and children under the age of 6 years would take half the adult dosage.

Avenoc

What is it? This is a combination remedy produced by Boiron, a homeopathic pharmaceutical supply house. *Avenoc* tablets contain the following ingredients in very low potencies: *Aesculus hippocastanum, Hamamelis virginiana, Lachesis mutus* and *Nux vomica*, in lactose-based tablets. *Avenoc* suppositories contain the following ingredients in very low potencies: *Aesculus hippocastanum, Collinsonia canadensis* and *Hamamelis virginiana* in a cocoa butter suppository. *Avenoc* ointment contains the same active homeopathic ingredients as *Avenoc* suppositories except that the inactive ingredient is white petrolatum.

When should you use it? The **keynote** symptoms leading you to choose *Avenoc* tablets, suppositories, or ointment are discomfort from hemorrhoids, such as soreness, itching, and burning.

How should you use it? When using *Avenoc* tablets, chew or allow to dissolve in the mouth 1 or 2 tablets depending on severity. This may be repeated every 2 hours, up to 6 times in one day. When using *Avenoc* suppositories, insert one suppository once or twice daily. When using *Avenoc* ointment, apply externally to the area with a finger up to 4 times daily. *Avenoc* suppositories and ointment are not intended for use by children.

Gasalia

What is it? This is a combination remedy produced by Boiron, a homeopathic pharmaceutical supply house. *Gasalia* contains the following ingredients in very low potencies: *Carbo vegetalis, Lycopodium clavatum, Nux moschata* and *Raphanus sativus*, in a lactose-based tablet.

When should you use it? The **keynote** symptoms leading you to choose *Gasalia* are abdominal gas and the associated bloating, pressure, and pain.

How should you use it? Chew or allow to dissolve in the mouth 1 or 2 tablets of *Gasalia* depending on severity of abdominal gas, repeating every 15 minutes for 3 more doses. For more chronic use, take 2 tablets 15 minutes before meals.

Kalium Aceticum Compound

What is it? This is a combination remedy produced by Weleda, a homeopathic pharmaceutical supply house. *Kalium Aceticum Compound* is a powder which contains the following ingredients in very low potency: *Kalium aceticum, Corallium rubrum* and *Antimonium crudum*.

When should you use it? The **keynote** symptoms leading you to choose *Kalium Aceticum Compound* are indigestion with burning or pressing pain in the area just below the sternum (epigastrium). This is homeopathy's "antacid."

How should you use it? The directions are to take ⅛ teaspoon of the powder 3-4 times daily, not to exceed one teaspoon daily. Since it is next to impossible to follow these directions, I suggest that you measure ¼ teaspoon of the powder with a cooking measuring ¼ teaspoon, take ½ of that amount and dissolve it in mineral or spring water, and drink. Repeat 3-4 times daily depending on severity, not exceeding one teaspoon of the powder

daily. This preparation may be used for young children, aged 2-7 years, who should take ½ the adult dose.

Hemorrhoid Relief

What is it? This is a combination remedy oral spray produced by King Bio (in their *SafeCareRx* line of products). The ingredients in *Hemorrhoid Relief* include: *Aesculus hippocastanum, Aloe socotrina, Collinsonia canadensis, Hamamelis virginiana, Muriaticum acidum, Nux vomica, Paeonia officinalis, Ratanhia, Sepia* and *Sulphur*, in pure water. Each ingredient comes in a broad spectrum of low to high potencies. This is an alcohol-free preparation.

When should you use it? The **keynote** symptoms leading you to choose *Hemorrhoid Reliever* are pain, burning, itching, bleeding, and oozing at the anal area associated with protruding hemorrhoids.

How should you use it? Spray 3 complete pump sprays onto or under the tongue 4-6 times daily until symptoms are relieved.

Guidelines for Consulting Your Health Care Provider

You should consult your health care provider if:
- the patient doesn't look right or act right (trust your instincts!)
- the patient is getting worse instead of better over the course of the illness
- the patient has a sustained high fever (103°F [39.5°C] to 104°F [40°C])
- the patient has persistent loss of weight
- the patient has persistent loss of appetite
- the patient is uninterested in eating or drinking or playing
- the patient has not had a wet diaper or urinated in the past 12 hours
- the patient's eyes look sunken into her head
- the patient has abdominal pain, holding or pointing to the lower right side of the abdomen
- the patient complains of a sudden severe pain in the abdomen

- the patient is less than one month old and has vomiting (especially projectile vomiting) or diarrhea
- the patient has had more than 1 day of frequent vomiting or more than 2 days of diarrhea with frequent watery stools
- there is fresh red blood in the vomit or the stool
- there is black coffee grounds in the vomit
- there is dark black blood in the stool
- there is constipation for more than 3-4 days along with pain in the abdomen
- there is reflux of gastric contents into the mouth for more than 2-3 months
- there is chronic abdominal pain lasting more than 2-3 months
- there has been a slow-down or cessation of growth in height (in growing children) over the past 6 months
- the patient is having trouble breathing or complaining of chest pains or there is mental confusion or lethargy or irritability

> Note: Do not discontinue taking any pharmaceutical medication that has been prescribed by your health care provider unless you or your family member is under the supervision of a physician.

Recommendations for Homeopathic Remedies

Chamomilla 30C—in pellets and liquid drops
Nux vomica 30C—in pellets and liquid drops
Ipecac 30C—in pellets and liquid
Colocynthis 30C—in pellets and liquid
Argentum nitricum 30C—in pellets and liquid
Sulphur 30C—in pellets and liquid
Lycopodium 30C—in pellets and liquid drops
Veratrum album 30C—in pellets and liquid drops
Camphor 30C—in pellets and liquid drops
Cuprum metallicum 30C—in pellets and liquid drops
China 30C—in pellets and liquid drops
Carbo vegetalis 30C—in pellets and liquid drops
Kali carbonicum 30C—in pellets and liquid drops
Arsenicum album 30C—in pellets and liquid drops
Anacardium 30C—in pellets and liquid drops
Natural Relief Indigestion—in chewable tablets
Acidil—in chewable/dissolvable tablets
Constipation—in chewable/dissolvable tablets

Avenoc—in chewable/dissolvable tablets, suppositories, and ointment
Gasalia—in chewable/dissolvable tablets
Kalium Aceticum Compound—liquid
Hemorrhoid Relief—oral spray

Guidelines for Administration of Homeopathic Remedies

Once you have chosen the homeopathic remedy and the potency that is likely to help you or your family member, you should try to give as few repetitions of the remedy as you can. You start off repeating it more frequently in a severe, acute situation, quickly decreasing the frequency once improvement has begun, stopping the remedy as soon as the problem has resolved.

> Note: For more information on *how often* to give the homeopathic remedy please see **Potency and Frequency**, in **Chapter 2: Basic Homeopathy**. For information on *how much* of the homeopathic remedy to give and the importance of a *"clean tongue*,*"* please see **How to take homeopathic remedies** in the same chapter.

Lower potency remedies, such as 30C and below, are used to treat acute ailments. They are usually repeated often, every $\frac{1}{2}$-2 or $\frac{1}{2}$-4 hours. You should notice improvement in symptoms after just one to perhaps a few repetitions. If you do not see improvement, it is wise to stop the remedy and try a different one, guiding yourself by the **keynote** symptoms. You may use different single remedies together or you may try a combination remedy. And you may use homeopathic remedies together with pharmaceutical prescription and non-prescription drugs without any effect of interference.

General guidelines to treat serious, chronic, relapsing ailments include using single remedies at potencies of 200C. These are generally administered once weekly to once monthly, but they may be used once or twice daily at first if the condition warrants it, quickly decreasing the frequency as you see improvement. Do not continue giving the remedy if it becomes apparent that it is not working. You may always stop one remedy and choose to administer another remedy on the basis of the **keynote** symptoms of the new remedy. In addition, you may administer more than one remedy at a time.

Putting It All Together

Coping with gastrointestinal tract disorders will generally require a multi-pronged approach incorporating all the essential natural alternatives, homeopathy, herbal remedies, and nutritional supplements.

It is a good idea to consider giving the sick person's homeopathic constitutional remedy (please refer to **Chapter 9: Homeopathic Remedies for Constitutional Problems in Infants, Children, and Adolescents** or to **Chapter 18: Homeopathic Constitutional Remedies** if you are dealing with an adult). Eating disorders and weight disorders are sometimes consequences of gastrointestinal ailments. Please refer to **Chapter 15: Homeopathy for Eating Disorders and Weight Control**.

Gastrointestinal tract ailments require all the vitamins and minerals necessary to repair and replenish tissues (please refer to **Chapter 23: Vitamins and Minerals**) as well as a general antioxidant supplement (please refer to **Chapter 24: Antioxidant Phytochemicals**).

You may want to investigate certain herbal remedies such as *Milk thistle* and *Psyllium* (please refer to **Chapter 20: Herbs You Need to Know**) as well as *omega-3 fatty acids* (please refer to **Chapter 31: Oils and Fats**). You will need to incorporate *probiotics* (please refer to **Chapter 30: Prebiotics and Probiotics**) into your daily supplements.

Healthy nutrition goes hand-in-hand with longevity. If you want to prevent or treat most of the chronic ailments that beset us in this century, you will need to learn about healthy nutrition. Please read the nutritional advice in **Chapter 27: Nutritional Supplements to Prevent Cancer and Augment Your Immune System; Chapter 26: Nutritional Supplements for Healthy Weight Control** and **Chapter 24: Antioxidant Phytochemicals**.

Chapter 12

Homeopathy for Urinary Tract Ailments

Urinary Tract Ailments in General

Ailment/Disorder/Symptom	Homeopathic Remedy
Sudden, burning pains on urination	*Aconitum napellus*
Burning, stinging pains on urination	*Apis mellifica*
Undescended testicles	*Aurum metallicum*
Kidney infections with back pains	*Berberis vulgaris*
Bladder infections with burning pains and urgency	*Cantharis*
Incontinence	*Causticum*
Hesitancy, dribbling, small stream caliber, and urinating frequently	*Lycopodium*
Frequent urgings to urinate with very little urine produced	*Nux vomica*
Sudden loss of erection or imperfect erection	*Phosphoric acid*
Hesitancy, dribbling, small stream caliber, and urinating frequently	*Sabal serrulata*
Pain at the end of urination	*Sarsaparilla*
Burning after urination due to medical procedures	*Staphysagria*
Pain during urination, urgency, bedwetting, and incontinence	*Uri-Control*
Bedwetting at night	*Bedwetting/Enuresis*

Guidelines for Consulting Your Health Care Provider
Putting It All Together

Urinary Tract Ailments in General

Urinary tract ailments include the following conditions:

> bedwetting (enuresis); incontinence or daytime wetting; obstructive disorders (usually from prostate enlargement, with hesitancy in starting the urinary stream and straining as the main symptoms); bladder infections (cystitis and interstitial cystitis) with pain on urination or after urination as the main symptom, along with frequency and urgency; stones (which may occur throughout the entire urinary tract, causing obstruction and severe pain called renal colic); and kidney infection (with pain in the flanks and fever as the main symptoms)
> (Adapted from *The Merck Manual* at www.merck.com)

Some urinary tract ailments lend themselves to self-care with homeopathy, such as bladder infections, bed-wetting and incontinence, and prostate enlargement (benign prostatic hypertrophy). However, even these ailments can become dangerous to health, so it is always important that you check the **Guidelines for Consulting Your Health Care Provider** at the end of this chapter. Urinary tract complaints that are accompanied by a slow-down or a cessation of growth in height (in children who are still supposed to be growing) may indicate a smoldering kidney disease, such as pyelonephritis or renal failure. The proper diagnosis is essential to good health. I recommend that you consult with your primary health care provider or your homeopath.

Patients who suffer from acute or chronic renal failure from any cause need to be extremely cautious about taking any medication, herbal remedy, or nutritional supplement. Therefore, for these patients, homeopathy is the only self-care alternative that I would recommend. For these patients, homeopathy may be effective adjunctive treatment in concert with their prescription pharmaceuticals. In these cases, herbal remedies and nutritional supplements must be prescribed by physicians (and homeopath physicians) who are conversant with the effects of herbal remedies and nutritional supplements on the medicines used to treat renal failure.

The same cautionary statement may be made for patients who have prostate cancer or any other cancer of the urinary tract. Self-care for persons with *any type of cancer* is also limited to homeopathy, but I strongly recommend that you use homeopathy together with oncology treatment. In that way, homeopathy can be expected to be effective adjunctive treatment in the hopes of cure. Before taking herbal remedies or nutritional supplements please consult with your health care provider, your oncology specialists, and with your homeopath.

Bladder infections are very common, especially in females, and these may occur and reoccur throughout the life cycle. The reason that bladder infections are so much more common in females than in males is that in females the urethra (the tube leading urine from the bladder to the outside of the body) is situated so close to the anus. This makes it possible for bacteria that naturally live in the intestinal tract to be swept into the urinary tract. The first stop for such bacteria is the bladder. Urine in the bladder is naturally sterile until bacterial contamination occurs. This means that it is essential to perform hygienic wiping up procedures after urination and bowel movements (defecation).

When the urinary tract infection is confined to the bladder, the situation is usually amenable to self-care with homeopathy. However, you it is important that you check the **Guidelines for Consulting Your Health Care Provider** at the end of this chapter in order to know when a urinary tract infection might be a kidney infection (pyelonephritis) which can be dangerous to health. Symptoms of bladder infection (cystitis) are: burning pain on urination or after urination, pain or cramping in the lower abdomen just above the pubic bone after urination, blood in the urine (hematuria), cloudy or putrid smelling urine, frequency of urination, dribbling of urine, and urgency.

Recurrent urinary tract infections are difficult to treat and very difficult to prevent, unless of course, you use homeopathy. If you or a person in your family suffers from recurrent urinary tract infections when each recurrence resolves after treatment with a certain homeopathic remedy, then you may wish to try to *prevent* recurrences by giving that remedy in a 200C potency. You would administer that remedy once weekly for 2 months and then once monthly for 6 months. If the urinary tract infection returns after that treatment, you may begin again, first treating the acute infection, and then preventing future infections with the 200C potency. However, at this point, I recommend that you continue with the once monthly remedy for one year.

A good place to start learning about how to treat infections with homeopathy is by reading **Chapter 7: Homeopathic Remedies for Infections**. The remedies listed in that chapter (especially *Mercurius solubilis* and *Pulsatilla*) also apply to the treatment of urinary tract infections, and can be used in conjunction with any of the remedies in this chapter.

As with any and all medical conditions, when dealing with urinary tract ailments you must pay strict attention to the **Guidelines for Consulting Your Health Care Provider** at the end of this chapter. You may want to refer to the last section **Putting It All Together** for ideas on how to integrate the essential natural alternatives, homeopathy, herbal remedies, and nutritional supplements.

Aconitum napellus

What is it? This homeopathic remedy, called in shorthand *Aconite*, is made from the plant commonly called *monkshood* or *wolfsbane*, a member of the *Ranunculaceae* botanical family.
When should you use it? The **keynote** symptoms urging you to use *Aconite* are sudden burning pains on urination, perhaps with bloody drops of urine at the beginning or end of urination, along with fear and restless agitation, all coming on suddenly. There is a hot feeling to the urine on the labia.
How should you use it? Give *Aconite* 30C every ½-2 hours until the acute pains have lessened, then decreasing the frequency, and then stopping when the pains have gone.

Apis mellifica

What is it? This is a homeopathic remedy from the animal kingdom, made from the whole, crushed *honeybee*.
When should you use it? The **keynote** symptoms leading towards trying *Apis mellifica* are burning, stinging pains on urination with thirstlessness. The pains are better with cold compresses to the bladder area. They are worse when the area is touched or with warm compresses. *Apis mellifica* is a remedy often used to treat and prevent cystitis or interstitial cystitis.
How should you use it? Give *Apis mellifica* 30C every ½-2 hours until the acute pains have lessened, then decreasing the frequency, then stopping when the pains have gone.

Aurum metallicum

When should you use it? This is the element *gold*, one of the metals in the periodic table of chemicals.
How should you use it? The **keynote** symptoms leading you to consider using *Aurum metallicum* are undescended testicle, especially on the right side, or for any inflammation of the testicle.
How should you use it? Give *Aurum metallicum* 200C once weekly until the testicle has descended into the scrotum. Then give *Aurum metallicum* 200C once monthly for 6 months. Then stop. Please be sure to consult your health care provider if you suspect undescended testicle in a young child because it must be corrected, either with homeopathy or surgery, for 2 reasons: 1) uncorrected undescended testicles are associated with a high rate of cancer developing in that testicle; and 2) uncorrected undescended testicles will not produce viable sperm and fertility may be seriously affected.

Berberis vulgaris

What is it? This is the plant *Berberis vulgaris*, common name *Barberry*, a member of the *Berberidaceae* botanical family.
When should you use it? The **keynote** symptoms helping you to choose *Berberis* are infections of the kidneys with tearing or piercing pains in the area of the kidneys which may be accompanied by back pains, or sticking pains in the bladder. The pains may extend from the kidneys down the ureters to the bladder. The urine may be cloudy or bloody. There may be pains in the thighs when urinating. This is a remedy for stones in the urinary tract.

How should you use it? Give *Berberis* 30C every ½-2 hours until the acute pains have lessened, then decreasing the frequency, then stopping when the pains have gone.

Cantharis

What is it? This is the homeopathic remedy made from the whole insect, the *Spanish fly, Cantharis vesicatoria*.

When should you use it? The **keynote** symptoms for which you would try *Cantharis* are severe burning pains and urgency, meaning the patient has the urge to urinate frequently even though only a few drops may come out. There is a burning feeling to the urine on the labia. The pains are lessened with warm compresses or by gently rubbing the area, which helps to distinguish *Cantharis* from *Apis*. *Cantharis* is the homeopathic remedy that is most often prescribed for acute and recurrent urinary tract infections such as cystitis and interstitial cystitis.

How should you use it? Give *Cantharis* 30C every ½-4 hours until the burning pains have receded, decreasing the frequency with improvement, stopping when they are gone.

Causticum

What is it? The homeopathic remedy is a chemical compound prepared from *calcium hydroxide (lime)* and *potassium bisulphate*.

When should you use it? The **keynote** symptoms leading you to give *Causticum* are involuntary loss of urine during coughing or sneezing, or during anything that increases abdominal pressure. *Causticum* is a remedy often used for urinary incontinence.

How should you use it? Give *Causticum* 200C once daily until the urinary incontinence symptoms have decreased, then once weekly until they have disappeared. Then stop.

Lycopodium

What is it? This plant is the primitive moss, *Lycopodium clavatum*, common name *Club moss*, a member of the *Lycopodiaceae* botanical family. The spores of the moss are used to produce the homeopathic remedy.

When should you use it? The **keynote** symptoms encouraging you to try *Lycopodium* are urinary stream obstructive problems commonly seen with prostate enlargement (benign prostatic hypertrophy), namely, hesitancy, dribbling, small stream caliber, and urinating frequently at night. *Lycopodium* also has a positive effect on lagging libido. These symptoms may occur in a person who appears to be arrogant in order to cover a deficiency of self-esteem, a feeling he or she may never be good enough to succeed. *Lycopodium* is sometimes used to treat bloody or red-tinged gravel in the urine, as well as impotence.

How should you use it? Give *Lycopodium* 200C once daily until the urinary obstructive symptoms are decreased, then once weekly until urination has reverted to normal. Then stop.

Nux vomica

What is it? This is a poisonous plant, *Nux vomica*, containing strychnine, common name *Poison nut*, a member of the *Loganiaceae* botanical family. The homeopathic remedy is non-toxic.

When should you use it? The **keynote** symptoms helping you to choose *Nux vomica* are frequent urgings to urinate with very little urine produced, along with pain on urination. These symptoms may occur in a person who is considered by his family to be a workaholic. He or she may over-indulge in alcohol, cigarettes, and coffee and have gastrointestinal and insomnia complaints directly stemming from this.

How should you use it? Give *Nux vomica* 30C every ½-2 hours until the frequency and urgency have lessened, then decreasing the frequency of administrations, then stopping when the symptoms have gone.

Phosphoric acid

What is it? *Phosphoric acid* is a chemical compound that is produced from *Phosphorus* containing minerals.
When should you use it? The **keynote** symptoms for which you would consider using *Phosphoric acid* are sudden loss of erection during sexual intercourse, or imperfect erection that does not allow intercourse to continue. This is the main remedy for erectile dysfunction.
How should you use it? Give *Phosphoric acid* 200C once nightly until symptoms of erectile dysfunction abate. Then give *Phosphoric acid* 200C once weekly for 4 weeks, then once monthly for 6 months. Then stop. If symptoms of erectile dysfunction do not disappear, it is wisest to consult with your health care provider because there may be a serious underlying disease that requires medical attention.

Sabal serrulata

What is it? This is the plant *Sabal serrulata* (also called *Sarenoa serrulata*), common name *Saw palmetto*, a member of the *Palmaceae* botanical family. *Saw Palmetto* is a commonly used herbal remedy to treat the symptoms of prostatic enlargement.
When should you use it? The **keynote** symptoms indicating the use of *Sabal Serrulata* are urinary stream obstructive problems commonly seen with prostate enlargement (benign prostatic hypertrophy), namely, hesitancy, dribbling, small stream caliber, and urinating frequently at night.
How should you use it? Give *Sabal Serrulata* 200C once daily until the urinary obstructive symptoms are decreased, then once weekly until urination has reverted to normal. Then you may wish to continue in a preventive manner, by giving *Sabal Serrulata* 200C once monthly for 6 months.

Sarsaparilla

What is it? This is the plant *Smilax ornata*, common names *Wild liquorice*, and *Smilax Medica*, a member of the *Liliaceae* botanical family. *Smilax ornata* comes from Jamaica. The swollen root (actually called a rhizome) is dried and then prepared for the homeopathic remedy.
When should you use it? The **keynote** symptoms for which you might try *Sarsaparilla* are pain and discomfort which are worse at the end of urination, just as the urine stops. *Sarsaparilla* has been used effectively in cases of bladder stones and gravel as well as in bladder infections. Some serious genital infections, notably gonorrhea, may also present with the **keynote** symptoms for *Sarsaparilla* and I would recommend it in those situations as adjunctive therapy with antibiotics. *Sarsaparilla* may be helpful in preventing recurrences of sexually transmitted disease.
How should you use it? Give *Sarsaparilla* 30C every ½-4 hours until the pains at the end of urination have receded, decreasing the frequency with improvement, stopping when they are gone. If the patient (either male or female) who is being treated for gonorrhea of the genital tract responds to *Sarsaparilla*, then I recommend that *Sarsaparilla* 200C be given once weekly for one month and then once monthly for 6 months to help in preventing recurrences.

Staphysagria

What is it? This is the plant *Delphinium staphysagria*, common name *stavesacre*, a member of the *Ranunculaceae* botanical family.
When should you use it? The **keynote** symptoms for which you might try *Staphysagria* are burning during urination but also in the urethra while not urinating, especially after medical procedures. There is also urgency to urinate (but unproductive) and a feeling that it is impossible to empty the bladder. This is the main remedy for "honeymoon cystitis." These complaints may occur in a person who does not allow herself (or himself) to express the anger that is palpable just under the surface.
How should you use it? Give *Staphysagria* 30C every ½-4 hours until the burning has receded, decreasing the frequency with improvement, stopping when it has resolved.

Uri-Control

What is it? This is a combination remedy produced by Boericke & Tafel, a homeopathic pharmaceutical supply house. *Uri-Control* contains the following ingredients in very low potencies: *Belladonna, Apis mellifica, Argentum nitricum, Cantharis, Equisetum hymale, Pulsatilla, Sarsaparilla, Causticum, Petroselinum sativum* and *Terebinthina*, in a lactose-based tablet.

When should you use it? The **keynote** symptoms helping you to choose *Uri-Control* are pain during urination, urgency, bedwetting, and incontinence.

How should you use it? Dissolve one *Uri-Control* tablet in the mouth 3-4 times daily, depending on severity of symptoms. However, you may take one tablet as often as every 5 minutes, until the pain is relieved. As soon as improvement sets in, decrease the frequency. Stop when the problem has resolved.

Bedwetting/Enuresis

What is it? This is a combination remedy produced by Luyties homeopathic pharmaceutical supply house. *Bedwetting/Enuresis* contains the following ingredients in low potencies: *Ammonium carbonica, Belladonna* and *Equisetum verbascum*.

When should you use it? The **keynote** symptoms helping you to choose *Bedwetting/Enuresis* are bedwetting at night, especially if it occurs towards morning, sometimes accompanied by coughing at night.

How should you use it? Take 1 tablet onto or under the tongue before going to bed every night.

Guidelines for Consulting Your Health Care Provider

You should consult your health care provider if:
• the patient doesn't look right or act right (trust your instincts!)
• the patient is getting worse instead of better over the course of the illness

• the patient has a sustained high fever (103°F [39.5°C] to 104°F [40°C])
• the patient has persistent loss of weight
• the patient has persistent loss of appetite
• the patient is uninterested in eating or drinking or playing
• the patient has not had a wet diaper or urinated in the past 12 hours
• the patient's eyes look sunken into her head
• the patient has severe lower abdominal pain (over the bladder)
• the patient has severe flank pain (over the kidneys) with fever
• the patient has such severe pain that you must consider kidney or bladder stone (renal colic)
• the patient has cloudy urine or urine that smells like infection
• the patient has blood in the urine
• the patient has her *first* urinary tract infection
     Note: imaging studies of the urinary tract are often recommended with the first urinary tract infection in infants and young boys and depending on the severity in young girls
• the patient is a male with a urinary tract infection
     Note: urinary tract infections in young males are uncommon and often indicate an underlying abnormality of the urinary tract that must be diagnosed and corrected so as not to cause kidney failure
• the patient has recurrent bladder infections with severe symptoms
• the patient has persistent symptoms of erectile dysfunction
• the patient has persistent undescended testicle
• the patient has acute or chronic kidney (renal) failure
• the patient is having trouble breathing or complaining of chest pains or there is mental confusion or lethargy or irritability

Remember: Patients who suffer from acute or chronic kidney (renal) failure from any cause need to be extremely cautious about taking any medication, herbal remedy, or nutritional supplement. Therefore, for these patients, homeopathy is the only self-care alternative that I would recommend. Homeopathy should be taken along with the prescription pharmaceuticals.

The same cautionary statement may be made for patients who have prostate cancer or any other cancer of the urinary tract. Self-care for persons with *any type of cancer* is also limited to homeopathy, but I strongly recommend that you use homeopathy *together* with oncology treatment(s). In that way, homeopathy may be expected to be an adjunct to a long-lasting cure.

Note: For patients who have *any type of cancer*, before taking herbal remedies or nutritional supplements please consult your health care provider, your oncology specialists, and your homeopath.

Note: Do not discontinue taking any pharmaceutical medication that has been prescribed by your health care provider unless you or your family member is under the supervision of a physician.

Recommendations for Homeopathic Remedies

Aconitum napellus 30C—in pellets and liquid drops
Apis mellifica 30C—in pellets and liquid drops
Aurum metallicum 200C—in pellets and liquid drops
Berberis vulgaris 30C—in pellets and liquid drops
Cantharis 30C—in pellets and liquid drops
Causticum 200C—in pellets
Lycopodium 200C—in pellets
Nux vomica 30C—in pellets
Phosphoric acid 200C—in pellets
Sabal serrulata 200C—in pellets
Sarsaparilla 30C and 200C—in pellets and liquid drops
Staphysagria 30C—in pellets and liquid drops
Uri-Control—tablets
Bedwetting/Enuresis—tablets

Guidelines for Administration of Homeopathic Remedies

Once you have chosen the homeopathic remedy and the potency that is likely to help you or your family member, you should try to give as few repetitions of the remedy as you can. You start off repeating it more frequently in a severe, acute situation, quickly decreasing the frequency once improvement has begun, stopping the remedy as soon as the problem has resolved.

> **Note:** For more information on *how often* to give the homeopathic remedy please see **Potency and Frequency**, in **Chapter 2: Basic Homeopathy**. For information on *how much* of the homeopathic remedy to give and the importance of a "*clean tongue*," please see **How to take homeopathic remedies** in the same chapter.

Lower potency remedies, such as 30C and below, are used to treat acute ailments. They are usually repeated often, every $\frac{1}{2}$-2 or $\frac{1}{2}$-4 hours. You should notice improvement in symptoms after just one to perhaps a few repetitions. If you do not see improvement, it is wise to stop the remedy and try a different one, guiding yourself by the **keynote** symptoms. You may use different single remedies together or you may try a combination remedy. And you may use homeopathic remedies together with pharmaceutical prescription and non-prescription drugs without any effect of interference.

General guidelines to treat serious, chronic, relapsing ailments include using single remedies at potencies of 200C. These are generally administered once weekly to once monthly, but they may be used once or twice daily at first if the condition warrants it, quickly decreasing the frequency as you see improvement. Do not continue giving the remedy if it becomes apparent that it is not working. You may always stop one remedy and choose to administer another remedy on the basis of the **keynote** symptoms of the new remedy. In addition, you may administer more than one remedy at a time.

Putting It All Together

Coping with urinary tract disorders will generally require a multi-pronged approach incorporating all the essential natural alternatives, homeopathy, herbal remedies, and nutritional supplements.

It is a good idea to consider giving the sick person's homeopathic constitutional remedy (please refer to **Chapter 9: Homeopathic Remedies for Constitutional Problems in Infants, Children, and Adolescents** or to **Chapter 18: Homeopathic Constitutional Remedies** if you are dealing with an adult).

Urinary tract ailments require all the vitamins and minerals necessary to repair and replenish tissues (please refer to **Chapter 23: Vitamins and Minerals**) as well as a general antioxidant supplement (please refer to **Chapter 24: Antioxidant Phytochemicals**).

You may want to investigate certain herbal remedies such as *Saw Palmetto* (please refer to **Chapter 20: Herbs You Need to Know**) and *Cranberry* (please refer to **Chapter 21: Herbal Remedies for Women's Health**) as well as *omega-3 fatty acids* (please refer to **Chapter 31: Oils and Fats**). You may wish to incorporate *probiotics* (please refer to **Chapter 30: Prebiotics and Probiotics**) into your daily supplements because your may find your urinary tract problems to be sensitive to enhanced gastrointestinal health.

Chapter 13

Homeopathy for Elderly Persons

Ailments in the Elderly in General

Ailment/Disorder/Symptom	Homeopathic Remedy
Sluggishness and lethargy	*Alumina*
Intellectual impairment, forgetfulness, confusion	*Ambra grisea*
Severe depression	*Aurum metallicum*
Dementia symptoms, childish reactions	*Baryta carbonica*
Physical exhaustion and collapse	*Carbo vegetalis*
Stupor, inability to concentrate or pay attention	*Helleborus niger*
Insomnia with fears of death	*Lycopodium*
Drowsiness, memory deficiencies and confusion	*Nux moschata*
Depression, emaciation	*Secale cornutum*
Dementia, exhaustion	*Selenium*
Poor memory with forgetfulness, lack of concentration	*Cerebrum Compositum N*
Slow metabolism, fatigue, and exhaustion	*Coenzyme Compositum*
Edema, lymphedema, and problems with lymphatic drainage	*Lymphomyosot*
Detoxification, sluggish metabolism with fatigue	*Ubichinon Compositum*

Guidelines for Consulting Your Health Care Provider
Putting It All Together

Ailments in the Elderly in General

Homeopathic remedies for elderly persons are usually started in potencies under 200C (such as 15C and 30C) because they are less likely to cause a homeopathic aggravation. Homeopathic aggravations may affect the elderly more so than someone younger. After the elderly person responds positively to the remedy at the starting potency, you may then decide to try a higher potency (such as 200C), but do so cautiously. If you have any concerns about increasing potencies in an elderly person that you are caring for, I recommend that you seek the help of your homeopath.

The elderly come with a special set of problems because: 1) their cellular and metabolic processes are slowing down; and 2) they may more likely have developed chronic diseases which greatly compromise their health, vitality, and longevity. If you have any hesitation in treating the elderly person under your care, I strongly recommend that you consult your health care provider. You may first want to acquaint yourself with the **Guidelines for Consulting Your Health Care Provider** at the end of this chapter.

Ailments in the elderly all too often seem to be related to senile dementia or Alzheimer's disease. Assuming that the elderly person under your care has been given a diagnosis of senile dementia from any cause, then homeopathy may be able to work with whatever reserves the patient has left to blunt the harsh consequences of that disease. You may administer homeopathic remedies along with prescription pharmaceuticals.

Elderly patients who suffer from acute or chronic diseases from any cause need to be extremely cautious about taking any pharmaceutical medication, herbal remedy, or nutritional supplement. Therefore, for these patients, homeopathy is the only self-care alternative that I would recommend. For these patients, homeopathy may be effective adjunctive treatment in concert with their prescription pharmaceuticals. In these cases, herbal remedies and nutritional supplements must be prescribed by physicians (and homeopath physicians) who are conversant with the interactions of herbal remedies and nutritional supplements with the medicines used to treat elderly patients.

You may prefer to use a *combination homeopathic remedy* to treat any of the conditions discussed in this chapter. *Combination remedies* are certainly easier to use than single remedies and are very often effective. Combination remedies will likely include many of the single remedies listed below, but in very low potencies. Using combination remedies is like taking a stab in the dark.

However, many people find that combination remedies do not work well enough so it is important to be able to use single remedies according to their **keynote** symptoms. You may always give a remedy, gauge the reaction, and if necessary, give a different remedy. You may use more than one single remedy at one time. You should have on hand those remedies for treating those **keynote** symptoms that tend to recur in you or members of your family.

As with any and all medical conditions, and more especially when dealing with the ailments in elderly people, you must pay strict attention to the **Guidelines for Consulting Your Health Care Provider** at the end of this chapter. You may want to refer to the last section **Putting It All Together** for ideas on how to integrate the essential natural alternatives, homeopathy, herbal remedies, and nutritional supplements.

Alumina

What is it? This is the chemical compound, *Aluminum oxide. Aluminum silicate* is present in the earth's crust, then becoming part of the soil, then of plants, thereby entering all living organisms. Research has not yet determined a role for *Aluminum* even though it is present in all living matter. A high tissue level of *Aluminum* has been implicated in cases of Alzheimer's disease, but researchers now do not believe it plays a causative role. The homeopathic remedy is non-toxic.

When should you use it? The **keynote** symptoms helping you to decide on *Alumina* are sluggishness and lethargy in all functions (including intellectual) with dryness of the mucus membranes, skin, and stool (with severe constipation). There may be trembling and twitching of the muscles, face, or limbs. *Alumina* is used to treat senile dementia with confusion, lethargy, intellectual impairments, and a general slowing of all responses. All movements and thinking processes are slow and deliberate. The elderly person needing *Alumina* becomes tense and anxious when being hurried.

How should you use it? Give *Alumina* 30C once daily until some improvement is achieved. Then you may wish to try *Alumina* 200C once weekly until the symptoms are stable or have abated. Then stop.

Ambra grisea

What is it? This is *Ambergris*, a product of the *Sperm whale*.

When should you use it? The **keynote** symptoms helping you to decide on *Ambra grisea* are intellectual impairment with forgetfulness, confusion, and deficits in comprehension along with shyness, easy embarrassment, and a fear of strangers. *Ambra grisea* is useful to treat senile dementia. The patient needing *Ambra grisea* may be talkative but will ask questions and then jump to another subject without waiting to hear the answers.

How should you use it? Give *Ambra grisea* 30C once daily until some improvement is achieved. Then you may wish to try *Ambra grisea* 200C once weekly until the symptoms are stable or have abated. Then stop.

Aurum metallicum

What is it? This is the element *gold*, one of the metals in the periodic table of chemicals.

When should you use it? The **keynote** symptoms leading you to consider using *Aurum metallicum* are severe depression, especially in a person with cardiovascular disease symptoms such as angina pectoris and shortness of breath. An intention to commit suicide may be expressed.

How should you use it? Give *Aurum metallicum* 30C once daily until some improvement is achieved. Then you may wish to try *Aurum metallicum* 200C once weekly until the symptoms are stable or have abated. Then stop.

Baryta carbonica

What is it? This is the poisonous mineral compound *barium carbonate*. The homeopathic remedy is non-toxic.

When should you use it? The **keynote** symptoms telling you when to choose *Baryta carbonica* are inappropriate childish reactions (emotional immaturity), difficulties making decisions, mental impairments, and a deficiency of self-confidence. *Baryta carbonica* is useful to treat senile dementia and post-stroke dementia. The elderly patient is likely to be overweight, shy, passive, with great anxiety necessitating constant reassurance. *Baryta carbonica* is very useful at the two extremes of life, infants and children and the elderly.

How should you use it? Give *Baryta carbonica* 30C once daily until some improvement is achieved. Then you may wish to try *Baryta carbonica* 200C once weekly until the symptoms are stable or have abated. Then stop.

Carbo vegetalis

What is it? This is the homeopathic remedy made from *charcoal* that is made from partially burned wood.

When should you use it? The **keynote** symptoms pointing towards using *Carbo veg* (as it is called) are physical exhaustion and collapse with weakness and coldness. *Carbo veg* is called the "corpse reviver" because it has been known to help patients on their deathbeds. Elderly patients needing *Carbo veg* are likely to crave fresh air (or air conditioning), even though they are cold, and they must sit up to get enough air because they have shortness of breath (dyspnea). These are irritable old people and they are likely to display their irritability at family members. They may have attacks of indigestion accompanied by abdominal pain, flatulence, bloating, and burping. The elderly person is likely to be emotionally lethargic and physically sluggish.

How should you use it? Give *Carbo veg* 30C once daily until some improvement is achieved. Then you may wish to try *Carbo veg* 200C once weekly until the symptoms are stable or have abated. Then stop.

Helleborus niger

What is it? This is the plant *Helleborus niger*, common names *Christmas Rose* and *Black Hellebore*, a member of the *Ranunculaceae* botanical family.

When should you use it? The **keynote** symptoms pointing you in the direction of choosing *Helleborus niger* are a severe degree of mental dullness, perhaps even stupor, with inability to concentrate or pay attention, and weak memory along with depression and decreased vision and hearing. *Helleborus niger* is often prescribed for Alzheimer's disease or other forms of dementia.

How should you use it? Give *Helleborus niger* 30C once daily until some improvement is achieved. Then you may wish to try *Helleborus niger* 200C once weekly until the symptoms are stable or have abated. Then stop.

Lycopodium

What is it? This plant is the primitive moss, *Lycopodium clavatum*, common name *Club moss*, a member of the *Lycopodiaceae* botanical family.

When should you use it? The **keynote** symptoms helping you to choose *Lycopodium* are insomnia, especially when after falling asleep they awaken full of fears, such as fear of being alone, of failure, and of death. Depression, anxieties, and worries about everything are usually present. There may be mistakes in speaking, writing, or reading. It is likely that the patient's physical ailments will be worse from 4-8 p.m. The elderly person needing *Lycopodium* lacks self-confidence and can become tyrannical with family members.

How should you use it? Give *Lycopodium* 30C once daily until some improvement is achieved. Then you may wish to try *Lycopodium* 200C once weekly until the symptoms are stable or have abated. Then stop.

Nux moschata

What is it? This is the plant *Myristica fragrans*, common name *Nutmeg*, a member of the *Myristicaceae* botanical family.

When should you use it? The **keynote** symptoms helping you to choose *Nux moschata* are memory deficiencies and confusion associated with an overwhelming drowsiness, almost to the point of stupor. The patient who needs *Nux moschata* will likely have a dry mouth and eyes and dry mucus membranes in general. *Nux moschata* is useful to treat patients with narcolepsy, Alzheimer's disease, and other dementias such as organic brain syndrome.

How should you use it? Give *Nux moschata* 30C once daily until some improvement is achieved. Then you may wish to try *Nux moschata* 200C once weekly until the symptoms are stable or have abated. Then stop.

Secale cornutum

What is it? When the fungus *Claviceps purpurea* infests *Secale cereale*, common name *Rye*, a member of the *Gramineae* botanical family, the resulting product is called *Secale cornutum*, common name *Ergot of Rye*.

When should you use it? The **keynote** symptoms indicating the use of *Secale cornutum* are emaciation in irritable, depressed, anxious people who have cognitive impairments and sleepiness.

How should you use it? Give *Secale cornutum* 30C once daily until some improvement is achieved. Then you may wish to try *Secale cornutum* 200C once weekly until the symptoms are stable or have abated. Then stop.

Selenium

What is it? This is the chemical element *Selenium* (Se).

When should you use it? The **keynote** symptoms directing you towards trying *Selenium* are weakness of the entire body and mental weakness (poor memory, mispronunciation of words) with exhaustion and lethargy. *Selenium* is sometimes indicated to treat the liver enlargement that is the result of liver diseases.

How should you use it? Give *Selenium* 30C once daily until some improvement is achieved. Then you may wish to try *Selenium* 200C once weekly until the symptoms are stable or have abated. Then stop.

Cerebrum Compositum N

What is it? This is the homeopathic combination remedy manufactured by Heel, a homeopathic supply house. The ingredients are: *Aesculus hippocastanum, Cinchona officinalis, Cocculus indicus, Conium maculatum, Gelsemium sempervirens, Ruta graveolens, Aconitum napellus, Anacardium orientale, Hyoscyamus niger, Kali bichromicum, Kali phosphoricum, Thuja occidentalis, Cerebrum suis, Ignatia amara, Manganum phosphoricum, Ambra grisea, Bothrops lanceolatus, Embryo suis, Hepar suis, Magnesia phosphorica, Phosphoricum acidum, Placenta suis, Selenium metallicum, Sulphur, Medorrhinum* and *Arnica montana radix*, in low potencies in lactose-based tablets.
When should you use it? The **keynote** symptoms pointing you towards using *Cerebrum Compositum N* are poor memory with forgetfulness, lack of concentration, mental fatigue, along with anxiety.
How should you use it? Allow 2 tablets to dissolve in the mouth 1-3 times daily depending on severity of symptoms. Discontinue when symptoms have stablized or improved.

Coenzyme Compositum

What is it? This is the homeopathic combination remedy manufactured by Heel, a homeopathic supply house. The ingredients are: *Beta vulgaris, Ascorbicum acidum, Cysteinum, Magnesium oroticum, Manganum phosphoricum, Natrum oxalaceticum, Nicotinamidum, Pulsatilla, Pyridoxinum hydrochloricum, Riboflavinum, Thiaminum hydrochloricum, Alpha-lipoicum acidum, Alpha ketoglutaricum acidum, Cerium oxalcium, Aconitum acidum, Citricum acidum, Coenzyme A, Fumaricum acidum, Malicum acidum, Naddium, Natrum pyruvicum, Succinicum acidum, Adenosine5-triphosphate, Baryta oxasuccinicum, Hepar sulphuris calcareum* and *Sulphur*, in low potencies, in lactose-based tablets.
When should you use it? The **keynote** symptoms for which you would try *Coenzyme Compositum* are slow metabolism, fatigue, and exhaustion especially from stress.

How should you use it? Allow 1 tablet to dissolve in the mouth 1-3 times daily depending on severity of symptoms. Discontinue when symptoms have stablized or improved.

Lymphomyosot

What is it? This is the homeopathic combination remedy manufactured by Heel, a homeopathic supply house. The ingredients are: *Geranium robertianum, Nasturtium aquaticum, Ferrum iodatum, Juglans reglia, Myosotis arvensis, Scrophularia nodosa, Teucrium scorodonia, Veronica officinalis, Equisetum hymenale, Fumaria officinalis, Natrum sulphuricum, Opinus sylvestris, Gentiana lutea, Aranea diadema, Sarsaparilla, Calcarea phosphorica* and *Thyroidinum*, in low potencies, in lactose-based tablets or alcohol-based liquid.
When should you use it? The **keynote** symptoms urging you to try *Lymphomyosot* are edema, lymphedema, and problems with lymphatic drainage, especially after damage to the immune system.
How should you use it? Allow 1 tablet (or 10 drops) to dissolve in the mouth 1-3 times daily depending on severity of symptoms. Discontinue when symptoms have stablized or improved. The dose is halved for infants and children to age 6 years.

Ubichinon Compositum

What is it? This is the homeopathic combination remedy manufactured by Heel, a homeopathic supply house. The ingredients are: *Colchicum autumnale, Conium maculatum, Hydrastis canadensis, Vaccinum myritillus, Podophyllum pellatum, Ascorbicum acidum, Gallium aparine, Nicotinamidum, Pryidoxinum hydrochloricum, Riboflavinum, Sarcolacticum acidum, Thiaminum hydrochloricum, Hydroquinone, Manganum phosphoricum, Alpha-lipoicum acidum, Natrum oxalaceticum, Sulphur, Acetylsalicilicum acidum, Anthraquinone, Adenosine 5-triphosphate sodium salt, Benzoquoinone, Coenzyme A, Coenzyme Q10, Histaminum, Magnesia gluconicum, Naddium, Naphthoquinone* and *Trichinoyl*, all in low potencies in lactose-based tablets.
When should you use it? The **keynote** symptoms for using *Ubichinon Compositum* are sluggish metab-

olism with fatigue and build-up of toxins, perhaps as a result of environmental exposure to toxic substances, or from improper diet. This is a gentle yet effective detoxification method. All other (non-homeopathic) detox methods are likely to be dangerous for elderly persons (as well as for infants and children and frail or sick people).

How should you use it? Allow 1 tablet to dissolve in the mouth 1-3 times daily depending on severity of symptoms. Discontinue when symptoms have improved. You may take *Ubichinon Compositum* once daily for 3 months as a general, total body detoxification.

> **Note:** Another homeopathic detoxification remedy is the *Detox-Kit*, also manufactured by Heel. It consists of 3 components, *Lymphomyosot*, *Berberis Homaccord* and *Nux vomica Homaccord*, each in a 50 ml bottle. *Lymphomyosot* detoxifies the lymphatic system; *Berberis*, the excretory organs, specifically the kidneys, skin, and liver; and *Nux vomica*, the digestive system and liver. Thus, the *Detox-Kit* provides for the elimination of diverse toxins from most sources. The directions for use are to put 30 drops of each of the three solutions into one quart of water and drink it during the day.

> **Note:** For elderly persons suffering from insomnia, *Passiflora* is a gentle remedy. It is taken as the herbal tea at bedtime and is also given as the homeopathic rememdy in low potency (6C).

Guidelines for Consulting Your Health Care Provider

You should consult your health care provider if:
- the patient doesn't look right or act right (trust your instincts!)
- the patient is getting worse instead of better over the course of the illness

- the patient is having trouble breathing or complaining of chest pains or there is mental confusion or lethargy or irritability
- the patient has persistent loss of weight
- the patient has persistent loss of appetite
- the patient has become combative or aggressive
- the patient has become apathetic or indifferent or has lost interest in her surroundings
- the patient has developed difficulties with feeding him/herself or with eating
- the patient's medical condition(s) seems to be worsening
- the patient is having difficulties with insomnia or other vital functions

> **Remember:** Self-care for elderly persons with *any type of cancer* is also limited to homeopathy, but I strongly recommend that you use homeopathy *together* with oncology treatment(s). In that way, homeopathy may be expected to be an adjunct to a long-lasting cure.
>
> For patients who have *any type of cancer*, before taking herbal remedies or nutritional supplements please consult your health care provider, your oncology specialists, and your homeopath.

> **Note:** Do not discontinue taking any pharmaceutical medication that has been prescribed by your health care provider unless you or your family member is under the supervision of a physician.

> **Note:** Shingles, an infection with Herpes Zoster virus, can be painful and prolonged in elderly people. *Ranunculus bulbosus* is the main homeopathic remedy that treats the pain and itching of shingles and foreshortens the illness.

Recommendations For Homeopathic Remedies
Alumina 30C and 200C—in pellets and liquid drops
Ambra grisea 30C and 200C—in pellets and liquid drops
Aurum metallicum 30C and 200C—in pellets and liquid drops

Baryta carbonica 30C and 200C—in pellets and liquid drops

Carbo vegetalis 30C and 200C—in pellets and liquid drops

Helleborus niger 30C and 200C—in pellets and liquid drops

Lycopodium 30C and 200C—in pellets and liquid drops

Nux moschata 30C and 200C—in pellets and liquid drops

Secale cornutum 30C and 200C—in pellets and liquid drops

Selenium 30C and 200C—in pellets and liquid drops

Cerebrum Compositum N—in tablets

Coenzyme Compositum—in tablets

Lymphomyosot—in tablets and liquid drops

Ubichinon Compositum—in tablets

Guidelines for Administration of Homeopathic Remedies

The recommended potency of the constitutional homeopathic remedy will likely be 200C. I recommend that you start off once or twice weekly, depending on the severity of the situation or condition, and then quickly decrease the repetitions of the remedy once you notice improvement, stopping the remedy as soon as the problem has resolved and good health restored.

Once you have chosen the homeopathic remedy and the potency that is likely to help you or your family member, you should try to give as few repetitions of the remedy as you can. You start off repeating it more frequently in a severe, acute situation, quickly decreasing the frequency once improvement has begun, stopping the remedy as soon as the problem has resolved.

> **Note:** For more information on *how often* to give the homeopathic remedy please see **Potency and Frequency**, in **Chapter 2: Basic Homeopathy**. For information on *how much* of the homeopathic remedy to give and the importance of a *"clean tongue,"* please see **How to take homeopathic remedies** in the same chapter.

Lower potency remedies, such as 30C and below, are used to treat acute ailments. They are usually repeated often, every ½-2 or ½-4 hours. You should notice improvement in symptoms after just one to perhaps a few repetitions. If you do not see improvement, it is wise to stop the remedy and try a different one, guiding yourself by the **keynote** symptoms. You may use different single remedies together or you may try a combination remedy. And you may use homeopathic remedies together with pharmaceutical prescription and non-prescription drugs without any effect of interference.

General guidelines to treat serious, chronic, relapsing ailments include using single remedies at potencies of 200C. These are generally administered once weekly to once monthly, but they may be used once or twice daily at first if the condition warrants it, quickly decreasing the frequency as you see improvement. Do not continue giving the remedy if it becomes apparent that it is not working. You may always stop one remedy and choose to administer another remedy on the basis of the **keynote** symptoms of the new remedy. In addition, you may administer more than one remedy at a time.

Putting It All Together

Coping with problems of the elderly will generally require a multi-pronged approach incorporating all the essential natural alternatives, homeopathy, herbal remedies, and nutritional supplements.

It is a good idea to consider giving the sick person's homeopathic constitutional remedy (please refer to **Chapter 18: Homeopathic Constitutional Remedies**).

Sick elderly people generally require all the vitamins and minerals necessary to repair and replenish tissues (please refer to **Chapter 23: Vitamins and Minerals**) as well as a general antioxidant supplement (please refer to **Chapter 24: Antioxidant Phytochemicals**).

You may want to investigate certain herbal remedies such as *Ginkgo biloba* and *Ginseng* (please refer to **Chapter 20: Herbs You Need to Know**) as well as *omega-3 fatty acids* (please refer to **Chapter 31: Oils and Fats**). You will need to incorporate *probiotics* (please refer to **Chapter 30: Prebiotics and Probiotics**) into your daily supplements because most elderly people benefit from enhanced gastrointestinal health.

Healthy nutrition goes hand-in-hand with longevity. If you want to prevent or treat most of the chronic ailments that beset the elderly in this century, you will need to learn about healthy nutrition. Please read the nutritional advice in **Chapter 27: Nutritional Supplements to Prevent Cancer and Augment Your Immune System; Chapter 26: Nutritional Supplements for Healthy Weight Control** and **Chapter 24: Antioxidant Phytochemicals**.

Depending on the nature of the elderly person's ailment, you may need to consult the following chapters:

Chapter 14

Homeopathy for Problems in Joints, Bones and Muscles

Musculoskeletal Problems in General

Ailment/Disorder/Symptom	Homeopathic Remedy
Pains relieved by lying on the affected part	*Bryonia alba*
Joint pains and stiffness, low back pain	*Calcarea carbonica*
Osteoporosis with weak, brittle, soft bones	*Calcarea fluorica*
Growing pains, non-union of fractures	*Calcarea phosphorica*
Wandering joint pains	*Pulsatilla*
Joint pains worse in wet weather	*Rhododendron*
Joint pains and stiffness	*Rhus toxicodendron*
Muscle and joint pains and stiffness	*Pain Erase*
Pain and stiffness in muscles and joints	*Triflora Arthritis Gel*
Osteoarthritis, joint pain and stiffness	*Zeel*

Guidelines for Consulting Your Health Care Provider
Putting It All Together

Musculoskeletal Problems in General

The ailments that afflict joints, bones, and muscles are often responsive to treatment with homeopathic remedies, but usually will also require nutritional supplements to affect a long-lasting cure. This is a good example of how using essential natural alternatives from two domains together, namely homeopathy and nutritional supplements, may act in synergy to strengthen the positive treatment response.

Problems in joints, bones, and muscles are often categorized as musculoskeletal ailments. In this category you will find such ailments as: arthritis (including osteoarthritis, gout, and rheumatoid arthritis), osteoporosis (and bone decalcification that is less severe called osteopenia), bone spurs (exostoses), low back pain, fibromyalgia, and carpal tunnel syndrome, as well as many other less common problems.

Fibromyalgia is a poorly understood condition consisting of a debilitating constellation of symptoms affecting women six times more frequently than men. Due to the complex nature of fibromyalgia, it may be prudent to seek the services of your homeopath. However, be assured that medical research has found that fibromyalgia patients taking homeopathic treatment showed significantly greater improvements in pain and quality of life that those on placebo.

The symptoms that are associated with joint inflammation are pain and stiffness (sometimes worse in the morning) leading to decreased mobility, and hot, red, or swollen joints (sometimes with bony deformities). There is solid medical evidence that the homeopathic treatment of joint disorders is more effective when compared to placebo.

When dealing with problems in joints, bones, and muscles, it is probably wise to obtain a firm diagnosis first from your health care practitioner. Some life-threatening conditions (such as cancer) may masquerade as arthritic pain in joints, bones, and muscles.

Oftentimes patients are already using *NSAIDS* (nonsteroidal anti-inflammatory drugs, such as *ibuprofen*, or *naproxen*) or *COX-2 inhibitors* (*Celebrex*) to ease the pain of arthritis (as well as many other musculoskeletal problems). Homeopathic remedies may be used as adjunctive alternatives along with medications. When the homeopathic remedy (or remedies) takes effect the patient may be ready to stop the medication. (Tapering of *NSAIDs* or *COX-2 inhibitors* is not required).

Joints, bones, and muscles (along with tendons and ligaments) are the movers in our bodies that allow us to perform all our daily motor activities. It is not enough to use homeopathy, nutritional supplements, and prescription medications to treat the ailments of these organs. It is absolutely essential to perform daily physical activity. This, by itself, is the single most important thing you can do for the health of your musculoskeletal system.

If you are not a regular performer of daily physical activity, you must start now. Start slowly, just 5 minutes a day. Choose some form of low-impact physical activity that you enjoy, such as walking, dancing, aerobics, or swimming. Increase by one-minute intervals whenever you are able without feeling pain or becoming exhausted. After 3 or 4 months you will be able to perform $\frac{1}{2}$-1 hour of daily physical activity. Then you should begin to consider the various forms of physical activity, such as flexibility and balance exercises, aerobic exercises, and weight training. They should all have a place in your daily routine. For more information, visit The Arthritis Foundation at www.arthritis.org.

Although this book does not delve into the specifics of a healthy daily diet in each chapter, nutrition is of great importance in treating and preventing ailments of the musculoskeletal system. Elements of the *Mediterranean diet* are recommended by the *American Institute for Cancer Research* (*AICR*) for optimal health, not only for persons with cancer. The *Mediterranean diet*, when compared to the *Western diet*, contains less red meat and less animal protein in general, more fruits and vegetables, nuts, and legumes. The main protein source in the *Mediterranean diet* is legumes and whole grains. *Olive oil* is the preferred oil for cooking and salads.

You may prefer to use a *combination homeopathic remedy* to treat any of the conditions discussed in this chapter. *Combination remedies* are certainly easier to use than single remedies and are very often effective. Combination remedies will likely include many of the single remedies listed below, but in very low potencies. Using combination remedies is like taking a stab in the dark.

However, many people find that combination remedies do not work well enough so it is important to be able to use single remedies according to their **keynote** symptoms. You may always give a remedy, gauge the reaction, and if necessary, give a different remedy. You may use more than one single remedy at one time. You should have on hand those remedies for treating those **keynote** symptoms that tend to recur in you or members of your family.

As with any and all medical conditions, when dealing with joints, bones, and muscles you must pay strict attention to the **Guidelines for Consulting Your Health Care Provider** at the end of this chapter. You may want to refer to the last section **Putting It All Together** for ideas on how to integrate the essential natural alternatives, homeopathy, herbal remedies, and nutritional supplements.

Bryonia alba

What is it? This is the plant *Bryonia alba*, common name *wild hops*, a member of the *Cucurbitaceae* botanical family.

When should you use it? The **keynote** symptoms pointing the way towards trying *Bryonia* are pain (often severe and sharp or stabbing) that accompanies every movement and which may develop slowly over time. There may be some relief from firm pressure on the affected part (or lying still on the part). *Bryonia* is useful for acute joint pains from any cause that are aggravated by motion.

How should you use it? Give *Bryonia* 30C every 1-4 hours for acute pain, decreasing the frequency as soon as improvement is noted. Stop when the pains have resolved.

Calcarea carbonica

What is it? This is the chemical mineral compound *calcium carbonate* which is obtained from oyster shells.

When should you use it? The **keynote** symptoms guiding you towards trying *Calcarea carbonica* are pains and stiffness in joints or bones or slow development of bones or teeth. *Calcarea carbonica* is useful to treat low back pain, especially in overweight, fearful women who have a tendency towards constipation. It is also useful when a fracture is slow to heal, or when osteopenia (early thinning of bone) or

osteoporosis (more severe loss of bone density) has been diagnosed.

How should you use it? Give *Calcarea carbonica* 30C every 2-4 hours for acute joint, bone or teeth pain, rapidly decreasing the frequency to once daily with improvement. Then consider giving *Calcarea carbonica* 200C once weekly for 4 weeks, then once monthly for 6 months, to prevent recurrent episodes.

Calcarea fluorica

What is it? This is the chemical compound *calcium fluoride* present in bones and teeth.

When should you use it? The **keynote** symptoms suggesting that you consider using *Calcarea fluorica* are weak, brittle, or soft bones sometimes accompanied by curvatures and deformities. This is an important remedy to treat osteopenia and osteoporosis as well as bony spurs (exostoses) and scoliosis (curvature of the spine).

How should you use it? Give *Calcarea fluorica* 200C once weekly until some relief is noted, then once monthly for 6 months, to prevent recurrent episodes.

Calcarea phosphorica

What is it? This is the chemical mineral compound *calcium phosphate*, an essential component of bones and teeth, making them strong.

When should you use it? The **keynote** symptoms helping you to elect *Calcarea phosphorica* are pains and stiffness in the bones and joints, or tooth pain (from decay). *Calcarea phosphorica* is especially useful to treat "growing pains" and non-union of fractures. Infants and children who may need Calcarea phosphorica may have delayed, painful teeth eruption or delayed walking.

How should you use it? Give *Calcarea phosphorica* 30C every 2-4 hours for acute bone or teeth pain, rapidly decreasing the frequency to once daily with improvement. Then consider giving *Calcarea phosphorica* 200C once weekly for 4 weeks, then once monthly for 6 months, to prevent recurrent episodes.

Pulsatilla

What is it? This is the plant *Pulsatilla nigricans*, whose common name is *windflower*, a member of the *Ranunculaceae* botanical family.

When should you use it? The **keynote** symptoms signaling that *Pulsatilla* might be useful are wandering pains that go from joint to joint or side to side, especially when the pains are made worse from applications of warmth. A person needing *Pulsatilla* (usually but not always female) tends to have a shy, timid, yielding, gentle disposition.

How should you use it? Give *Pulsatilla* 30C every 2-4 hours for acute joint pain, rapidly decreasing the frequency to once daily with improvement. Then consider giving *Pulsatilla* 200C once weekly for 4 weeks, then once monthly for 6 months, to prevent recurrent episodes.

Rhododendron

What is it? This is the plant *Rhododendron chrysanthum*, common name *Snow Rose* a member of the *Ericaceae* botanical family.

When should you use it? The **keynote** symptoms guiding you towards trying *Rhododendron* are arthritic pains, especially when the pains are made worse before wet weather and thunderstorms, with swellings in the small joints. *Rhododendron* may be useful to treat gout and rheumatism.

How should you use it? Give *Rhododendron* 30C every 2-4 hours for acute bone or teeth pain, rapidly decreasing the frequency to once daily with improvement. Then consider giving *Rhododendron* 200C once weekly for 4 weeks, then once monthly for 6 months, to prevent recurrent episodes.

Rhus toxicodendron

What is it? The botanical name for this plant is *Rhus toxicodendron*, common name *poison ivy*, a member of the *Anacardiaceae* botanical family.

When should you use it? The **keynote** symptoms determining your use of *Rhus tox* (as it is commonly called) are joint pains and stiffness which are worse on first starting to move, then getting better after continued movement. *Rhus tox* is the most commonly prescribed homeopathic remedy for arthritic pains. Persons needing *Rhus tox* typically experience "morning stiffness" which reverts to improved mobility after moving around a bit. These people tend to need to change their position often, making them restless. *Rhus tox* may help arthritic pains and stiffness when they worsen in wet, cold weather. Sometimes people who need *Rhus tox* are irritable and depressed because of the long-standing pain.

How should you use it? The instructions for use of *Rhus tox*, either for joint and muscle or skin problems, are different from the others in this chapter. It is my experience that *Rhus tox* works best in the 200C potency, even for acute conditions. Administer *Rhus tox* 200C 2-4 times a day until the symptoms improve, rapidly decreasing the frequency to once daily, and then stop when the pain and stiffness are gone.

Pain Erase

What is it? This is a homeopathic combination remedy manufactured by Harbor Health (www.harborhealth.com or 1-888-851-9090). It consists of *Agaricus muscaris*, *Arnica montana*, *Nux vomica*, *Rhododendron* and *Rhus toxicodendron*, all in low 5C potency.

When should you use it? The **keynote** symptoms pointing you towards trying *Pain Erase* are joint pain and stiffness and/or muscles aches and pains.

How should you use it? *Pain Erase* comes in liquid drops for oral administration. Take 10 drops 3 times daily. *Pain Erase* also comes in a topical liquid but this preparation is not homeopathic but rather contains herbal remedies and medicinal oils. You may use both the topical and the oral forms together.

Triflora Arthritis Gel

What is it? This combination homeopathic remedy is a topical gel produced by Boericke & Tafel, a homeopathic pharmaceutical supply house. The ingredients are as follows, all in very low potency: *Symphytum officinale*, *Rhus toxicodendron* and *Ledum palustre*, in a witch hazel base with an herbal fragrance.

When should you use it? The **keynote** symptoms pointing you towards trying *Triflora Arthritis Gel* are stiffness in the muscles and joints with aches and pains. It is useful to treat backache, arthritis, and rheumatism.

How should you use it? Massage into the affected area 1-4 times daily. *Triflora Arthritis Gel* is not recommended for children under the age of 2 years.

Zeel

What is it? This combination homeopathic remedy is manufactured by Heel, a homeopathic pharmaceutical supply house. The ingredients in Zeel are: *Silicea, Rhus toxicodendron, Arnica montana, Dulcamara, Symphytum officinale, Sanguinaria canadensis, Sulphur, Acidum silicicum, Natrum oxalaceticum, Cartilago suis, Embryo totalis suis, Funiculus umbilicalis suis, Placenta suis, Alpha Lipoicum acidum* and *Coenzyme A*, all in low potencies.

When should you use it? The **keynote** symptoms pointing you towards trying *Zeel* are the pain and stiffness characteristic of osteoarthritis of the knee, hip, or fingers. The German medical literature contains research that shows that *Zeel* works as well as pharmaceutical anti-inflammatory medicines like NSAIDs and COX-2 inhibitors. *Zeel* probably specifically affects joint cartilage.

How should you use it? Allow one tablet of *Zeel* to dissolve on or under your tongue 3-4 times daily for acute pain, decreasing the frequency when you have less pain and stiffness. You may want to take one tablet once daily for a few weeks after the acute episode. *Zeel* also comes in ointment form for topical use.

Guidelines for Consulting Your Health Care Provider

You should consult your health care provider if:
- the patient doesn't look right or act right (trust your instincts!)
- the patient is getting worse instead of better over the course of the illness
- the patient is having trouble breathing or complaining of chest pains or there is mental confusion or lethargy or irritability
- the patient has not yet had a diagnostic evaluation and only assumes that the pains in joints, bones, or muscles are due to arthritis or "growing pains"
- the patient has persistent loss of weight
- the patient has persistent loss of appetite

> **Note:** Do not discontinue taking any pharmaceutical medication that has been prescribed by your health care provider unless you or your family member is under the supervision of a physician.

Recommendations for Homeopathic Remedies
Bryonia alba 30C—pellets
Calcarea carbonica 30C and 200C—pellets
Calcarea fluorica 200C—pellets
Calcarea phosphorica 30C and 200C—pellets
Pulsatilla 30C and 200C—pellets
Rhododendron 30C and 200C—pellets
Rhus toxicodendron 200C—pellets
Triflora Arthritis Gel—topical gel
Zeel—combination remedy by Heel, tablets and
    topical ointment

Guidelines for Administration of Homeopathic Remedies
Once you have chosen the homeopathic remedy and the potency that is likely to help you or your family member, you should try to give as few repetitions of the remedy as you can. You start off repeating it more frequently in a severe, acute situation, quickly decreasing the frequency once improvement has begun, stopping the remedy as soon as the problem has resolved.

> **Note:** For more information on *how often* to give the homeopathic remedy please see **Potency and Frequency**, in **Chapter 2: Basic Homeopathy**. For information on how much of the homeopathic remedy to give and the importance of a "*clean*

tongue," please see **How to take homeo-pathic remedies** in the same chapter.

Lower potency remedies, such as 30C and below, are used to treat acute ailments. They are usually repeated often, every ½-2 or ½-4 hours. You should notice improvement in symptoms after just one to perhaps a few repetitions. If you do not see improvement, it is wise to stop the remedy and try a different one, guiding yourself by the **keynote** symptoms. You may use different single remedies together or you may try a combination remedy. And you may use homeopathic remedies together with pharmaceutical prescription and non-prescription drugs without any effect of interference.

General guidelines to treat serious, chronic, relapsing ailments include using single remedies at potencies of 200C. These are generally administered once weekly to once monthly, but they may be used once or twice daily at first if the condition warrants it, quickly decreasing the frequency as you see improvement. Do not continue giving the remedy if it becomes apparent that it is not working. You may always stop one remedy and choose to administer another remedy on the basis of the **keynote** symptoms of the new remedy. In addition, you may administer more than one remedy at a time.

Putting It All Together

Coping with diseases of joints, bones, and muscles will generally require a multi-pronged approach incorporating all the essential natural alternatives, homeopathy, herbal remedies, and nutritional supplements.

It is a good idea to consider giving the sick person's homeopathic constitutional remedy (please refer to **Chapter 9: Homeopathic Remedies for Constitutional Problems in Infants, Children, and Adolescents** or to **Chapter 18: Homeopathic Constitutional Remedies** if you are dealing with an adult).

Ailments of joints, bones, and muscles require all the vitamins and minerals necessary to repair and replenish tissues (please refer to **Chapter 23: Vitamins and Minerals**) as well as a general antioxidant supplement (please refer to **Chapter 24: Antioxidant Phytochemicals**).

Please read **Chapter 28: Nutritional Supplements for Diseases of Joints, Bones and Muscles** and decide if you want to incorporate any of these nutritional supplements into your daily life.

You may want to investigate certain herbal remedies such as *Green tea* (please refer to **Chapter 20: Herbs You Need to Know**) as well as *omega-3 fatty acids* (please refer to **Chapter 31: Oils and Fats**). You may wish to incorporate *probiotics* (please refer to **Chapter 30: Prebiotics and Probiotics**) into your daily supplements because your may find your joints, bones, and muscle problems to be sensitive to enhanced gastrointestinal and immune systems health.

Diseases of joints, bones, and muscles sometimes overlap with neurologic diseases. If this is true for you, then you may want to investigate **Chapter 16: Homeopathy for Neurologic Disorders** and **Chapter 29: Nutritional Supplements for Neurologic Disorders**.

Chapter 15

Homeopathy for Eating Disorders and Weight Control

Eating Disorders in General

Ailment/Disorder/Symptom	Homeopathic Remedy
Overweight, obesity, excessive appetite	*Antimonium crudum*
Refusal to eat normal amount, perfectionism	*Arsenicum album*
Abdominal obesity	*Calcarea carbonica*
Obesity, binge eating disorder	*Capsicum annuum*
Bingeing in young children	*Carcinosin*
Bingeing on large quantities of food alternating with loss of appetite, and periodic vomiting	*Ferrum metallicum*
Overweight, obesity, sluggish metabolism	*Graphites*
Intentional caloric restriction with exhaustion	*Ignatia*
Overeating, craving sweets	*Lycopodium*
Bingeing after sadness	*Natrum muriaticum*
Night eating with insomnia and depression	*Phosphorus*
Bulimia nervosa and anorexia nervosa	*Phytolacca decandra*
Refusal to eat after sadness	*Platina*
Food cravings	*Appetite and Weight Control*
Overeating, binge eating, bingeing and then vomiting	*Eating Disorders*
Overeating, overweight, obesity	*Weight Loss XL*

Guidelines for Consulting Your Health Care Provider
Putting It All Together

Eating Disorders in General

Feeding and eating are vital functions of the human being, necessary for survival. Yet, in today's world, there are many people who have lost control of the whole process, so much so that their feeding and eating habits are *disordered*. Disordered eating is one of the prerequisites of an eating disorder. Disordered eating occurs when a person eats too much (or too little), too often (or too infrequently), too fast (or too slowly), while eating in secret and making unhealthy food choices.

All too frequently disordered eating becomes an eating disorder. Eating disorders, considered psychiatric ailments, come in at least 4 forms: anorexia nervosa, bulimia nervosa, binge eating disorder and night eating disorder. Eating disorders are not really about food. Rather, food abuse is a proxy for a different problem. It's most often that something serious has gone awry in one's emotional life. All too often she (or he) feels a loss of control. This translates into controlling one's food intake or body weight and shape. Food abuse becomes a coping mechanism (and a particularly poor one) for emotional trauma of most any nature.

Obesity is sometimes considered to be another form of eating disorder (although it is not included in psychiatric ailments). Obesity is often times the unhappy outcome of certain eating disorders, most especially binge eating disorder (or compulsive overeating). Obesity tends to occur in the fertile interplay of our out-of-control, food-based culture, our sedentary lifestyles, and our incessant media messages about food. Obesity most often becomes a chronic, relapsing disease with frequent exacerbations over a lifetime.

Eating disorders and obesity share a common causality. Any of these ailments may occur in a person when three basic factors converge:
1) there is an inherited tendency or vulnerability in the brain neurotransmitter chemistry (called serotonin dysfunction) that predisposes towards an eating disorder or obesity;
2) there are environmental or cultural factors encouraging or triggering disordered eating, eating disorders, and obesity;
3) there are psychological factors in the

person's personal history that predispose towards disordered eating, eating disorders, and obesity.

Sometimes the disordered eating, or the eating disorder, or the overweight or even the obesity is not yet ingrained and can be corrected with heeding the proper (*ordered*) eating rules of behavior along with *daily physical activity*. It is at these times that homeopathy can be of most help.

Disordered eating, the eating disorders, as well as overweight and obesity can be helped by lifestyle changes. First and foremost, a program of *daily physical activity* is required. If you are not a regular performer of daily physical activity, you must start now. Start slowly, just 5 minutes a day. Choose some form of low-impact physical activity that you enjoy, such as walking, dancing, aerobics, or swimming. Increase by one-minute intervals whenever you are able without feeling pain or becoming exhausted. After 3 or 4 months you will be able to perform $1/2$-1 hour (goal) of *daily physical activity*. Then you should begin to consider the various forms of physical activity, such as flexibility and coordination exercises, aerobic exercises, and weight training. They should all have a place in your daily routine.

The second most important lifestyle change is *daily nutrition. Healthy eating* over the long-term is the only option because dieting does not work. In fact, diets tend to make the dieter fatter and fatter over the long-term. The widespread dieting of the American public is one of the reasons that every time a survey is taken it shows that we along with our children are gaining in girth and unhealthy fat.

In addition, if you are attempting to alter one family member's daily nutrition program towards healthier eating, it is imperative that the entire family adopts the new routine. Otherwise, the lone person's quest for healthy eating is likely doomed to failure.

The third most important factor helping to make changes that will influence feeding and eating behaviors as well lead towards a healthy body weight is homeopathy. Homeopathic remedies are useful to help prevent food cravings and increase metabolism. They are also employed to prevent relapse which, in the case of the treatment of obesity, is known to occur in as much as 95% of persons who have lost weight.

Disorders of feeding and eating are an example of how combining homeopathy with nutritional supplements and herbal remedies will be more effective than using only one of those three essential natural alternatives alone.

You may prefer to use a *combination homeopathic remedy* to treat any of the conditions discussed in this chapter. *Combination remedies* are certainly easier to use than single remedies and are very often effective. Combination remedies will likely include many of the single remedies listed below, but in very low potencies. Using combination remedies is like taking a stab in the dark.

Do not attempt to treat persons with well-established eating disorders by yourself. You will need diagnostic testing and supervision from your health care provider. You may choose to supplement your health care provider's suggestions with recommendation from this chapter and **Chapter 26: Nutritional Supplements for Healthy Weight Control**.

If you or your family member has a well-established eating disorder, I recommend that you familiarize yourself with the signs and symptoms of eating disorders. It is also important that you seek consultation from a licensed psychologist and certified nutritionist and that you check to make sure that their subspecialty is the treatment of eating disorders.

As with any and all medical conditions, when dealing with overweight, obesity, or eating disorders you must pay strict attention to the **Guidelines for Consulting Your Health Care Provider** at the end of this chapter. You may want to refer to the last section **Putting It All Together** for ideas on how to integrate the essential natural alternatives, homeopathy, herbal remedies, and nutritional supplements.

Antimonium crudum

What is it? This is the chemical compound *sulphide of antimony*, occurring naturally as *stibnite*. The chemical symbol is Sb.

When should you use it? The **keynote** symptoms recommending the use of *Antimonium crudum* are overweight or obesity in persons whose excessive appetites may be caused by emotional upsets. *Antimonium crudum* is often called the remedy for "the greedy pig," although persons who need *Antimonium crudum* tend not to overeat on sweets. They tend to have a thickly coated white tongue.

How should you use it? Give *Antimonium crudum* 200C once weekly until some improvement in overeating is seen. Then give *Antimonium crudum* 200C once monthly for 6 months to help prevent relapse. Then stop.

Arsenicum album

What is it? This is the homeopathic remedy made from the chemical compound *arsenic oxide* which is highly poisonous if not given in homeopathic dilution. *Arsenicum album* is one of homeopathy's often-used polychrests or constitutional remedies. *Arsenicum album* is also useful to treat emotional disorders.

When should you use it? The **keynote** symptoms leading you to choose *Arsenicum album* is refusal to eat a normal amount and/or variety of food with perfectionism as the prominent personality trait. This is often present in persons with anorexia nervosa.

How should you use it? Give *Arsenicum album* 200C once weekly until some improvement in refusal to eat is seen. Then give *Arsenicum album* 200C once monthly for 6 months to help prevent relapse. Then stop.

Calcarea carbonica

What is it? This is the chemical mineral compound *calcium carbonate* which is obtained from oyster shells. *Calcarea carbonica* is a polychrest constitutional remedy and is also an important homeopathic remedy for emotional ailments and for ailments in infants, children, and adolescents.

When should you use it? The **keynote** symptoms of *Calcarea carbonica* are overweight or obesity in both men and women who tend to have relatively large heads and wide abdominal girths. Persons needing *Calcarea carbonica* are likely to be clumsy, plodding, sluggish and lethargic, not very interested in physical activity. They may have cravings for chocolate, carbohydrates, and sweets. They tend to have many fears, such as fear of death, cancer, going insane, poverty, and the dark.

How should you use it? Give *Calcarea carbonica* 200C once weekly until some improvement in overweight or obesity is seen. Then give *Calcarea carbonica* 200C once monthly for 6 months to help prevent relapse. Then stop.

Capsicum annuum

What is it? This is the plant *Capsicum annuum*, common name *chili pepper* or *red cayenne pepper*, a member of the *Solanaceae* botanical family.

When should you use it? The **keynote** symptoms recommending that you choose *Capsicum* are overweight or obesity in persons who have a tendency to overeat to the point of feeling the abdomen is so distended so as to be "bursting," something that is common in binge eating disorder. *Capsicum* helps people who favor eating spicy foods and consequently suffer burning pains from heartburn and reflux. *Capsicum* may be useful for people who do not engage in physical activity. One of the peculiar symptoms that *Capsicum* may help to alleviate is homesickness.

How should you use it? Give *Capsicum* 200C once weekly until some improvement in control of eating occurs. Then give *Capsicum* 200C once monthly for 6 months to help prevent relapse. Then stop.

Carcinosin

What is it? This is a homeopathic remedy prepared from cancerous breast tissue. However, as a homeopathic remedy, it is useful for many different ailments beyond cancer, for which it is commonly used.

When should you use it? The **keynote** symptoms indicating the use of *Carcinosin* are bingeing on food in young children. *Carcinosin* is the prime homeopathic remedy to think of whenever bingeing occurs at such a tender, young age that it startles you.

How should you use it? Give *Carcinosin* 200C once weekly until some improvement in control of bingeing behavior occurs. Then give *Carcinosin* 200C once

monthly for 6 months to help prevent relapse. Then stop.

Ferrum metallicum

What is it? This is the chemical metal element, iron, also called *ferrous*. The chemical symbol is Fe.

When should you use it? The **keynote** symptoms signaling the use of *Ferrum metallicum* are emaciation, weakness, coldness, anemia, bingeing on large quantities of food alternating with loss of appetite, and periodic vomiting. *Ferrum metallicum* may be useful to treat bulimia and anorexia nervosa alternating with bulimia.

How should you use it? Give *Ferrum metallicum* 200C once weekly until some improvement in symptoms is seen. Then give *Ferrum metallicum* 200C once monthly for 6 months to help prevent relapse. Then stop.

Graphites

What is it? This is the homeopathic remedy made from *graphite*, also called *plumbago* or *black lead*, used to make lead pencils and as a lubricant. It is a naturally occurring soft carbon, a mineral.

When should you use it? The **keynote** symptoms suggesting the use of *Graphites* are overweight females (occasionally males) with excessive appetites, sluggish metabolism, lethargic, indecisive temperaments, and dry, cracked skin. For persons with cracking behind the ears, there may be oozing of honey-like discharges.

How should you use it? Give *Graphites* 200C once weekly until general energy is improved and eating is under control. Then give *Graphites* 200C once monthly for 6 months to help prevent relapse. Then stop.

Ignatia

What is it? This is the plant *Ignatia amara*, common name *St. Ignatius's bean*, a member of the *Loganiaceae* botanical family.

When should you use it? The **keynote** symptoms indicating the use of *Ignatia* are starving from intentional restriction of calories along with exhaustion. This is commonly seen in patients with anorexia nervosa.

How should you use it? Give *Ignatia* 200C once weekly until general energy is improved and caloric restriction has improved. Then give *Ignatia* 200C once monthly for 6 months to help prevent relapse. Then stop.

Lycopodium

What is it? This plant is the primitive moss, *Lycopodium clavatum*, common name *Club moss*, a member of the *Lycopodiaceae* botanical family.

When should you use it? The **keynote** symptoms helping you to choose *Lycopodium* are irritability when kept waiting for their food, with complaints of feeling empty even after finishing a meal. Persons needing *Lycopodium* may eat two (or more) full meals at a sitting. These people are likely to suffer from a large amount of abdominal gas. The person who may need *Lycopodium* tends to be arrogant to cover his/her sense of inferiority. They crave sweets.

How should you use it? Give *Lycopodium* 200C once weekly until the overeating has improved. Then give *Lycopodium* 200C once monthly for 6 months to help prevent relapse. Then stop.

Natrum muriaticum

What is it? This is the polychrest *Natrum muriaticum*, a homeopathic remedy made from common table salt. *Natrum muriaticum* is a polychrest constitutional remedy.

When should you use it? The **keynote** symptoms pointing towards the use of *Natrum muriaticum* are bingeing on large quantities of food with sadness as the trigger for bingeing.

How should you use it? Give *Natrum muriaticum* 200C once weekly until the bingeing has improved. Then give *Natrum muriaticum* 200C once monthly for 6 months to help prevent relapse. Then stop.

Phosphorus

What is it? This is the homeopathic remedy that is made from the non-metallic chemical element *Phosphorus*. It is one of the commonest elements in the human body because it makes up part of ATP (adenosine triphosphate), the chemical that stores our energy. *Phosphorus* is a polychrest constitutional remedy.

When should you use it? The **keynote** symptoms for homeopathic *Phosphorus* is elements of the night eating syndrome, such as consuming most of one's calories during nighttime hours, awakening in the early morning hours to eat, not eating breakfast, insomnia, and depression.

How should you use it? Give *Phosphorus* 200C once weekly until the elements night eating syndrome have improved. Then give *Phosphorus* 200C once monthly for 6 months to help prevent relapse. Then stop.

Phytolacca decandra

What is it? This is the plant *Phytolacca decandra*, common name *Pokeroot*, a member of the *Phytolaccaceae* family.

When should you use it? The **keynote** symptoms guiding you towards trying *Phytolacca* are enlargements of the parotid and submaxillary glands as is seen in patients with bulimia nervosa. *Phytolacca* may be helpful in cases of emaciation due to refusal to eat, such as occurs in anorexia nervosa. When *Phytolacca* berries are eaten by birds they tend to become emaciated. This observation has led to using *Phytolacca* as the homeopathic remedy to cause slimming in persons who are obese. *Phytolacca* is an important homeopathic remedy for any and all breast problems.

How should you use it? Give *Phytolacca* 200C once weekly until the bulimia or emaciation has improved. Then give *Phytolacca* 200C once monthly for 6 months to help prevent relapse. Then stop.

Platina

What is it? This is homeopathic *Platinum metallicum*, commonly called *Platina*. As the homeopathic remedy, it is most commonly used for ailments of the female reproductive tract.

When should you use it? The **keynote** symptoms of *Platina* are refusal to eat and easy satiety after just a few bites with sadness as the trigger. This constellation of symptoms may be found in persons with anorexia nervosa.

How should you use it? Give *Platina* 200C once weekly until the refusal to eat, easy satiety, and sadness have improved. Then give *Platina* 200C once monthly for 6 months to help prevent relapse. Then stop.

Appetite and Weight Control

What is it? This is a combination homeopathic remedy manufactured by King Bio (in their *SafeCareRx* line of products), a homeopathic pharmaceuticals supply house. The ingredients in *Appetite and Weight Control* are: *Abies canadensis, Ammonium bromatum, Ammonium muriaticum, Anacardium orientale, Antimonium crudum, Argentum metallicum, Calcarea carbonica, Capsicum annuum, Cinchona officinalis, Ferrum metallicum, Fucus vesiculosus, Ignatia amara, Kali bichromicum, Lycopodium clavatum, Mercurius solubilis, Natrum sulphuricum, Oleander, Phosphorus, Phytolacca decandra, Sabadilla, Staphysagria, Sulphur, Thyroidinum* and *Veratrum album*, in pure water base. Each ingredient comes in a broad spectrum of low to high potencies.

When should you use it? The **keynote** symptoms indicating the use of *Appetite and Weight Control* are food cravings in persons who have excessive appetites and who have a tendency to gain weight.

How should you use it? Take 2-3 sprays onto or under the tongue twice daily. This may be used long-term, especially to prevent food cravings in persons trying to lose weight.

Eating Disorders

What is it? This is a combination homeopathic remedy manufactured by King Bio (in their *SafeCareRx* line of products), a homeopathic pharmaceuticals supply house. The ingredients in *Eating Disorders* are: *Antimonium crudum, Cinchona officinalis, Ferrum metallicum, Hyoscyamus niger, Ignatia amara, Natrum muriaticum, Nux vomica, Phosphoricum acidum, Pulsatilla, Staphysagria, Thuja occidentalis* and *Veratrum album*, in pure water base. Each ingredient comes in a broad spectrum of low to high potencies.

When should you use it? The **keynote** symptoms directing you towards trying *Eating Disorders* are overeating, binge eating, bingeing and then vomiting, and any of the symptoms associated with disordered eating.

How should you use it? Take 2-3 sprays onto or under the tongue twice daily. This may be used long-term, especially to prevent disordered eating in persons with binge eating disorder or bulimia nervosa and in persons trying to lose weight.

Weight Loss XL

What is it? This is a combination homeopathic remedy manufactured by Liddell Laboratories a homeopathic pharmaceuticals supply house. You may call 1-800-460-7733 to order. The ingredients in *Weight Loss XL* are: *Thyroidinum* 30C, *Antimonium crudum* 30C, *Apis mellifica* 3X, *Badiaga* 5X, *Calcarea carbonica* 30C, *Fucus vesiculosus* 1X, *Hydrocotyle asiatica* 1X, *Ignatia amara* 30C, *Lycopodium clavatum* 200C, *Lycopus virginicus* 3X, *Nux vomica* 6X, *Boldo* 1X, *Phytolacca decandra* 1X, *Rhus toxicodendron* 200C and *Spongia tosta* 3X. The potencies are listed here because some of them are very low, some intermediary, and some are high.

When should you use it? The **keynote** symptoms helping you to choose *Weight Loss XL* are overeating and uncontrolled appetite in persons who need to loose weight for health reasons.

How should you use it? Take 2 sprays under the tongue three times daily. This product is not recommended for children under the age of 12 years.

Guidelines for Consulting Your Health Care Provider

You should consult your health care provider if:
• the patient doesn't look right or act right (trust your instincts!)

- the patient is getting worse instead of better over the course of the illness
- the patient has untreated high blood pressure
- the patient has untreated diabetes
- the patient has untreated high blood cholesterol
- the patient is depressed or talks about suicide
- the patient is apathetic or indifferent to his/her surroundings
- the patient has persistent vomiting after meals
- the patient has a sustained rapid weight loss (more than 2 lbs per week, sustained for more than a month)
- the patient abuses laxatives, ipecac, or diuretics
- the patient has a well-established eating disorder
- the patient has a sustained weight gain
- the patient is having trouble breathing or complaining of chest pains or there is mental confusion or lethargy or irritability

> **Note:** Do not discontinue taking any pharmaceutical medication that has been prescribed by your health care provider unless you or your family member is under the supervision of a physician.

> **Note:** For persons seeking abstinence from substance abuse and/or alcoholism, as well as freedom from eating disorders, I recommend that you investigate *Desert Canyon*'s nutritional program. *Desert Canyon*, located in Sedona, Arizona, is a non-twelve step program. You may want to read the book *End Your Addiction Now: The Proven Nutritional Supplement Program That Can Set You Free* by Charles Gant and Greg Lewis, published by Warner Books, 2002.

Recommendations for Homeopathic Remedies

Antimonium crudum 200C—in pellets
Arsenicum album 200C—in pellets
Calcarea carbonica 200C—in pellets
Capsicum annuum 200C—in pellets
Carcinosin 200C—in pellets
Ferrum metallicum 200C—in pellets
Graphites 200C—in pellets
Ignatia 200C—in pellets

Lycopodium 200C—in pellets
Natrum muriaticum 200C—in pellets
Phosphorus 200C—in pellets
Phytolacca decandra 200C—in pellets
Platina 200C—in pellets
Appetite and Weight Control—combination remedy from King Bio
Eating Disorders—combination remedy from King Bio
Weight Loss XL—combination remedy from Liddell Laboratories

Guidelines for Administration of Homeopathic Remedies

Once you have chosen the homeopathic remedy and the potency that is likely to help you or your family member, you should try to give as few repetitions of the remedy as you can. You start off repeating it more frequently in a severe, acute situation, quickly decreasing the frequency once improvement has begun, stopping the remedy as soon as the problem has resolved.

> **Note:** For more information on *how often* to give the homeopathic remedy please see **Potency and Frequency**, in **Chapter 2: Basic Homeopathy**. For information on *how much* of the homeopathic remedy to give and the importance of a "*clean tongue*," please see **How to take homeopathic remedies** in the same chapter.

Lower potency remedies, such as 30C and below, are used to treat acute ailments. They are usually repeated often, every ½-2 or ½-4 hours. You should notice improvement in symptoms after just one to perhaps a few repetitions. If you do not see improvement, it is wise to stop the remedy and try a different one, guiding yourself by the **keynote** symptoms. You may use different single remedies together or you may try a combination remedy. And you may use homeopathic remedies together with pharmaceutical prescription and non-prescription drugs without any effect of interference.

General guidelines to treat serious, chronic, relapsing ailments include using single remedies at potencies of 200C. These are generally administered once weekly to once monthly, but they may be used once or twice daily at first if the condition warrants it, quickly decreasing the frequency as you see improvement. Do not continue giving the remedy if it becomes apparent that it is not working. You may always stop one remedy and choose to administer another remedy on the basis of the **keynote** symptoms of the new remedy. In addition, you may administer more than one remedy at a time.

Putting It All Together

Coping with diseases of feeding and eating will generally require a multi-pronged approach incorporating all the essential natural alternatives, homeopathy, herbal remedies, and nutritional supplements.

It is a good idea to consider giving the sick person's homeopathic constitutional remedy (please refer to **Chapter 9: Homeopathic Remedies for Constitutional Problems in Infants, Children, and Adolescents** or to **Chapter 18: Homeopathic Constitutional Remedies** if you are dealing with an adult).

Ailments of feeding and eating require all the vitamins and minerals necessary to repair and replenish tissues (please refer to **Chapter 23: Vitamins and Minerals**) as well as a general antioxidant supplement (please refer to **Chapter 24: Antioxidant Phytochemicals**).

Please read **Chapter 26: Nutritional Supplements for Healthy Weight Control** and decide if you want to incorporate any of these nutritional supplements into your daily life.

You may want to investigate certain herbal remedies such as *Green tea* (please refer to **Chapter 20: Herbs You Need to Know**) as well as *omega-3 fatty acids* (please refer to **Chapter 31: Oils and Fats**). You may wish to incorporate *probiotics* (please refer to **Chapter 30: Prebiotics and Probiotics**) into your daily supplements because you may find feeding and eating problems to be sensitive to enhanced gastrointestinal health.

Diseases of feeding and eating sometimes overlap with emotional and neurological diseases. If this is true for you, then you may want to investigate **Chapter 8: Homeopathic Remedies for Emotional Problems; Chapter 16: Homeopathy for Neurologic Disorders** and **Chapter 29: Nutritional Supplements for Neurologic Disorders**.

Chapter 16

Homeopathy for Neurologic Disorders

Neurologic Disorders in General

Ailment/Disorder/Symptom	Homeopathic Remedy
Sudden severe headaches with throbbing pains	*Belladonna*
Vertigo, dizziness, with nausea and vomiting	*Cocculus indicus*
Insomnia with agitation and racing thoughts	*Coffea cruda*
Migraine headaches	*Cyclamen*
Headaches with onset of menstruation	*Cimicifuga racemosa*
Migraine headaches, feeling the head is enlarged	*Gelsemium*
Violent throbbing headaches	*Glonoinum*
Right-sided headaches	*Iris versicolor*
Headaches starting in the neck	*Sanguinaria*
Restless legs syndrome	*Zincum metallicum*
Insomnia	*Insomnia*
Migraine headaches	*Migraide*
Sciatica and back pain	*Sciatic-Aide*
Insomnia	*Sleepaid*
Insomnia	*Avena Sativa Compound*
Nicotine addiction	*Nico-Rx*

Guidelines for Consulting Your Health Care Provider
Putting It All Together

Neurologic Disorders in General

Neurologic disorders range in severity from headaches and insomnia to autism and coma. It is the purpose of this chapter to discuss those homeopathic remedies that are useful to treat the less severe neurologic disorders (non-life threatening), such as: headache (tension, migraine, cluster), insomnia (and other sleep disorders), tics, tremors, sciatica, and restless legs syndrome. In these disorders, the proper homeopathic remedy may be all that is required.

However, even for these non-life threatening neurologic disorders, it is always a good idea to get a definite diagnosis first from your health care provider before you embark on self-care and administer a homeopathic remedy. If you find that the homeopathic remedies in this chapter are not helpful to you or your family member, then I recommend that you consider a *constitutional homeopathic remedy*.

> **Note:** Although Attention Deficit/Hyperactivity Disorder (ADD/ADHD) and developmental delay are neurologic disorders they are more completely discussed in **Chapter 9: Homeopathic Remedies for Constitutional Problems in Infants, Children, and Adolescents** and **Chapter 29: Nutritional Supplements for Neurologic Disorders**.

The more severe neurologic disorders include: brain and spinal cord infections and tumors, chronic pain syndromes, autism and other pervasive developmental disorders, coma, amnesia, multiple sclerosis, seizures and epilepsy, paralysis, stroke, Parkinson's disease, myasthenia gravis, muscular dystrophy, peripheral polyneuropathy, Alzheimer's disease and other dementias, as well as other less common disorders.
[Adapted from *The Merck Manual* at www.merck.com]

It is essential for the patient with one of these neurologic diseases to be under the care of a specialist physician. Please refer to the **Guidelines for Consulting Your Health Care Provider** at the end of this chapter.

The more severe neurologic disorders (listed above) are best treated with the patient's *constitutional homeopathic remedy*, integrating it along with conventional pharmaceutical medicines. In the case of severe neurologic disorders, homeopathy will enhance the effectiveness of conventional therapies. Homeopathic remedies may be given along with prescription pharmaceuticals without interference or interaction.

Determining the patient's *constitutional homeopathic remedy* may be possible for you to do, but it is sometimes difficult for an untrained person to find the appropriate *constitutional homeopathic remedy*. Finding the proper *constitutional homeopathic remedy* may require the services of a homeopath. In addition, if you find you have achieved only partial results after administering the *constitutional homeopathic remedy* that you have prescribed, I recommend that you consult with a homeopath.

Neurologic disorders are sometimes best treated with all three essential natural alternative health care practices, namely, homeopathy, herbal remedies, and nutritional supplements. I recommend that you first master using homeopathy to treat or prevent the ailments that concern you. Homeopathy is the safest of the three alternative health care practices because it has no significant side effects or interactions with prescription medications. Then you should investigate the nutritional supplements specifically for neurologic disorders that are used to augment the homeopathic remedies you have chosen. Then I urge you to learn about the use of the appropriate herbal remedies for the neurologic health issue that concerns you.

You may prefer to use a *combination homeopathic remedy* to treat any of the conditions discussed in this chapter. *Combination remedies* are certainly easier to use than single remedies and are very often effective. Combination remedies will likely include many of the single remedies listed below, but in very low potency. Using combination remedies is like taking a stab in the dark.

However, many people find that combination remedies do not work well enough so it is important to be able to use single remedies according to their **keynote** symptoms. You may always give a remedy, gauge the reaction, and if necessary, give a different remedy. You may use more than one single remedy at one time. You should have on hand those remedies for treating those **keynote** symptoms that tend to recur in you or members of your family.

As with any and all medical conditions, when dealing with neurologic disorders you must pay strict attention to the **Guidelines for Consulting Your Health Care Provider** at the end of this chapter. You may want to refer to the last section **Putting It All Together** for ideas on how to integrate the essential natural alternatives, homeopathy, herbal remedies, and nutritional supplements.

Belladonna

What is it? This is the homeopathic remedy made from the plant, *Atropa belladonna*, common name *deadly nightshade*, a member of the *Solanaceae* botanical family.

When should you use it? The **keynote** symptoms encouraging you to use *Belladonna* are sudden onset, severe headaches with throbbing pain. The patient needing *Belladonna* may have facial flushing and dilated pupils as well. The headache may come from exposure to sun, colds, sinus infections, or as a side effect of pharmaceuticals.

How should you use it? Give *Belladonna* 30C every ½-4 hours, depending on severity, quickly decreasing the frequency as soon as the headache is improved, stopping when the headache is gone.

Cocculus indicus

What is it? This is the poisonous climbing plant *Cocculus indicus*, common name *Levant nut* or *Fish Berry*, a member of the *Menispermaceae* botanical family. The seeds contain the poison *picrotoxine*. The homeopathic remedy is non-toxic.

When should you use it? The **keynote** symptoms helping you to choose *Cocculus indicus* are dizziness (vertigo) that is described as though everything in the room is spinning accompanied by nausea and vomiting. The dizziness in persons needing *Cocculus* is worse when riding in a motor vehicle and even when looking at one drive by.

How should you use it? Give *Cocculus* 30C every

½-4 hours, depending on severity, quickly decreasing the frequency as soon as the dizziness is improved, stopping when the dizziness is gone.

Coffea cruda

What is it? This is the plant *Coffea cruda*, common name *coffee*, a member of the *Rubiaceae* botanical family.

When should you use it? The **keynote** symptoms helping you to choose *Coffea* are restless agitation (tossing and turning) at bedtime with inability to sleep, alert wakefulness and racing thoughts. Remember that whatever the symptoms that *coffee* (with caffeine) can cause, those are the symptoms that homeopathic *Coffea* can cure.

How should you use it? Give *Coffea* 30C 2-4 hours before bedtime, repeat just before going to bed. This may be repeated in the middle of the night if necessary.

Cyclamen

What is it? This is the plant *Cyclamen europaeum*, common name *Sowbread*, a member of the *Primulaceae* botanical family.

When should you use it? The **keynote** symptoms suggesting the use of *Cyclamen* are migraine headaches with bursting pains that come on with flickering before the eyes (scintillation).

How should you use it? Give *Cyclamen* 30C every ½-4 hours, depending on severity, quickly decreasing the frequency as soon as the headache is improved, stopping when the headache is gone.

Cimicifuga racemosa

What is it? This is the plant *Cimicifuga racemosa*, common name *Black cohosh*, a member of the *Ranunculaceae* botanical family. The homeopathic remedy is abbreviated as *Cimic*.

When should you use it? The **keynote** symptoms leading you to choose to try *Cimic* are severely painful headaches with a waving sensation in the brain, made worse by movement and by the onset of menstruation. The headache may either begin at or extend to the nape of the neck.

How should you use it? Give *Cimic* 30C every ½-4 hours, depending on severity, quickly decreasing the frequency as soon as the headache is improved, stopping when the headache is gone.

Gelsemium

What is it? This is the plant *Gelsemium sempervirens* whose common name is *yellow jasmine*, a member of the *Loganiaceae* botanical family.

When should you use it? The **keynote** symptoms pointing towards the use of *Gelsemium* are painful migraine headaches coming on with visual disturbances (scotomata). The migraine sufferer may feel a sense of heaviness, confusion, and feel that the head is enlarged.

How should you use it? Give *Gelsemium* 30C every ½-4 hours, depending on severity, quickly decreasing the frequency as soon as the headache is improved, stopping when the headache is gone.

Glonoinum

What is it? This is the chemical compound *glyceryl trinitrate*, known as *Nitroglycerine*. This is the compound that Alfred Nobel used to make dynamite.

When should you use it? The **keynote** symptoms prompting you to try *Glonoinum* are sudden onset of severe and violent headache pains, which are characterized as bursting, throbbing, pulsating, or explosive. The pain is made worse from the least movement, made better by firm pressure. There may be a feeling of blood rushing to the head. *Glonoinum* is often used to treat angina pectoris.

How should you use it? Give *Glonoinum* 30C every ½-4 hours, depending on severity, quickly decreasing the frequency as soon as the headache is improved, stopping when the headache is gone.

Iris versicolor

What is it? This is the plant *Iris versicolor*, common name *Iris*, a member of the *Iridaceae* botanical family.

When should you use it? The **keynote** symptoms pointing in the direction of *Iris* are right-sided migraine headaches, usually over the right eyes that are severe and throbbing. The headache may be accompanied by visual and/or gastrointestinal disturbances. Vomiting may lessen the severity of the headache.

How should you use it? Give *Iris* 30C every ½-4 hours, depending on severity, quickly decreasing the frequency as soon as the headache is improved, stopping when the headache is gone.

Sanguinaria

What is it? This is the plant *Sanguinaria canadensis*, common name *Blood root*, a member of the *Papaveraceae* botanical family.

When should you use it? The **keynote** symptoms suggesting the use of *Sanguinaria* are periodic (every 7-8 days) headaches starting in the nape of the neck then extending over the right eye. Headaches for which *Sanguinaria* may be helpful are made better after sleep.

How should you use it? Give *Sanguinaria* 30C every ½-4 hours, depending on severity, quickly decreasing the frequency as soon as the headache is improved, stopping when the headache is gone.

Zincum metallicum

What is it? This is the metal element *Zinc* (Zn).

When should you use it? The **keynote** symptoms leading you to choose *Zincum metallicum* are restless, sometimes violent, involuntary movements of the legs that may awaken the sleeping person. *Zincum metallicum* is a homeopathic remedy for restless legs syndrome. *Zincum metallicum* is also helpful to treat movements characterized as tremors, trembling, jerking, and twitching.

How should you use it? Give *Zincum metallicum* 30C 2-4 hours before bedtime; repeat just before going to bed. This may be repeated in the middle of the night if necessary.

Insomnia

What is it? This is a combination homeopathic remedy produced by Boericke & Tafel, a homeopathic pharmaceutical supply house. The ingredients are: *Eschscholtzia californica, Humulus lupulus, Passiflora incarnata* and *Zincum metallicum*, in a lactose based-tablet with sorbitol. Since the first three ingredients are in "*Mother Tincture*" strength (they have not been diluted), they are actually herbal remedies. However, the *Zincum metallicum* is homeopathic, low potency.

When should you use it? The **keynote** symptoms helping you to choose *Insomnia* are difficulties falling asleep.

How should you use it? Chew 2 tablets or let dissolve in mouth, once every hour for 2-3 doses before bedtime and again if you awaken in the middle of the night. This product is not for children under age 12 years.

Migraide

What is it? This is a combination homeopathic remedy produced by Boericke & Tafel, a homeopathic pharmaceutical supply house. The ingredients are: *Cyclamen europaeum, Cimicifuga racemosa, Gelsemium sempervirens, Iris versicolor* and *Sanguinaria canadensis*, all in low potencies.

When should you use it? The **keynote** symptoms encouraging you to choose *Migraide* are typical migraine headache symptoms: visual disturbances or nausea and vomiting at the outset, severe throbbing pain usually on one side of the head, sometimes relieved by sleep.

How should you use it? Take 3 tablets under the tongue (sublingual) every 1-2 hours until the pain is relieved. Children aged 2-12 years should take one-half the adult dose.

Sciatic-Aide

What is it? This is a combination homeopathic remedy produced by Boericke & Tafel, a homeopathic pharmaceutical supply house. The ingredients are: *Arsenicum album, Chamomilla, Colocynthis* and *Sulphur* in low potencies, in lactose-based tablets.

When should you use it? The **keynote** symptoms leading you to try *Sciatic-Aide* are the characteristic pains associated with irritation of the sciatic nerve, such as dull, aching lower back pain, often radiating to the buttocks, sometimes extending down the back of the thigh to the calf.

How should you use it? Give *Sciatic-Aide* 2 tablets under the tongue (sublingual) every 2 hours until some relief is noted. Then decrease the frequency until the pain is gone. Then stop.

Sleepaid

What is it? This is a combination homeopathic remedy produced by Nelson Bach, a homeopathic pharmaceutical supply house. The ingredients are: *Kali bromatum, Coffea cruda, Passiflora, Avena, Alfalfa* and *Valeriana*, all in 30C potency, with lactose and sucrose in the pellets.

When should you use it? The **keynote** symptoms for which you may use *Sleepaid* are occasional sleeplessness with restlessness and irritability.

How should you use it? Let 2 pellets of *Sleepaid* dissolve in the mouth (or they can be chewed), 4 hours before bedtime, repeating immediately before going to bed. This may be repeated in the middle of the night if needed.

Avena Sativa Compound and Sedative Pilules

What is it? These are combination homeopathic remedies produced by Weleda, a homeopathic pharmaceutical supply house. The ingredients are: *Avena sativa, Passiflora incarnata, Valeriana officinalis, Coffea tosta* and *Humulus lupulus*. All except for *Coffea tosta* are in mother tincture or 1X potency that makes the preparation, technically speaking, an herbal remedy. *Coffea tosta* is in 60X potency, a low potency homeopathic remedy.

When should you use it? The **keynote** symptoms for which you may use *Avena Sativa Compound* and *Sedative Pilules* are sleeplessness with nervous agitation.

How should you use it? Take 10-20 drops at bedtime of *Avena Sativa Compound*. Repeat dose again in one hour if needed. *Sedative Pilules* (granules) is the same formulation as *Avena Sativa Compound*. Take 15 pilules of *Sedative Pilules* before bedtime and 3-4 times daily if needed.

Nico-Rx

What is it? *Nico-Rx* is a homeopathic, nicotine-free, smoking cessation preparation manufactured by NatraBio. *Nico-Rx* contains: *Caladium seguinum, Daphne indica, Plantago major, Cinchona officinalis, Lobelia inflate, Nux vomica, Staphysagria, Calcarea phosphorica* and *Ignatia amara* in low potencies. Other ingredients include: sorbitol, gum base, maltitol syrup, natural *Peppermint oil*, lecithin titanium dioxide, glaze, and carnauba wax. It is peculiar that a homeopathic remedy would be made with peppermint oil that is often said to interfere with the action of homeopathic remedies. Nevertheless, the *Nico-Rx* Program appears to be effective in many cases.

When should you use it? The **keynote** symptoms for which you should consider *Nico-Rx* are nicotine addiction along with cravings for cigarettes and other forms of tobacco. *Nico-Rx* is also helpful to combat the irritability, moodiness, and anxiety that may be experienced during withdrawal from tobacco products.

How should you use it? The *Nico-Rx* Program is designed to take 3 months. It consists of *Nico-Rx* Anti-Craving Gum (chew 1 piece every 1-2 hours as needed for the first month, decreasing thereafter) and *Nico-Rx* Detox Tablets (chew 2 tablets 4 times daily, for the first month, decreasing thereafter).

> **Note:** The two homeopathic remedies often used to help detoxify the body from nicotine addiction are *Tabacum* and *Caladium*, each used in 6X or 12X potencies. These are also used to reduce cravings for nicotine. They may be used together. Take *Tabacum* (*Nicotiana tabacum*) or *Caladium* (*Caladium seguinum*), or both, every time you experience craving for cigarettes (or any other nicotine-based product). Decrease the frequency of use as soon as nicotine addiction symptoms improve and discontinue when they resolve. Nicotine addiction often resolves imper-

fectly, with stops and starts, common to all addictions. Don't worry; you may always restart homeopathic remedies.

Guidelines for Consulting Your Health Care Provider

You should consult your health care provider if:
• the patient doesn't look right or act right (trust your instincts!)
• the patient is getting worse instead of better over the course of the illness
• the patient is having trouble breathing or complaining of chest pains or there is mental confusion or lethargy or irritability
• the patient is experiencing *new onset* paralysis, weakness, tingling, inability to focus or concentrate, blurred or double vision or blindness, slurred speech, severe headaches, seizures, irritability, dizziness, disorientation, memory loss, anxiety, depression, insomnia, blackouts, fainting, or the person complains of not feeling like himself
• the patient has been diagnosed with any of the following neurologic disorders:
concussion, brain and spinal cord infections and tumors, chronic pain syndromes, autism and other pervasive developmental disorders, coma, amnesia, multiple sclerosis, seizures and epilepsy, paralysis, stroke, Parkinson's disease, myasthenia gravis, muscular dystrophy, peripheral polyneuropathy, Alzheimer's disease and other dementias, as well as other less common disorders.

Note: Do not discontinue taking any pharmaceutical medication that has been prescribed by your health care provider unless you or your family member is under the supervision of a physician.

Note: For more information on how to get the proper amount and quality of sleep, contact the National Sleep Foundation at www.sleepfoundation. org. You will find sound advice for sound sleep.

Note: If your child has been diagnosed with autism, please read Amy Lansky's book, *Impossible Cure, the Promise of Homeopathy*, published by R. L. Ranch Press, California, 2003. It is the story of how her son Max was cured from autism by homeopathy. Yes, cured. After reading this book you will have new respect for homeopathy and understand it better too.

But, please skip all the malarkey about vaccinations causing autism. Dr. Andrew Wakefield (and colleagues) published a study supposedly linking autism and MMR (measles-mumps-rubella) vaccine in 1998 in the *Lancet*. Since then any association of autism and vaccines has been soundly disproved not only by our foremost scientific agency the *Institute of Medicine*, but also a gigantic Scandinavian study of approximately 500,000 children. The prestigious British medical journal *Lancet* has since discovered Dr. Wakefield's study to have serious methodological flaws. Worse than that, Dr. Wakefield did not reveal a conflict of interest. While performing the study, he was also financially involved in the legal battle of parents against the MMR vaccine companies. Ten of the original 13 authors of that paper have since retracted their conclusions.

You will also want to use the information and services of Cure Autism Now at www.cureautismnow.org.

Note: You may want to investigate the link between exposure to mercury and autism by reading David Kirby's book, *Evidence of Harm*. Since childhood immunizations no longer contain mercury (except for some brands of influen-

za vaccine), this link may now be moot. Medical researchers did not find high-quality evidence to support the link between mercury and autism. If you are convinced of the link in your child, please be very careful of having mercury in teeth fillings or otherwise removed because the detoxification process, called chelation, is likely itself to be harmful to health.

Note: It is very difficult, even for properly trained homeopaths, to treat youngsters with autism spectrum diseases (ASD), so I don't recommend that you attempt this on your own. It is important that you become familiar with the alternatives available for treatment by reading *A Drug-Free Approach to Asperger Syndrome and Autism* by Judyth Reichenberg-Ullman, Robert Ullman, and Ian Leupker. You may order at 800-398-1151 or www.drugfreeasperger.com.

Note: If you or your family member has any neurologic disease, especially autism, it is wise to aim for zero exposure to heavy metals such as mercury, lead, aluminum, and cadmium. Ingestion of seafood contaminated with mercury exposes us to undesirably high levels. Pregnant women must be careful to avoid mercury-contaminated seafood so as not to inadvertently expose the developing fetus.

Note: A small subset of children with autism may benefit from a wheat- and milk-free diet called the *gluten-free-casein-free diet*. Some children with autism may actually have an increased intestinal permeability that, in theory, would allow certain absorbed compounds to affect behavior. Your child may need to remain on this diet for 8 months before you would be able to judge whether behavioral benefits occurred or not. I recommend that you do not attempt this diet on your own, but rather work with a nutritionist, because of the opportunity for calcium and protein deficiencies to develop in your child.

You may also be interested in experimenting with a sugar-free and artificial-sugar-free diet (called *sugar avoidance diet*) for your child with autism because of the beneficial behavioral changes noted by both parents and clinicians.

Note: For more information on ADHD, visit online www.kidsmeds.org/adhd. In addition to Western medicine approach to ADHD, you will find some alternative therapy options. Pediatric OnCall at www.pediatriconcall.com is another excellent site for information on ADHD (and all the other pediatric ailments). The information on alternative medicine is rudimentary.

A small subset of children with ADHD may respond to the *Feingold Diet* (not a relative of this author!) that eliminates certain chemicals in food. You can find information on the *Feingold Association* at www.feingold.org. [For more information on nutritional supplements for children and adults with ADHD, please see **Chapter 29: Nutritional Supplements for Neurologic Disorder**s.]

Recommendations for Homeopathic Remedies
Belladonna 30C—pellets
Cocculus indicus 30C—pellets
Coffea cruda 30C—pellets
Cyclamen 30C—pellets
Cimicifuga racemosa 30C—pellets
Gelsemium 30C—pellets
Glonoinum 30C—pellets
Iris versicolor 30C—pellets
Sanguinaria 30C—pellets
Zincum metallicum 30C—pellets
Insomnia—combination remedy, chewable tablets
Migraide—combination remedy, tablets
Sciatic-Aide—combination remedy, tablets

Sleepaid—combination remedy, pellets
Avena Sativa Compound—drops and granules (called *Sedative Pilules*)

Guidelines for Administration of Homeopathic Remedies
Once you have chosen the homeopathic remedy and the potency that is likely to help you or your family member, you should try to give as few repetitions of the remedy as you can. You start off repeating it more frequently in a severe, acute situation, quickly decreasing the frequency once improvement has begun, stopping the remedy as soon as the problem has resolved.

> **Note:** For more information on *how often* to give the homeopathic remedy please see **Potency and Frequency**, in **Chapter 2: Basic Homeopathy**. For information on *how much* of the homeopathic remedy to give and the importance of a "*clean tongue*," please see **How to take homeopathic remedies** in the same chapter.

Lower potency remedies, such as 30C and below, are used to treat acute ailments. They are usually repeated often, every $\frac{1}{2}$-2 or $\frac{1}{2}$-4 hours. You should notice improvement in symptoms after just one to perhaps a few repetitions. If you do not see improvement, it is wise to stop the remedy and try a different one, guiding yourself by the **keynote** symptoms. You may use different single remedies together or you may try a combination remedy. And you may use homeopathic remedies together with pharmaceutical prescription and non-prescription drugs without any effect of interference.

General guidelines to treat serious, chronic, relapsing ailments include using single remedies at potencies of 200C. These are generally administered once weekly to once monthly, but they may be used once or twice daily at first if the condition warrants it, quickly decreasing the frequency as you see improvement. Do not continue giving the remedy if it becomes apparent that it is not working. You may always stop one remedy and choose to administer another remedy on the basis of the **keynote** symptoms of the new remedy. In addition, you may administer more than one remedy at a time.

Putting It All Together

Coping with neurologic diseases will generally require a multi-pronged approach incorporating all the essential natural alternatives, homeopathy, herbal remedies, and nutritional supplements.

It is a good idea to consider giving the sick person's homeopathic constitutional remedy (please refer to **Chapter 9: Homeopathic Remedies for Constitutional Problems in Infants, Children, and Adolescents** or to **Chapter 18: Homeopathic Constitutional Remedies** if you are dealing with an adult). Neurologic problems often occur among elderly people (please refer to **Chapter 13: Homeopathy for Elderly Persons**).

Please read **Chapter 29: Nutritional Supplements for Neurologic Disorders** to decide if you want to incorporate any of the recommended nutritional supplements and for information on ADD/ADHD.

Neurologic ailments require all the vitamins and minerals necessary to repair and replenish tissues (please refer to **Chapter 23: Vitamins and Minerals**) as well as a general antioxidant supplement (please refer to **Chapter 24: Antioxidant Phytochemicals**).

You may want to investigate certain herbal remedies such as *Ginkgo biloba* and *Feverfew* (please refer to **Chapter 20: Herbs You Need to Know**) as well as *omega-3 fatty acids* (please refer to **Chapter 31: Oils and Fats**). You may wish to incorporate *probiotics* (please refer to **Chapter 30: Prebiotics and Probiotics**) into your daily supplements because you may find neurologic problems to be sensitive to enhanced gastrointestinal health.

Neurologic diseases often overlap with emotional ailments. If this is true for you, then you may want to investigate **Chapter 8: Homeopathic Remedies for Emotional Problems**.

Chapter 17

Homeopathy for Persons with Cancer

Cancer in General

Ailment/Disorder/Symptom	Homeopathic Remedy
Cancer with family history	*Carcinosin*
Stony hard cancers	*Scirrhinum*
Terminal cancer with pain	*Arsenicum album*
Cancer with bone metastases	*Conium*
Cancerous tumors	*Thuja*

Guidelines for Consulting Your Health Care Provider
Putting It All Together

Cancer in General

Cancer is such a life-threatening condition that it does not make sense to consider self-care for its treatment. It is essential that you obtain oncology health care services from a M.D. or D.O. specialist in the cancer you are trying to treat or the recurrences you are trying to prevent. It is irresponsible to "go it alone" when the diagnosis is cancer. The patient with cancer needs an exact diagnosis, then the proper surgery, chemotherapy and/or radiation therapy, and then the proper follow-up care designed to prevent recurrences and metastases. It is these last two steps where homeopathy fits into the scheme. And it is at this point that homeopathy may do its best and deepest work in the body.

However, for the homeopathic adjunctive treatment of cancer, I urge you to consult with a homeopath who is specifically knowledgeable in the homeopathic treatment of cancer. After reading this chapter, you will have a preliminary understanding of what kind of homeopathic treatment is available for persons with cancer and this may empower you to seek a homeopath who will help you attain this kind of treatment.

There are *essential natural alternatives* that can help you or your family member recover from cancer, even if metastases exist, even if chemotherapy or radiation has failed. Cancers and metastases are best treated with all three *essential natural alternative* health care practices, namely, *homeopathy, herbal remedies* and *nutritional supplements*. I recommend that you first master using homeopathy prescribed by your homeopath to treat or prevent the cancer that concerns you. Homeopathy is the safest of the three alternative health care practices because it has no significant side effects or interactions with prescription medications. Then you should investigate the nutritional supplements specifically for persons with cancer that are used to augment the homeopathic remedies you have chosen. Then I urge you to learn about the use of the appropriate herbal remedies for cancer.

The most important thing to understand about using *homeopathy, herbal remedies* and *nutritional supplements* for the treatment of cancer is that these must **not** be given during chemotherapy or radiation therapy. This is because the effects of *homeopathy, herbal remedies* and *nutritional supplements* may actually go against the action of chemotherapy or radiation therapy. For this reason *homeopathy, herbal remedies* and *nutritional supplements* are taken after the chemotherapy or radiation therapy sessions are finished, or during the respite between sessions.

> **Note:** As we go to press, these recommendations are undergoing profound changes due to medical research results. Ask your homeopath and oncologist to update you.

When considering the treatment or prevention of cancer, it is imperative that you and your family members heed the **good health practices**:
>—no smoking, moderate alcohol, nutritionally healthy diet, adequate daily physical exercise, adequate sleep, time for daily relaxation techniques, seeking humor and love in everyday life, engaging in activities for intellectual stimulation, doing things for other people, and participating in preventive health testing.

You cannot expect to erase the effects of nicotine addiction, or a diet high in saturated fats, or a sedentary lifestyle by taking homeopathic remedies, herbal remedies, and nutritional supplements. You and the members of your family must practice the **good health practices** at the same time that you institute the **essential alternative health practices** to treat or prevent cancer.

If you are unsure about a nutritional program to treat and/or prevent cancer, you may obtain further information from the *American Institute for Cancer Research (AICR)* 202-328-7744 or www.aicr.org. They are the leading nonprofit organization doing research (and translating it into consumer-friendly terms) into nutritional ways to treat and prevent cancer. The *AICR* publishes a free, worthwhile newsletter *AICR Science Now*, that has always been helpful to me. You may order toll-free at 1-800-843-8114.

You may also find that the reader-friendly *How to Prevent and Treat Cancer with Natural Medicine* by Murray, Birdsall, Pizzorno and Reilly (published by Riverhead Books, 2002) to have all the nutritional information you need. It's a good investment.

In 2001 Dr. A. U. Ramakrishnan and Catherine R. Coulter published much of what we know about the homeopathic treatment of persons with cancer, in a book titled *A Homeopathic Approach to Cancer*. If you are considering obtaining cancer treatment or prevention of relapse in yourself or a family member you should purchase this book. I strongly recommend that you choose a homeopath to help you choose the appropriate homeopathic remedies for yourself or your family member and to supervise its administration.

Cancer and its life-threatening metastases are sometimes treated with the patient's *constitutional homeopathic remedy* (taken just after chemotherapy and/or radiation therapy). In the case of cancer and metastases, homeopathy will enhance the effectiveness of chemotherapy and/or radiation therapy. Homeopathic remedies may be given along with prescription pharmaceuticals (but wait until after chemotherapy and/or radiation therapy) without interference or interaction.

Determining the patient's *constitutional homeopathic remedy* may be possible for you to do, but it is sometimes difficult for an untrained person to find the appropriate *constitutional homeopathic remedy*. Finding the proper *constitutional homeopathic remedy* may require the services of a homeopath. In addition, if you find you have achieved only partial results after administering the *constitutional homeopathic remedy* that you have prescribed, I recommend that you consult with a homeopath.

This chapter will describe two "cancer specific" remedies (*Carcinosin Scirrhinum*) and three wide-spectrum cancer remedies *Arsenicum album, Conium* and *Thuja*). There are many more homeopathic remedies that are useful to treat and prevent cancer. You may read about those in *A Homeopathic Approach to Cancer*.

As with any and all medical conditions, when dealing with persons with cancer you must pay strict attention to the **Guidelines for Consulting Your Health Care Provider** at the end of this chapter. You may want to refer to the last section **Putting It All Together** for ideas on how to integrate the essential natural alternatives, homeopathy, herbal remedies, and nutritional supplements.

Note: If you or someone in your family requires homeopathic treatment for

cancer or prevention of recurrences, it is a good idea to read this chapter as well as the book by Dr. A. U. Ramakrishnan and Catherine Coulter, *A Homeopathic Approach to Cancer*. Most of the information on remedies and the 'plussing method' is derived from that book.

Carcinosin

What is it? This is a homeopathic remedy prepared from cancerous breast tissue.

When should you use it? The **keynote** symptoms indicating the use of *Carcinosin* are having a family history of cancer, and for cancerous tumors that are not stony hard. *Carcinosin* and *Scirrhinum* are sometimes used alternately, especially when the patient is not responding to one.

How should you use it? This is administered by the "plussing method" (see below).

Scirrhinum

What is it? This is a homeopathic remedy prepared from cancerous liver tissue.

When should you use it? The **keynote** symptoms indicating the use of *Scirrhinum* are stony hard cancerous tumors, especially of the breast, lungs, liver, rectum, and prostate. *Carcinosin* and *Scirrhinum* are sometimes used alternately, especially when the patient is not responding to one.

How should you use it? This is administered by the "plussing method" (see below).

Arsenicum album

What is it? This is the homeopathic remedy made from the chemical compound *arsenic oxide* which is highly poisonous if not given in homeopathic dilution. *Arsenicum album* is one of homeopathy's often-used polychrests or constitutional remedies.

When should you use it? The **keynote** symptoms indicating the use of *Arsenicum album* are pain during early, advanced, and terminal cases of cancer, as well as to treat the stressful challenges that malignancies present to the body.

How should you use it? This is administered by the "plussing method" (see below).

Conium

What is it? This is the plant *Conium maculatum*, common name *Hemlock*, a member of the *Umbelliferae* botanical family. Drinking the poisonous juice of this plant was the method that the Ancient Greeks used to put Socrates to death.

When should you use it? The **keynote** symptoms indicating the use of *Conium* are stony hard cancerous tumors of the esophagus, breast, stomach, liver, and prostate, as well as for metastases to bones.

How should you use it? This is administered by the "plussing method" (see below).

Thuja

What is it? This is the plant *Thuja occidentalis*, common name *Arbor vitae* or *Tree of Life*, a member of the *Coniferae* botanical family. The new green twigs are used to make the homeopathic remedy.

When should you use it? The **keynote** symptoms indicating the use of *Thuja* are cancerous tumors especially of the stomach, colon, rectum, bladder, ovaries, uterus, and prostate.

How should you use it? This is administered by the "plussing method" (see below).

Guidelines for Consulting Your Health Care Provider

Note: Never self-prescribe homeopathy, herbal remedies, or nutritional supplements for a person with cancer. You must have the expert guidance of a health care provider or homeopath.

You should consult your health care provider if any of the following occurs during a course of treatment for cancer:

- the patient doesn't look right or act right (trust your instincts!)
- the patient is getting worse instead of better over the course of the illness
- the patient is having trouble breathing or complaining of chest pains or there is mental confusion or lethargy or irritability
- the patient has a new onset growth, tumor, or lump
- the patient is experiencing new onset bleeding or severe pain
- the patient has complications of conventional therapy (chemotherapy and radiation therapy) such as uncontrolled vomiting leading to dehydration, prostration, exhaustion, extreme weakness, bleeding, or severe pain
- the patient has any untoward effect after taking any treatment, either conventional or alternative.

Note: If you attempt self-care of persons with cancer without the guidance of a qualified health care provider, you do so at considerable peril.

Note: All types of cancers have a better cure rate the earlier they are detected and treated. It is important to become familiar with the cancer screening tests that are recommended (according to age and gender) by the American Cancer Society for yourself and for your family members.

Note: Do not discontinue taking any pharmaceutical medication that has been prescribed by your health care provider unless you or your family member is under the supervision of a physician.

Note: For more information please visit www.annieappleseedproject.org and www.nfam.org. Both the Annie Appleseed Project and The National Foundation for Alternative Medicine have alternative medicine cancer care links.

Recommendations for Homeopathic Remedies

Carcinosin 200C—in pellets, plussing method
Scirrhinum 200C—in pellets, plussing method
Arsenicum album 200C—in pellets, plussing method
Conium 200C—in pellets, plussing method
Thuja 200C—in pellets, plussing method

Guidelines for Administration of Homeopathic Remedies

Treatment of cancer and prevention of relapses are generally treated with two remedies at potencies of 200C, alternating one every week. These are generally administered using the *plussing method*. The details of the plussing method are found in the book *A Homeopathic Approach to Cancer*.

A summary of the plussing method follows below:

Week 1 Day 1

Dissolve 5 granules of *Week 1* homeopathic remedy in 11 teaspoons (11 X 5 cc.) of spring water in a glass bottle. Sip one teaspoon (using a plastic teaspoon that measures 5 cc.) every 15 minutes for 2½ hrs. (10 teaspoons), shaking once between doses, or gently stirring between each dose, reserving the 11ᵗʰ teaspoon for the next day.

> **Note:** you may use the same glass bottle for each day of the same week. However, you must change glass bottles and plastic teaspoon measurers between weeks (between remedies).

Week 1 Day 2

Add 10 teaspoons of fresh spring water, but no remedy, and now you begin the same routine as for *Day 1*. The process continues for 7 days after which the remedy is changed and the same procedure is repeated with the new homeopathic remedy for *Week 2*. The homeopathic remedy for *Week 3* will be the same remedy as for *Week 1*; the homeopathic remedy for *Week 4* will be the same remedy as for *Week 2*, and so on.

Putting It All Together

Coping with cancer will generally require a multi-pronged approach incorporating all the essential natural alternatives, homeopathy, herbal remedies, and nutritional supplements.

It is a good idea to consider giving the sick person's homeopathic constitutional remedy (please refer to **Chapter 9: Homeopathic Remedies for Constitutional Problems in Infants, Children, and Adolescents** or to **Chapter 18: Homeopathic Constitutional Remedies** if you are dealing with an adult). Cancer often occurs among elderly people (please refer to **Chapter 13: Homeopathy for Elderly Persons**). It makes sense to consult with a homeopath to determine the proper constitutional remedy. Please be sure you understand when to discontinue taking homeopathic remedies during chemotherapy and radiation treatments.

Cancer requires all the vitamins and minerals necessary to repair and replenish tissues (please refer to **Chapter 23: Vitamins and Minerals**) as well as a general antioxidant supplement (please refer to **Chapter 24: Antioxidant Phytochemicals**). Please be sure you understand when to discontinue taking antioxidants during chemotherapy and radiation treatments.

Please read **Chapter 27: Nutritional Supplements to Prevent Cancer and Augment Your Immune System** and decide if you want to incorporate any of these nutritional supplements, especially *medicinal mushrooms*, into your daily life.

You may want to investigate certain herbal remedies such as *Cat's Claw* (please refer to **Chapter 20: Herbs You Need to Know**) as well as *omega-3 fatty acid*s (please refer to **Chapter 31: Oils and Fats**). You may wish to incorporate *probiotics* (please refer to **Chapter 30: Prebiotics and Probiotics**) into your daily supplements because you may find cancer to be sensitive to enhanced gastrointestinal health. It is essential that you check with your oncologist before embarking on nutritional supplements. Please be sure you understand when to discontinue taking nutritional supplements during chemotherapy and radiation treatments.

Chapter 18

Homeopathic Constitutional Remedies

Constitutional Disorders in Adults in General

Ailment/Disorder/Symptom	Homeopathic Remedy
Fastidiousness, perfectionism, chilliness, fearfulness	*Arsenicum album*
Slowness, sluggishness, chilliness, fearfulness	*Calcarea carbonica*
Jealousy, talkativeness, clairvoyance, menopausal women	*Lachesis*
Insecurity, arrogance, depression	*Lycopodium*
Silent grief, abandoned	*Natrum muriaticum*
Workaholism, perfectionism, chilliness, prone to addictions	*Nux vomica*
Sensitivity, needs company of others, expressivity	*Phosphorus*
Emotional lability with weepiness, self-pitying	*Pulsatilla*
Overwhelmed by responsibilities, apathy	*Sepia*
Eccentricity, hoarding, argumentativeness	*Sulphur*

Guidelines for Consulting Your Health Care Provider
Putting It All Together

Constitutional Disorders in Adults in General

Finding and administering the patient's *constitutional homeopathic remedy* is prescribing for the entire person, synthesizing in one remedy all the parts of that person, physical, emotional, intellectual (mental), spiritual, and sexual. This is the miracle of homeopathy and this is where homeopathy differs most completely from Western medicine.

The *constitutional homeopathic remedy* may be given to treat serious, chronic, relapsing diseases, usually as an adjunct to conventional pharmaceutical medications. The *constitutional homeopathic remedy* acts to enhance the effectiveness of conventional therapies and may help the patient to taper or discontinue these as well. In many cases, the proper *constitutional homeopathic remedy* may take the place of pharmaceutical treatments and may act to prevent recurrences, even in chronic diseases.

Here is a list of some of the more common serious, chronic, relapsing diseases that are amenable to treatment with the patient's *constitutional homeopathic remedy*:

> adult attention deficit disorder, arthritis, autism, cancer, HIV and AIDS, multiple sclerosis, coronary artery disease, heart attack (myocardial infarction), congestive heart failure, diabetes mellitus, obesity, thyroid disorders, high blood pressure (hypertension), stroke, seizures, acute and chronic kidney (renal) failure, schizophrenia, bipolar disorder, borderline personality disorder, eating disorders, fibromyalgia, chronic fatigue syndrome, Crohn's disease, ulcerative colitis, celiac disease, mental deficiency disorders, chromosomal disorders, infertility, frequent miscarriages, polyneuropathy.
> [Adapted from
> *The Merck Manual*
> at www.merck.com]

In homeopathic philosophy, *polychrest* remedies are considered to be *constitutional homeopathic remedies*. Determining the patient's *constitutional homeopathic remedy* (from the list of *polychrest* remedies) may be possible for you to do, but it is sometimes difficult for an untrained person to find the appropriate *constitutional homeopathic remedy*. Finding the proper *constitutional homeopathic remedy* may require the services of a homeopath. In addition, if you find you have achieved only partial results after administering the *constitutional homeopathic remedy* that you have prescribed, I recommend that you consult with a homeopath.

The **keynote** symptoms of the polychrest remedies in this chapter are divided into the five spheres of functioning of the human being: physical, emotional, intellectual (mental), spiritual, and sexual. Remember that the long lists of **keynote** symptoms under each remedy are not absolutes, rather they are tendencies. Remember that you or your family member does not need to match each and every remedy characteristic, rather the overall remedy picture.

If you wish to read more about *constitutional homeopathic remedies*, you may order the three volume set of *Portraits of Homeopathic Medicines, Psychophysical Analyses of Selected Constitutional Types* by Catherine R. Coulter. If you prefer a less comprehensive and easier to read book, then order *The Complete Guide to Homeopathy, The Principles and Practice of Treatment* by Lockie and Geddes or *Homeopathic Psychology, Personality Profiles of the Major Constitutional Remedies* by Philip M. Bailey, M.D.

As with any and all medical conditions, when dealing with *constitutional homeopathic remedies* you must pay strict attention to the **Guidelines for Consulting Your Health Care Provider** at the end of this chapter. You may want to refer to the last section **Putting It All Together** for ideas on how to integrate the essential natural alternatives, home-opathy, herbal remedies, and nutritional supplements.

Arsenicum album

What is it? This is the homeopathic remedy made from the chemical compound *arsenic oxide* which is highly poisonous if not given in homeopathic dilution. *Arsenicum album* is one of homeopathy's often-used polychrests or constitutional remedies.

When should you use it? The **keynote** characteristics guiding you towards using *Arsenicum album* as the patient's *constitutional homeopathic remedy* are divided into the five spheres of functioning:

Physical: chilly, cold, burning pains, thirsty for small sips of water often, weakness, exhaustion, often used for certain ailments (food poisoning, asthma, allergies, cancer), everything tends to become worse after midnight, everything tends to become better for warmth.

Emotional: anxious, restless, many fears (of his own health, death, poverty, something bad will happen), neat, organized, perfectionistic, fastidious, meticulous, fussy, conscientious, many worries (his health, his family's health, financial matters, germs), selfish, intolerant, domineering, commanding, critical of others, arrogant, worried about his health, extreme sensitivity to his environment, hypersensitive to music, odors.

Intellectual (mental): bright, intelligent, ambitious, competitive, responsible, likes to be in control, may have an artistic career, but intellectualizes performance in the arts, tends towards teaching.

Spiritual: sometimes religious, morally superior.

Sexual: loss of libido.

How should you use it? Take *Arsenicum album* 200C as the *constitutional homeopathic remedy* once or twice a week until improvement in symptoms. As soon as there is some improvement it is prudent to discontinue taking the remedy. It will continue exerting its deep action in the body. You may return to taking the remedy if a relapse occurs.

Calcarea carbonica

What is it? This is the chemical mineral compound *calcium carbonate* which is obtained from oyster shells.

When should you use it? The **keynote** characteristics guiding you towards using *Calcarea carbonica* as the patient's *constitutional homeopathic remedy* are divided into the five spheres of functioning:

Physical: "fat, fair, and flabby," cold, sweaty (profuse perspiration about the head), clumsy, short stature, large head, tendency towards obesity (slow metabolism), easily overextended, poor stamina, fatigue, weakness, sluggish, lethargic,

dislikes clothing tight around waist, useful for ailments of bones and teeth, used to treat constipation, depression.

Emotional: fearful, many fears (of insanity, poverty, darkness, ghosts, cancer, heart disease), easily overwhelmed, diligent, placid, calm, depressed, dislikes change, fair-minded, craving for sweets and eggs, dairy, ice-cream.

Intellectual (mental): slow (in developmental milestones), poor concentration, dull intellect, postpones mental work.

Spiritual: clairvoyance; ailments aggravated at full moon.

Sexual: weakness and irritability after sexual intercourse.

How should you use it? Take *Calcarea carbonica* 200C as the *constitutional homeopathic remedy* once or twice a week until improvement in symptoms. As soon as there is some improvement it is prudent to discontinue taking the remedy. It will continue exerting its deep action in the body. You may return to taking the remedy if a relapse occurs.

Lachesis

What is it? This is *Trigonocephalus lachesis*, common name *Surukuku snake* or the *Bushmaster snake*. The homeopathic remedy is made from the venom of the snake. It is non-toxic.

When should you use it? The **keynote** characteristics guiding you towards using *Lachesis* as the patient's *constitutional homeopathic remedy* are divided into the five spheres of functioning:

Physical: dislikes clothing around neck, symptoms worse after sleep, bingeing (food and alcohol), the most frequently used remedy for premenstrual and menstrual disorders and menopausal complaints, ailments are worse before menstrual flow begins and worse for light touch but better for firm pressure, complaints predominately left-sided.

Emotional: talkative (can be incessant or obsessive), jumps from topic to topic, suspicious, jealous, egocentric, cynical, quarrelsome, cunning, malicious, vindictive, emotional, intense emotional life, vital, erratic, passionate, easily changeable, manipulative, hypercritical.

Intellectual (mental): intelligent, highly creative

(especially at night).

Spiritual: mystical, interested in mysticism, dreams of her own death, perceptive, insightful, clairvoyant, religious.

Sexual: passionate sexual life, sensual, secures sexual gratification, tendency towards sexual disorders.

How should you use it? Take *Lachesis* 200C as the *constitutional homeopathic remedy* once or twice a week until improvement in symptoms. As soon as there is some improvement it is prudent to discontinue taking the remedy. It will continue exerting its deep action in the body. You may return to taking the remedy if a relapse occurs.

Lycopodium

What is it? This plant is the primitive moss, *Lycopodium clavatum*, common name *Club moss*, a member of the *Lycopodiaceae* botanical family.

When should you use it? The **keynote** characteristics guiding you towards using *Lycopodium* as the patient's *constitutional homeopathic remedy* are divided into the five spheres of functioning:

Physical: cold, appear older than they are, balding, useful for digestive ailments, symptoms worse 4-8 a.m. and 4-8 p.m., symptoms tend to be right-sided, craves sweets.

Emotional: depressed, irritable, cowardly, arrogant, self-righteous, patronizing, dictatorial (especially in the home), fears (of failure, of the future), conservative, evasive, low self-confidence, low self-esteem, insecurity, inadequacy, detached emotional life, difficulties with close relationships and commitment, resiliency, stable, seeks power and control, tolerant of mediocrity, underestimates others' abilities, diplomatic, responsible, respectful, political, moody, mistrustful of medicine and doctors.

Intellectual (mental): mediocre intellect,

Spiritual: may be either religious or non-religious, limited insight.

Sexual: may be promiscuous, marital infidelities, high libido with impotence.

How should you use it? Take *Lycopodium* 200C as the *constitutional homeopathic remedy* once or twice a week until improvement in symptoms. As soon as there is some improvement it is prudent to discon-

tinue taking the remedy. It will continue exerting its deep action in the body. You may return to taking the remedy if a relapse occurs.

Natrum muriaticum

What is it? This is the polychrest *Natrum muriaticum*, a homeopathic remedy made from common table *salt*. Ionized *salt* is the electrochemical method of communication between every cell in the body. *Salt* is a major component of all of the body's fluids, semen, urine, sweat, and tears.

When should you use it? The **keynote** characteristics guiding you towards using *Natrum muriaticum* as the patient's *constitutional homeopathic remedy* are divided into the five spheres of functioning:

Physical: craving for salt and salty foods, thirsty, constipated, dry or oily skin, sinus infections, ailments caused by exposure to hot sun.

Emotional: useful for emotional ailments that plague our society, sad, depressed, hopeless, despondent, desire to be alone, aversion to sympathy, empathic, lonely, isolated, feeling forsaken or abandoned or unloved, socially awkward, brutally honest, abrupt, self-reliant, stoic, ailments that are caused by profound grief or disappointed love (of parents, siblings, or sexual partners), difficulties with intimate relationships (often celibate), idealistic, strong moral sense, unconventional, resentful, fear of insanity, crowds, and being late, self-absorbed, sincere, hypersensitive to criticism and insults, tries to reform others, exaggerates grievances, responsible, conscientious, loyal, monogamous, holds grudges, moody, repressed emotions, weepy (can have hysterical sobbing), sensitive to the "existential dilemma."

Intellectual (mental): unconventionally intelligent, articulate, natural teachers.

Spiritual: concern for the spiritual well-being of self and others.

Sexual: weakness after sexual intercourse, aversion to sexual intercourse.

How should you use it? Take *Natrum muriaticum* 200C as the *constitutional homeopathic remedy* once or twice a week until improvement in symptoms. As soon as there is some improvement it is prudent to discontinue taking the remedy. It will continue exerting its deep action in the body. You may return to taking the remedy if a relapse occurs.

Nux vomica

What is it? This is a poisonous plant, *Nux vomica*, containing strychnine, common name *Poison nut*, a member of the *Loganiaceae* botanical family.
When should you use it? The **keynote** characteristics guiding you towards using *Nux vomica* as the patient's *constitutional homeopathic remedy* are divided into the five spheres of functioning:
Physical: cold, disturbances in digestive system, allergies, fatigue with insomnia (with rush of ideas), hypertension, bad breath, bad taste in mouth, strains to vomit, strains at stool (constipation) (straining is called "ineffectual urgings"), craving for spicy and fatty food, tics and twitches.
Emotional: prone to excesses of all kinds, over-stimulated, craves stimulation of all types (prone to alcoholism and other addictions such as caffeine, nicotine, licit and illicit drugs), angry, explodes with anger, "road-rage," impatient, suppressed anger, tense, irritable, business-like, "workaholic," pragmatic, complaining, critical, abusive, perfectionistic, quarrelsome, ambitious, driven, competitive, calculating, manipulating on his own behalf, needs to be in control, fear of marriage and intimacy, Type A personality.
Intellectual (mental): superior intelligence, logical, intellectual, witty, verbally expressive.
Spiritual: deficient spiritual life.
Sexual: high libido.
How should you use it? Take *Nux vomica* 200C as the *constitutional homeopathic remedy* once or twice a week until improvement in symptoms. As soon as there is some improvement it is prudent to discontinue taking the remedy. It will continue exerting its deep action in the body. You may return to taking the remedy if a relapse occurs

Phosphorus

What is it? This is the homeopathic remedy that is made from the non-metallic chemical element *Phosphorus*. It is one of the commonest elements in the human body because it makes up part of ATP (adenosine triphosphate), the chemical that stores our energy. *Phosphorus* is part of DNA, the genetic material present in every living cell. *Phosphorus* forms part of *phospholipids* that give cell membranes their permeability.
When should you use it? The **keynote** characteristics guiding you towards using *Phosphorus* as the patient's *constitutional homeopathic remedy* are divided into the five spheres of functioning:
Physical: sleeps on right side, left-sided ailments, symptoms better for being stroked and massage, symptoms worse at twilight, hypersensitive to noise and touch, thirsty for cold water, craves chocolate and ice-cream, sudden extreme growth spurts in children (tall and thin people), used for bleeding, respiratory diseases and burning pains.
Emotional: sympathetic, empathetic, needs affection and returns affection, needs company, sociable, artistic, creative, imaginative, impressionable, expressive, effervescent, extroverted, enthusiastic, sensitive, responsive, supportive, optimistic, cheerful, friendly, resilient, center of attention, energetic, dramatic, self-centered, easily distracted, generous, does not bear grudges or resentments, fears thunderstorms, twilight, business failure, cancer, illness.
Intellectual (mental): bright, verbally expressive.
Spiritual: clairvoyant, inner life revolves around intimate interpersonal relationships, sensitive to auras, experience déjà vu, telepathic.
Sexual: passionate, heightened sexuality.
How should you use it? Take *Phosphorus* 200C as the *constitutional homeopathic remedy* once or twice a week until improvement in symptoms. As soon as there is some improvement it is prudent to discontinue taking the remedy. It will continue exerting its deep action in the body. You may return to taking the remedy if a relapse occurs.

Pulsatilla

What is it? This is the plant *Pulsatilla nigricans*, whose common name is *windflower*, a member of the *Ranunculaceae* botanical family.
When should you use it? The **keynote** characteristics guiding you towards using *Pulsatilla* as the

patient's *constitutional homeopathic remedy* are divided into the five spheres of functioning:

Physical: hypersensitive to heat, thirstless despite dry mouth, changes in location of pains (wandering pains), ailments better for being in open air and after crying, ailments tend to be worse for heat or warmth, used for infections (with yellow-green discharges), reproductive tract ailments in women and as a constitutional remedy for children.

Emotional: labile emotions, desires to please, sweet-natured, mild, kind, gentle, unassertive, tearful, cries easily, changes moods easily, indecisive, irresolute, dependent, sadness, needs company and sympathy, needs affection, loving, demanding, needs attention, needs encouragement, manipulative, sulky, whiny, self-pity, easily hurt and insulted, avoids confrontation, peacemaking, suppressed anger, ailments better after crying and consolation.

Intellectual (mental): non-intellectual, personalizes and concretizes abstractions.

Spiritual: religious, intuitive.

Sexual: aversion to sexual intercourse, but desires marriage and children.

How should you use it? Take *Pulsatilla* 200C as the *constitutional homeopathic remedy* once or twice a week until improvement in symptoms. As soon as there is some improvement it is prudent to discontinue taking the remedy. It will continue exerting its deep action in the body. You may return to taking the remedy if a relapse occurs.

Sepia

What is it? The homeopathic remedy *Sepia* is made from the black ink sac of *Sepia officinalis*, the *cuttlefish*, a species of mollusk found in the Mediterranean Sea and the Atlantic Ocean.

When should you use it? The **keynote** characteristics guiding you towards using *Sepia* as the patient's *constitutional homeopathic remedy* are divided into the five spheres of functioning:

Physical: blue-black under eyes, yellow spots on the face, sallow complexion, tall and slim with narrow hips, ailments with downward pressure in the pelvis (bearing down pains), dislikes being touched, profuse perspiration with strong

smell (especially feet and hands), weariness, exhaustion, cravings for pickles, ailments better in the open air, better for warmth and heat, useful for reproductive tract ailments (especially left-sided) and sagging organs (prolapse and ptosis).

Emotional: apathetic, indifferent to business concerns, family (even one's own children), feels alienated from family and friends, fulfils her homemaker tasks from a sense of duty, organized, fastidious, overwhelmed by responsibilities (the typical overworked housewife), resentful, dissatisfied, complaining, contempt for people, averse to company, negative, irritable, moody, outspoken, easily offended, intolerant of contradiction, suppressed anger, ailments better when busy or occupied, career woman, loves dancing, reject sympathy, difficulties giving sympathy and affection.

Intellectual (mental): concentration and thinking difficult.

Spiritual: closed off spiritual life.

Sexual: painful sexual intercourse, diminished libido, non-orgasmic, infertility.

How should you use it? Take *Sepia* 200C as the *constitutional homeopathic remedy* once or twice a week until improvement in symptoms. As soon as there is some improvement it is prudent to discontinue taking the remedy. It will continue exerting its deep action in the body. You may return to taking the remedy if a relapse occurs.

Sulphur

What is it? The mineral element *Sulphur*, common name *brimstone*, is present in every cell of the human body. *Sulphur* without a doubt had been the most frequently used *constitutional homeopathic remedy* for more than a century, but in the latter part of the twentieth century, perhaps *Natrum muriaticum* and *Nux vomica* are prescribed more often.

When should you use it? The **keynote** characteristics guiding you towards using *Sulphur* as the patient's *constitutional homeopathic remedy* are divided into the five spheres of functioning:

Physical: cold, dry itchy skin, offensive perspiration, reddened body orifices, ailments worse for water, heat, wearing wool, cyclic or periodic changes in pains and ailments, gets weak from hunger (especially at 11 a.m.), used for skin diseases and burning pains.

Emotional: emotionally insensitive, untidy, unwashed, unorganized, aversion to washing, unclean, self-centered, eccentric, spouts philosophical obscurities ("absent-minded professor"), unfocused, extroverted, enthusiastic talker about his own concerns but lacks action and averse to follow-up, lazy, leaves projects unfinished, collects junk and clutter ("pack rat"), hoarding, collects books and music, practical, tight-fisted in money matters, averse to waste, critical, unsatisfied, argumentative, provokes controversy, monopolizes the conversation, unskilled socially, opinionated, forgets proper names, withdraws from society, sadness.

Intellectual (mental): superior intellectual ability, intellectual curiosity, inquisitive, many ideas, great ideas, prolific interests, inventive, enjoy debate but listens mostly to himself, excellent memory.

Spiritual: may be very religious or non-religious, spiritual realm is no comfort, bored by religion.

Sexual: robust sexual life, marital infidelities.

How should you use it? Take *Sulphur* 200C as the *constitutional homeopathic remedy* once or twice a week until improvement in symptoms. As soon as there is some improvement it is prudent to discontinue taking the remedy. It will continue exerting its deep action in the body. You may return to taking the remedy if a relapse occurs.

Guidelines for Consulting Your Health Care Provider

You should consult your health care provider if the following occurs during a course of treatment for cancer:

- the patient doesn't look right or act right (trust your instincts!)
- the patient is getting worse instead of better over the course of the illness
- the patient is having trouble breathing or complaining of chest pains or there is mental confusion or lethargy or irritability
- the patient develops new symptoms while taking the *constitutional homeopathic remedy*

> **Note:** Do not discontinue taking any pharmaceutical medication that has been prescribed by your health care provider unless you or your family member is under the supervision of a physician.

Recommendations for Homeopathic Remedies

Arsenicum album 200C—pellets or liquid drops
Calcarea carbonica 200C—pellets or liquid drops
Lachesis 200C—pellets or liquid drops
Lycopodium 200C—pellets or liquid drops
Natrum muriaticum 200C—pellets or liquid drops
Nux vomica 200C—pellets or liquid drops
Phosphorus 200C—pellets or liquid drops
Pulsatilla 200C—pellets or liquid drops
Sepia 200C—pellets or liquid drops
Sulphur 200C—pellets or liquid drops

Guidelines for Administration of Homeopathic Remedies

General guidelines to treat serious, chronic, relapsing ailments with the patient's *constitutional homeopathic remedy* include using single remedies at potencies of 200C (or higher, but only when prescribed by a homeopath). These are generally administered once weekly to once monthly, but they may be used once or twice daily at first if the condition warrants it, quickly decreasing the frequency as you see improvement. Remember in homeopathy, less is more. Some homeopaths have been trained to give the *constitutional homeopathic remedy* only once and do not repeat it unless the patient's symptoms return.

Do not continue giving the *constitutional homeopathic remedy* if it becomes apparent after 1-3 months that it is not working. You may always stop one remedy and choose to administer another remedy on the basis of the **keynote** symptoms of the new remedy. When administering the *constitutional homeopathic remedy*, generally only one remedy is given at a time, but this is not an absolute rule.

Note: For more information on *how often* to give the homeopathic remedy please see **Potency and Frequency**, in **Chapter 2: Basic Homeopathy**. For information on *how much* of the homeopathic remedy to give and the importance of a *"clean tongue,"* please see **How to take homeopathic remedie**s in the same chapter.

Lower potency remedies, such as 30C and below, are used to treat acute ailments. They are usually repeated often, every ½-2 or ½-4 hours. You should notice improvement in symptoms after just one to perhaps a few repetitions. If you do not see improvement, it is wise to stop the remedy and try a different one, guiding yourself by the **keynote** symptoms. You may use different single remedies together or you may try a combination remedy. And you may use homeopathic remedies together with pharmaceutical prescription and non-prescription drugs without any effect of interference.

General guidelines to treat serious, chronic, relapsing ailments include using single remedies at potencies of 200C. These are generally administered once weekly to once monthly, but they may be used once or twice daily at first if the condition warrants it, quickly decreasing the frequency as you see improvement. Do not continue giving the remedy if it becomes apparent that it is not working. You may always stop one remedy and choose to administer another remedy on the basis of the **keynote** symptoms of the new remedy. In addition, you may administer more than one remedy at a time.

Putting It All Together

Coping with difficult ailments requiring homeopathic constitutional remedies is best done utilizing a multi-pronged approach incorporating all the essential natural alternatives, homeopathy, herbal remedies, and nutritional supplements.

Depending on the chronicity of the problems you may decide to incorporate certain homeopathic remedies in **Chapter 16: Homeopathy for Neurologic Disorders** and **Chapter 8: Homeopathic**

Remedies for Emotional Problems. Constitutional problems often occur among the elderly (please refer to **Chapter 13: Homeopathy for Elderly Persons**).

Note: A homeopathic detoxification remedy is the *Detox-Kit*, manufactured by Heel. It consists of 3 components: *Lymphomyosot, Berberis Homaccord* and *Nux vomica Homaccord*, each in a 50 ml bottle. *Lymphomyosot* detoxifies the lymphatic system; *Berberis*, the excretory organs, specifically the kidneys, skin, and liver; and *Nux vomica*, the digestive system and liver. Thus, the *Detox-Kit* provides for the elimination of diverse toxins from most sources. The directions for use are to put 30 drops of each of the three solutions into one quart of water and drink it during the day.

People with problems of a constitutional type require all the vitamins and minerals necessary to repair and replenish tissues (please refer to **Chapter 23: Vitamins and Minerals**) as well as a general antioxidant supplement (please refer to **Chapter 24: Antioxidant Phytochemicals**).

You may want to investigate certain herbal remedies such as *Valerian* and *St. John's Wort* (please refer to **Chapter 20: Herbs You Need to Know**) as well as *omega-3 fatty acids* (please refer to **Chapter 31: Oils and Fats**). In addition, it is a good idea to incorporate *probiotics* (please refer to **Chapter 30: Prebiotics and Probiotics**) into your daily supplements because your may find your constitutional problems to be sensitive to enhanced gastrointestinal health.

Depending on the nature of the constitutional ailment you are trying to prevent or treat, you may need to consult the following chapters:

Chapter 12: **Homeopathy for Urinary Tract Ailments**

Chapter 11: **Homeopathy for Digestive Tract Ailments**

Chapter 25: **Heart Healthy Nutritional Supplements**

Chapter 17: **Homeopathy for Persons with Cancer**

PART TWO

Herbal Remedies

Chapter 19

Introduction to Herbal Medicine

What are herbal remedies?
Advantages and disadvantages of taking herbal remedies
The top ten herbal remedies in the United States
Herbs to stay away from
Detoxification the gentle way

What are herbal remedies?

Herbal medicine has a long history, perhaps as long as humankind itself. It is the most ancient of all forms of health care. The word "drug" comes from the Old Dutch word, dragge, which means "to dry." In order to make herbal medicines, plants need to be dried.

Herbal remedies are *phytomedicines* or *phytochemicals* that have been extracted from plants or parts of plants. If these same compounds would be purified and synthesized in a laboratory they would be called drugs. So, herbal remedies are drugs without a patent. And if the big pharmaceutical corporations could obtain patents on these plants, they would become pharmaceutical drugs and they would enter the armamentarium of conventional medicine.

Herbal medicines are **not** homeopathic remedies (although some herbal remedies may go through the processes of dilution and potentization to become homeopathic remedies). Herbal remedies have side effects (in direct contradistinction to homeopathic remedies). They have contraindications. They may interfere with your conventional medicines.

Note: How to distinguish herbal medicine from homeopathy:

Here we should note three profound differences be-tween herbal medicine and homeopathy that will help you to distinguish one from the other.

The first difference is that herbal medicine uses undiluted natural plants as medicines, which can have side effects just like Western medicines. Homeopathy uses only extremely dilute natural substances, which do not have side effects and are safe for all people, even including pregnant women, newborn babies, and the very elderly.

The second difference is that herbal remedies use only plant substances whereas homeopathic remedies use materials from all three kingdoms, plant, animal, and mineral.

The third difference is that herbal remedies are prescribed on the basis of Western medicine principles, for example, using an anti-diarrheal herbal remedy to treat diarrhea. Homeopathic remedies are prescribed on the basis of the principle of Like Cures Like, for example, using an extremely dilute remedy that would cause diarrhea (if given in full strength) to treat diarrhea.

Since herbal remedies are medicines, they must be used cautiously. You must check the list of side effects and contraindications before taking any herbal remedy. In order to check side effects and contraindications, you will need access to a comprehensive book on herbal remedies. Two good books for this purpose are: *PDR for Herbal Medicines* and *The Complete German Commission E Monographs Therapeutic Guide to Herbal Medicines*. A listing of recommended books appears in the **Appendix** under **Book Resources for Herbal Remedies**.

Always check herb-drug interactions before using an herbal remedy.

Using caution in self-care with herbal remedies means that you are especially wary of prescribing for anyone who is pregnant or lactating, or for infants or the elderly. Herbal remedies are a different kettle of fish from homeopathy, which is safe for everyone.

Chapter 20: Herbs You Need to Know and **Chapter 21: Herbal Remedies for Women's Health** contain advice on using herbs that are commonly used by Western doctors. Many other herbal remedies exist, some belonging to *Traditional Chinese Medicine* and some to *Ayurvedic Medicine*. Although some herbal remedies in Western medicine lend themselves to self-care, I strongly recommend that you do not self-prescribe those herbal remedies in *Traditional Chinese Medicine* or *Ayurvedic Medicine* because their side effects and contraindications are not as well delineated.

Note: A recent article in the respected medical *Journal of American Medical Association* revealed that 20% of 70 *Ayurvedic* herbal remedies made in India and Pakistan were contaminated with heavy metals, such as lead, mercury, or arsenic. This is a very serious potential problem. The safest thing is not to take any imported *Ayurvedic* herbal remedies.

Herbal remedies are the most commonly used forms of alternative medicine (possibly excluding prayer) with sales of about $600 million in 2002. Herbal remedies are so popular because they are available without a physician's prescription and their low cost is within many families' health care budget.

Herbal remedies may be combined with homeopathy and/or nutritional supplements when the combination is likely to produce a level of healing deeper than would be expected if only the herbal remedy were to be used. When herbal remedies are used in conjunction with homeopathic remedies, the effects may be synergistic, that is, greater than when only the herbal or homeopathic remedy is used alone. In this instance, the homeopathic remedy acts as the potentiating agent. The homeopathic remedy may act to allow you to use lesser amounts and for a shorter period of time of the herbal remedy to effect a deep healing. The same is true when nutritional supplements are used along with a homeopathic and/or herbal remedy. This phenomenon is one of the reasons why I encourage you to concentrate on learning how to use the three *essential natural alternatives* in healing: homeopathy, herbal remedies, and nutritional supplements.

For most ailments, I recommend using homeopathic remedies first (since there are no side effects and they have a good chance to be effective), then instituting the appropriate nutritional supplements (to augment the homeopathic remedies). Then, only if needed, begin the recommended herbal remedies (but only after carefully checking the herb-drug interactions and possible side effects). In this manner, most of the time, you will find yourself using herbal remedies only when homeopathic remedies have not given you the relief you seek.

Herbal remedies may be used in conjunction with Western medicines, but you must always check on the side effects and contraindications to determine whether any interactions with pharmaceuticals are likely to occur. A good place to start checking is the National Institutes of Health's herbal remedies website http://www.nlm.nih.gov/medlineplus/druginfo/herb_All.html.

When using herbal remedies for self-care you must pay strict attention to the **Guidelines for Consulting Your Health Care Provider** at the end of every chapter. If you or your family member is pregnant, lactating, or is very young or very old, you will need to take even more stringent precautions. Make sure that the herbal remedy you have selected is appropriate for pregnant or lactating females, infants, or elderly persons. Make sure that you have checked the herb-drub interactions. You may want to refer to the last section **Putting It All Together** for ideas on how to integrate the essential natural alternatives, homeopathy, herbal remedies, and nutritional supplements.

Advantages and disadvantages of taking herbal remedies

Herbal remedies offer certain advantages over pharmaceutical medicines. Herbal remedies can be gentler in action, although this is not a fixed attribute because often their action is the same or even more pronounced. However, there are certain herbs which act in a more gentle manner, that is, they have fewer uncomfortable or serious side effects, than their drug counterparts.

A good example is *St. John's Wort*. This herbal remedy may be used to treat mild to moderate depression and can eliminate the need for one of the SSRI drugs, such as Prozac, Paxil and Zoloft. However, *St. John's Wort* is rarely effective in moderate-severe depression. This fact may be an expression of its "gentleness."

Sometimes there are herbal remedies that treat certain conditions for which there is no Western medicine drug. A good example is the adaptogenic herb *Ginseng*, used to treat physical and emotional fatigue and exhaustion.

Western drugs do not prevent the onset of any condition; rather they are useful only once the condition becomes manifest as a disease. Herbal remedies may prevent certain conditions from becoming full-blown diseases. A good example is the use of *Echinacea* and *Goldenseal* at the very first symptom of an upper respiratory illness in order to prevent a cold or sore throat. *Cranberry* is a preventive against urinary tract infections. *Astragalus* is used to prevent immune system fatigue after a serious illness, and may prevent viral infections.

Herbal remedies are labeled as supplements, not drugs. Supplements do not fall within the purview of the *Food and Drug Administration (FDA)*. According to the Dietary Supplement Health and Education Act of 1994, as long as the herbal remedy manufacturer does not make any health claims for cure of any condition on the label, that remedy may be sold without *FDA* controls.

However, despite the advantages of not having *FDA* supervision (low cost and easy availability), there are many disadvantages, namely quality, safety, and effectiveness may be compromised. Quality and potency of herbal products are not uniform between manufacturers. And herbal remedies may be sold without proof that they work (efficacy) or that they are safe.

In 2007, a new law was enacted that would make supplement manufacturers responsible for quality control assurance. This will ensure batch-to-batch uniformity of all the ingredients that go into their products and would go a long way to eliminating contaminants. The new law still would not ensure the consumer that the herbal remedy is safe or effective when taken as directed. The law goes into effect in 2010. A system for enforcement has to be worked out.

> **Note:** The Dietary Supplement and Non-Prescription Drug Consumer Protection Act of 2006 requires that all serious adverse events occurring with dietary supplements and over-the-counter drugs be reported directly to the *FDA*. This is a big step towards protecting consumers. It will help to pin-point dangerous interactions and contaminations.

Meanwhile, until the new law goes into effect, the consumer shoulders the burden of quality assurance. My recommendation is to buy herbal remedies only from reputable companies. Dr. Andrew Weil's list is as follows: *Eclectic Institute, Enzymatic Therapy, Herbal Fortress, Mariposa Botanicals, Nature's Way, PhytoPharmica, Solaray* and *Zand*. I would enlarge this list by adding *The Vitamin Shoppe* brand, *Twin Lab,* and *Nature's Plus*.

ConsumerLab.com is an independent testing laboratory. It has been certifying herbal remedies and nutritional supplements, making sure that the ingredients are present in the dosages that are claimed on the label and that the formulation is free from contaminants. You may view their results online at www.ConsumerLab.com. ConsumerLab.com reports that approximately 15% of tested supplements fail their standards for both having: 1) exact correspondence of amount of active ingredients on label vs actually determined by testing; and 2) finding that the preparation is free from contaminants. You will need to pay a fee to view their listing of brands that passed and those that failed. Or you may prefer to read the book, *ConsumerLab.com's Guide to Buying Vitamins and Supplements: What's Really in the Bottle?*

I strongly recommend that you purchase only recommended brands of herbal and nutritional supplements. If you see the *USP mark* (United States Pharmacopeia) on the label you know that the supplement has been tested for release and dissolution of its ingredients. And you are assured that label claims for potency and amount are actually true and that there are no harmful levels of contaminants. In addition, the company's plant has been inspected for good manufacturing practices.

When you buy herbal remedies, check the label for certification that the manufacturer follows the *Food Good Manufacturing Practices (Food GMPs)* or the even higher standards, *Drug Good Manufacturing Practices (Drug GMPs)*.

The *FDA* has recently proposed new manufacturing standards for all dietary supplements including herbal remedies. This may reduce the number of contaminated and poor quality herbal products on the market, but will not go so far as to begin to answer questions of safety and effectiveness. Only high-quality medical research will be able to answer those questions.

Certain herbal remedies, such as *Dong quai, Ginkgo biloba, Garlic, Ginseng* and *St. John's Wort,* should be discontinued at least 2 weeks before a surgical procedure because of their effects on coagulation. Whenever you decide to use a herbal remedy, you must familiarize yourself with its side effects and herb-drug interactions.

Note: Some nutritional supplements, like *Vitamin E* and *Coenzyme Q10* may also affect blood coagulation.

Do not delude yourself into believing that herbal remedies somehow are not medicines. They are. You must disclose the herbal medicines you or your family member are taking to your health care provider.

The top ten herbal remedies in the United States

Herbal remedies lose or gain popularity over the years based on many factors, such as the publication of research findings and toxic side effects. The recent trend in the increasing popularity of *soy* and *garlic* is probably due, at least in part, to the amount of published positive research reaching the public. The declining popularity of certain herbs has been ascribed to negative research findings.

The top ten herbal remedies in the United States for 2002*, in decreasing market share are:

Garlic, Ginkgo, Echinacea, Soy, Saw palmetto, Ginseng, St. John's Wort, Black cohosh, Cranberry and *Valerian*.

*From *Quantification of the Scientific Research in the United States About Popular Herbal Remedies Referenced on Pubmed* by Hall M and Nazir N, published in *Alternative Therapies Health and Medicine*, May/June 2005.

Herbs to stay away from

Just because herbal remedies are "natural," does not mean that they are safe. Some herbal remedies are dangerous and should not be used under any circumstances. A good example is *Ephedra sinica*, also called *Ma Huang*. *Ephedra* (containing the active components *ephedrine* and *pseudoephedrine*, amphetamine-like alkaloids) was once used to treat asthma but has since been supplanted by other, less cardiotoxic drugs. Some people abuse *Ephedra*-contain-

ing herbal remedies by substituting it for the illegal drug, *Ecstasy*, to which it is chemically related.

Ephedra had once been a prominent component in some weight loss remedies, but because of the number of deaths attributed to it from disturbances in heart rhythm, the *FDA* ordered it removed from all products sold in the U.S. early in 2004. *Ephedra* had once accounted for between $500 million and $1 billion in sales revenue each year.

Metabolife is a weight loss product containing *Ephedra* (together with *caffeine* which potentiates the weight loss and also the cardiotoxicity) that had been linked to reports of approximately 80 deaths and more than one thousand other adverse effects through the *FDA*'s *MedWatch* system. I strongly recommend that you avoid any product containing *Ephedra*.

Kava Kava (*Piper methysticum*) is an herbal remedy that has been used to treat anxiety, stress, and insomnia. It was a best-selling herbal remedy in this country, with sales of more than $50 million per year. But reports of liver failure associated with the use of *Kava Kava* have come to light in the past few years. *Kava Kava* has been associated with more than 2 dozen cases of liver failure with one death and at least 4 persons requiring liver transplant.

Kava Kava has been used for centuries among the inhabitants of the Polynesian Islands where it occurs naturally. It is possible that liver failure occurred in certain people because they exceeded an intake of 240mg of *Kava Kava* daily (or 60-120mg of *kavalactone*, the active ingredient). But remember, due to the rules and regulations of the *FDA* governing herbal remedies, it is possible to think you are taking a certain amount of herbal remedy (as labeled on the bottle), or a certain concentration of active ingredient, when in reality you are inadvertently taking more, perhaps much more.

Note: When testing results do not correspond to the amount on the label, the more common situation is that the labeled amount is greater than the amount actually found in the tablet. But the problem with *FDA* non-regulation is that the consumer has no quality assurance of what is in the capsule. Until the

FDA regulates herbal remedies, I strongly recommend that you avoid any product containing *Kava Kava*.

Ephedra and *Kava Kava* are two examples of herbal remedies whose safety records indicate that they are best not taken. Certain other herbs, due to their toxic effects or interactions with drugs, do not lend themselves to self-care but rather need to be taken under the supervision of a health care provider. **Chapter 20: Herbs You Need to Know** and **Chapter 21: Herbal Remedies for Women's Health** present only those herbal remedies that have an established safety record. However, you will still need to carefully check side effects, contraindications, and herb-drug interactions before taking any herbal remedy.

The *ConsumerReports.org* has published a list of 12 supplements you should avoid which they call their "dirty dozen." *Aristolochic acid*, Latin name *Asarum canadensis*, also called *Aristolochia* or *snakeweed*, is the only herb in their "definitely hazardous" category. This herb is toxic to the liver and may cause death. It is banned in many European countries and will likely become banned in America soon.

In their "very likely hazardous" category there are 4 herbs and 1 nutritional supplement (*androstenedione*). *Androstenedione*, now banned by sports associations, had been used to increase endurance. It is known to increase cancer risk and decrease HDL ("good") cholesterol. The herbal remedy *comfrey* (*Symphytum officinalis*), also called *knitbone*, has been known to cause liver failure and death.

> **Note:** When *Symphytum* is made into a homeopathic remedy, it has no side effects and no toxicity. As a homeopathic remedy, *Symphytum* is used to aid in the healing of broken bones.

Chaparral, Latin name *Larrea divaricata*, also called *creosote bush*, has been used to "cleanse the bowel." It is known to cause liver failure and death. The same is true for *Germander*, Latin name *Teucrium chamaedrys*. *Kava Kava* (*Piper methysticum*) is also in this category.

In their "likely hazardous" category there are 5 herbs and 1 nutritional supplement (organ and glandular extracts). Organ and glandular extracts, especially bovine brain extracts, may be dangerous on the basis of the theoretical risk of mad cow disease.

The prudent person will avoid all weight loss products made with *Bitter orange* from the flowers of the plant *Citrus aurantium* because the active compound, *synephrine*, is similar to *Ephedra*. The safety record on *Bitter orange* is just not known. *Bitter orange* is on *Consumer Reports'* list of supplements that may cause cancer, kidney or liver damage, or even death.

Lobelia, Latin name *Lobelia inflata*, common name *pukeweed*, or *wild tobacco*, has been used to treat asthma. It is known to cause respiratory distress, low blood pressure, dizziness, tremors, and even death. *Pennyroyal oil* (*Hedeoma pulegoidides*) may cause liver and kidney failure as well as death. *Scullcap* (*Scutellaria lateriflora*) is known to cause liver damage. *Yohimbe* (*Pausinystalia yohimbe*), used as an aphrodisiac for men, is known to cause heart arrhythmias, heart attack, and death.

Detoxification the gentle way

Homeopathy is the only gentle and yet effective way to achieve detoxification from environmental poisons, such as pesticides, herbicides, insecticides, fungicides, pollutants, nicotine addiction, substances of abuse, alcohol addiction, and prescription pharmaceuticals.

> **Note:** Please do not consider other methods of detoxification, such as fasting, purging, chelation or colonic irrigation. These methods are likely to be harmful, dangerous, and invasive. They surely are unnatural and they all come with side effects. Homeopathic detoxification does not.

For detoxification purposes, you may want to consider the homeopathic combination remedy called *Ubichinon Compositum*, which is manufactured by Heel, a homeopathic supply house.

Note: You will find more information on *Ubichinon Compositum* in **Chapter 13: Homeopathy for Elderly Persons**.

Note: Another homeopathic detoxification remedy is the *Detox-Kit*, also manufactured by Heel. It consists of 3 components: *Lymphomyosot, Berberis Homaccord* and *Nux vomica Homaccord*, each in a 50 ml bottle. *Lymphomyosot* detoxifies the lymphatic system; *Berberis*, the excretory organs, specifically the kidneys, skin, and liver; and *Nux vomica*, the digestive system and liver. Thus, the *Detox-Kit* provides for the elimination of diverse toxins from most sources. The directions for use are to put 30 drops of each of the three solutions into one quart of water and drink it during the day.

When using herbal remedies for self-care you must pay strict attention to the **Guidelines for Consulting Your Health Care Provider** at the end of every chapter. You may want to refer to the last section **Putting It All Together** for ideas on how to integrate the essential natural alternatives, homeopathy, herbal remedies, and nutritional supplements.

Note: Do not discontinue taking any pharmaceutical medication that has been prescribed by your health care provider unless you or your family member is under the supervision of a physician.

Chapter 20

Herbs You Need to Know

Herbal Remedies in General

Ailment/Disorder/Symptom	Herbal Remedy
Upper respiratory infections, influenza	*Echinacea*
Upper respiratory infections, fungal infections	*Goldenseal*
Immune system stimulation	*Astragalus*
Immune system stimulation, anti-cancer activity	*Cat's Claw*
Migraine prevention	*Feverfew*
Anti-bacterial agent, cholesterol, blood pressure	*Garlic*
Cognitive and memory functions of the brain	*Ginkgo biloba*
Enhance libido, sexual function, and ability to cope with stress	*Ginseng*
Powerful antioxidant, weight control	*Green Tea*
Heart disease	*Hawthorn*
Liver disease, liver cell regeneration	*Milk thistle*
Dietary fiber, irritable bowel syndrome, ulcerative colitis	*Psyllium*
Benign prostatic hypertrophy	*Saw Palmetto*
Depression	*St. John's Wort*
Anti-fungal topical	*Tea Tree*
Insomnia	*Valerian*

Guidelines for Consulting Your Health Care Provider
Putting It All Together

Herbal Remedies in General

For most ailments, I recommend using homeopathic remedies first (since there are no side effects and they have a good chance to be effective), then instituting the appropriate nutritional supplements (to augment the homeopathic remedies), and then, only if needed, begin the recommended herbal remedies. In this manner, most of the time, you will find yourself using herbal remedies only when homeopathic remedies have not given you the relief you seek.

When dealing with certain other serious diseases I strongly recommend that you use the services of a health care provider or homeopath for diagnosis and supervision, even if you have decided to try homeopathy, herbal remedies, and nutritional supplements. The following is a partial list of such diseases:

> adult attention deficit disorder, arthritis, autism, cancer, HIV and AIDS, multiple sclerosis, coronary artery disease, heart attack (myocardial infarction), blood dyscrasia, cancer (of any type), congestive heart failure, diabetes mellitus, obesity, thyroid disorders, high blood pressure (hypertension), stroke, seizures, acute and chronic kidney (renal) failure, schizophrenia, bipolar disorder, borderline personality disorder, eating disorders, fibromyalgia, chronic fatigue syndrome, Crohn's disease, ulcerative colitis, celiac disease, mental deficiency disorders, chromosomal disorders, infertility, frequent miscarriages, polyneuropathy, cystic fibrosis.   [Adapted from *The Merck Manual* at www.merck.com]

This chapter and **Chapter 21: Herbal Remedies for Women's Health** presents herbal remedies that have an established safety record so that they lend themselves to self-care. However, you will still need to carefully check side effects, contraindications, and herb-drug interactions before beginning to take any herbal remedy.

If you or your family member is pregnant, breastfeeding, or is very young or very old, you will need to take even more stringent precautions. You yourself should make sure that the herbal remedy you have selected is not contraindicated for pregnant or lactating females, infants, or elderly persons by reading this chapter. Then you should check with your health care provider before taking any herbal remedy.

The large number of different preparations of an herb (teas, tablets, capsules, tinctures, combinations) along with many nonstandardized dosage forms, containing any combination of the active ingredients, precludes any definite dosage recommendations. If you can find the *tincture* form of the herbal remedy you require, then the safest thing to do is to follow the directions on the bottle.

The herbal remedies discussed below are those most commonly used by me in my clinical practice of alternative medicine. I have included important information on prescription drug-herbal interactions, some of which is taken from *Consumer Reports on Health* (November 2002, page 10), a publication I recommend highly to you.

When using herbal remedies for self-care of any and all ailments you must pay strict attention to the **Guidelines for Consulting Your Health Care Provider** at the end of this chapter. You may want to refer to the last section **Putting It All Together** for ideas on how to integrate the essential natural alternatives, homeopathy, herbal remedies, and nutritional supplements.

Echinacea

What is it? *Echinacea* is a perennial herb, a Native American medicinal plant, common name *purple coneflower*, a member of the *Asteraceae* (*Compositae*) botanical family. *Echinacea purpurea, Echinacea angustifolia* and *Echinacea pallida* have somewhat different actions. Many preparations include all 3 species. Make sure you buy a preparation that contains *Echinacea purpurea*.

The medicinal parts of the plant are the fresh or dried roots (harvested in autumn), leaves, or the whole plant (harvested at flowering), depending upon the species that is being harvested.

When should you use it? *Echinacea* stimulates the immune system to produce certain chemicals (*cytokines*) which increase the body's healing abilities after the invasion of some foreign material, such as a virus or a bacterium. The net effect is to increase the activity of cells which engulf foreign particles (macrophages) or produce interferon (T lymphocytes) or mobilize infection-fighting white blood cells from the bone marrow (polymorphonuclear cells). *Echinacea* is used most commonly to treat the symptoms of the common cold and flu. Administration of *Echinacea* has been proven to lessen the duration as well as the severity of those symptoms. It is also effective in the treatment of bronchitis, sore throats, ear infections, sinus infections, flu (influenza infection), urinary tract infections, wounds and burns. The evidence that *Echinacea* can prevent the occurrence of a cold or flu is less robust, but it is effective in my experience so I recommend it for this purpose.

How should you use it? The large number of different *Echinacea* preparations (teas, tablets, capsules, tinctures, combinations) with many nonstandardized dosage forms, containing any combination of the three *Echinacea* species, precludes any definite dosage recommendations. The safest thing to do is to follow the directions on the bottle. Most herbal references give the dose for *Echinacea* as up to 900mg daily, but I sometimes recommend twice that dose, but just for 1-2 days.

The *German Commission E Monograph* states that use of *Echinacea* should not be longer than six consecutive weeks. Then you may take a one-week herb-free interval and begin again, if needed.

Here are my recommendations for preventing an upper respiratory illness with *Echinacea* in combination with *Goldenseal* (please see below, and remember that *Goldenseal* is contraindicated during pregnancy).

Buy *Echinacea* and *Goldenseal* together in one capsule from a reputable manufacturer of herbal remedies (a good choice is *The Vitamin Shoppe*), totaling approximately 450-500mg of both herbs. As soon as you feel the *very first* symptoms of becoming ill with an upper respiratory infection (which will be at least 24 hours before the full-blown symptoms appear) take 3 capsules along with 2000mg of *Vitamin C*. Repeat the 3 capsules every 4 hours for one day (along with 2000mg of *Vitamin C*) until the symptoms are relieved. Stop as soon as you no longer feel those first symptoms like you are coming down with a cold or flu. If you get sick anyway, you may continue with 2 capsules 3 times daily for 3 days (along with 2000mg of *Vitamin C*). This regimen will help to reduce the severity of the upper respiratory infection.

The effectiveness of this regimen in preventing upper respiratory infections depends upon beginning the first dose as soon as you feel the *very first* symptoms. Those *very first* symptoms could be something as fleeting as a headache, or a tickle in the throat, or tiredness, or perhaps crankiness or loss of appetite in a child. Whatever those *very first* symptoms are for you or for your family member, they generally tend to recur every time. The trick is to be in tune with your body and to note those *very first* symptoms so you have a chance to prevent an illness.

If you were not able to take this regimen at the *very first* symptoms, you still might try it because it may decrease the duration and severity of your upper respiratory infection (common cold).

Another way to achieve the same results is to take the liquid *tincture* form of *Echinacea* and *Goldenseal*. This form is generally more concentrated. Follow the directions on the bottle but always begin prevention at the *very first* symptom for maximal results.

> **Note:** For pregnant and lactating women take *Echinacea* without *Goldenseal* in the same dosage schedule, together with *Vitamin C*.

Some negative results from medical research: You should be aware that medical researchers in a recent study funded by the *National Center for Complementary and Alternative Medicine* (*NCCAM*) found that *Echinacea* administered to children did not decrease the number of days an upper respiratory infection lasted nor did it decrease the severity of symptoms. However, it is likely that these children did not receive exhortations to begin the use of *Echinacea* at the *very first* symptoms. And the study children did not get *Echinacea* combined with *Goldenseal*, which is more effective than either alone. It may be found in future studies that *Echinacea* does prevent the onset or if given early enough, decrease the duration and severity of symptoms. Another possibility is that *Echinacea* does work with certain cold viruses but not others.

> **Note:** Using homeopathic remedies to prevent or treat upper respiratory infec-

tions is another way to accomplish the same goal. In some cases, you may want to combine homeopathy and herbal remedies to achieve the results you want.

What are the side effects, contraindications, and herb-drug interactions? *Echinacea* is not recommended to treat any condition in persons with autoimmune diseases, HIV/AIDS (although studies are underway to determine the effects of treatment with *Echinacea*), tuberculosis, multiple sclerosis, or taking drugs to suppress the immune system (such as transplantation patients who take *cyclosporine*) or patients taking *corticosteroids*. In addition, according to the *Consumer Reports on Health* (November 2002), *Echinacea* may interact with the following drugs to increase their effects to potentially dangerous levels: *Allegra* (*fexofenadine* for allergies), *Halcion* (*triazolam* for anxiety), *Dilantin* (*phenytoin* for convulsions), *Nizoral* (*ketoconazole* for fungal infections), *Sporanox* (*itraconazole* for fungal infections), *Theo-Dur* (*theophylline* for asthma), *Coumadin* (*warfarin* for blood thinning), *Orinase* (*tolbutaminde* for diabetes), and the "statin" drugs to lower cholesterol such as *pravastatin* (*Pravachol*), *simvastatin* (*Zocor*) and *atorvastatin* (*Lipitor*). People with these conditions are safer taking homeopathic remedies to prevent colds along with frequent doses of 2000mg of *Vitamin C*.

There have been rare reports of allergy to *Echinacea*. There is cross-reactivity with other members of the *Compositae* botanical family, such as: *daisy, chrysanthemum, marigold, chamomile, calendula, yarrow* and *ragweed*.

> Note: Another safe herbal remedy alternative to *Echinacea* and *Goldenseal* to treat/prevent colds is *Sambucus nigra* or *Black Elderberry* extract, specifically a product called *Sambucol* by Nature's Way (follow the directions on the package). Daily use of *Sambucol* according to the directions on the package has been proven to shorten the illness with influenza virus by an average of four days compared to not using it. *Sambucol, Echinacea* and *Goldenseal* may be used in conjunction with antibiotics.

The *German Commission E Monograph* states that there are no effects of *Echinacea* (administered by mouth) on pregnancy and lactation. Tests done (only on *Echinacea purpurea*) showed no cancer-forming ability (carcinogenicity).

Sometimes *Echinacea* may be combined with *Propolis*, an immune stimulant harvested from beehives. *Propolis* has anti-inflammatory, antiviral, antimicrobial, and anticancer properties. A clinical research study of illness prevention using a combination of *Echinacea, Propolis* and *Vitamin C*, showed a significant reduction in the number of episodes of upper respiratory illnesses compared to persons taking placebo.

> **Note:** *Airborne* effervescent tablets are to be taken at the very first cold symptom. *Airborne* contains vitamins and minerals (vitamins A, C, E and riboflavin and minerals magnesium, selenium, manganese, and potassium), herbal extracts (several including *Echinacea*) and amino acids (glutamine and lysine). Data on safety and effectiveness is lacking, so pregnant and lactating women should not use it (especially because the dose of Vitamin A in just 2 *Airborne* tablets is 10,000 IU, the upper limit when fetal malformations may occur).

> **Note:** For more information on *Echinacea* please visit the National Center for Complementary and Alternative Medicine (*NCCAM*) at http://nccam.nih.gov/health/echinacea/ and for research results on *Echinacea* please visit http://nccam.nih gov/clinicaltrials/echinacea_rr.htm.

> **Note:** *Andrographis*, an herbal remedy from the plant *Andrographis paniculata*, common name *Kan jang* or *Indian echinacea*, has been shown to be helpful in the treatment of colds and flu. Use a preparation with 4% *andrographolides* (the active component). Follow the directions on the bottle. Do not take this herb if you are taking anticoagulants.

Goldenseal

What is it? This is the perennial plant *Hydrastis canadensis*, a member of the *Ranunculaceae* botanical family. It is a woodland plant, growing in Canada, the eastern United States, the Ohio Valley, and the Blue Ridge Mountains. The dried root is used to make the herbal remedy. The active constituents of *Goldenseal* are *hydrastine* and *berberine*.

When should you use it? *Goldenseal* stimulates the immune system and has broad-spectrum anti-microbial actions as well on fungi, parasites, and many types of bacteria. *Goldenseal* increases macrophage activity. It is useful as an antiseptic to prevent wounds from becoming infected. *Goldenseal* is also useful as an antidiarrheal agent. Although many people (myself included) believe (based upon clinical evidence) that *Goldenseal* acts synergistically with *Echinacea*, there is no medical evidence to prove this. The most effective way to use *Goldenseal* is to combine it with *Echinacea* (see above) to treat/prevent upper respiratory infections. However, it is also used topically as a wound dressing, eye wash (for conjunctivitis), and as a treatment for acne and ringworm.

How should you use it? The large number of different *Goldenseal* preparations (teas, tablets, capsules, tinctures, combinations) with many nonstandardized dosage forms, precludes any definite dosage recommendations. The safest thing to do is to follow the directions on the bottle. When using *Goldenseal* in combination with *Echinacea*, please follow the dosage recommendations under *Echinacea* above.

What are the side effects, contraindications, and herb-drug interactions? *Goldenseal* is contraindicated during pregnancy because it may increase uterine contractions. There is no data on the safety of *Goldenseal* during lactation, and for this reason, I do not recommend it for breastfeeding women until their infants are more than six months old. *Goldenseal* is contraindicated in newborn infants because it may cause or potentiate newborn jaundice. It is also contraindicated in persons with jaundice, high blood pressure (because in large doses it causes an increase in blood pressure), and in persons who have an inherited enzyme deficiency (called glucose-6-phosphate-dehydrogenase). Since it interferes with the action of chemotherapeutic agents, it is contraindicated in persons undergoing chemotherapy for cancer, although *berberine* is being investigated as a treatment for cancer.

Side effects can occur when *Goldenseal* is taken above the recommended daily dose (500mg of *berberine*). The side effects are irritation of the skin, eyes, and kidney, with shortness of breath and lethargy.

> **Note:** Some *Echinacea* combination herbal remedies substitute *Oregon Grape Root* (*Mahonia aquifolium*) for *Goldenseal* because the latter is considered to be an endangered species. Both *Oregon Grape Root* and *Goldenseal* contain *berberine* and *hydrastine*. Both have similar actions, side effects, and warnings not for use during pregnancy and lactation.

Astragalus

What is it? This is the perennial shrub, *Astragalus membranaceus*, called *Huang Qi* or *Huang Se* (*yellow energy builder*) in Chinese, a member of the *Leguminosae* botanical family. The medicinal parts are the roots.

When should you use it? *Astragalus* has been proven in medical research to modulate and enhance the function of the immune system possibly by increasing the number and maturation of stem cells in the bone marrow which then transform, when called into action, into infection-fighting cells. *Astragalus* is also involved in the production of interferon and interleukin, *cytokines* that fight bacterial and viral infections. In Chinese medicine, *Astragalus* is considered to be a *Qi* (vital force in homeopathy) restorer. *Astragalus* is used to increase physical and emotional stamina.

When given to adults or children with repeated infections (such as colds and flu), it acts to stimulate the immune system and helps to prevent recurrences. *Astragalus* is effective against certain viruses. Currently *Astragalus* is used to treat acute and chronic respiratory tract infections, viral infections, debilitated immune system functioning, organ failure (kidney, liver, heart), and cancer. Research on *Astragalus* as an adjunctive therapy for cancer is promising, especially for patients undergoing chemotherapy or radiation.

Research is being conducted on the effects of *Astragalus* on persons infected with HIV as well as persons with autoimmune diseases. *Astragalus* is often used to treat persons with chronic fatigue syndrome.

How should you use it? There are many forms of *Astragalus* on the market. *Astragalus* tea is delicious and is an easy way to get your daily dose during an acute episode. The dose for *Astragalus* is 400-500mg, one or two capsules three times daily. The Chinese tend to use *Astragalus* on a daily basis for just 4-8 weeks, although Americans use it for longer periods of time. Try to find the *tincture* form of *Astragalus* and give the recommended drops every day to either fight an infection or to build up general immunity. You may discontinue *Astragalus* when your infection has resolved or when you no longer get recurrent episodes, thereby inferring that your immune system has been strengthened.

What are the side effects, contraindications, and herb-drug interactions? At this time, *Astragalus* is contraindicated in persons who take drugs to suppress their immune systems (autoimmune diseases) and in patients who are candidates for or who are taking drugs for transplantation. Do not use *Astragalus* in persons who take anticoagulant drugs (*Coumadin* or *warfarin*) because it may increase the risk for bleeding. Persons who are scheduled for surgery should not take *Astragalus*. Persons taking drugs for diabetes, phenobarbital, or beta-blockers (propranolol, atenolol) should not take *Astragalus* until new research data become available.

Cat's Claw

What is it? This is the plant *Uncaria tomentosa*, common name *Una de gato*, a member of the *Rubiaceae* botanical family. *Cat's Claw* is harvested from the Peruvian rain forest along the Amazon River. The medicinal part is the root bark. There has been confusion reported in identifying this plant in the wild because evidently several different plants have the common name *una de gato*.
When should you use it? *Cat's Claw* stimulates the immune system and shows activity against viral infections as well as having antioxidant properties.

Cat's Claw is used to bolster a weakened immune system. Research is continuing on the effects of *Cat's Claw* in the treatment of cancer as well as HIV infection. *Cat's Claw* may function to protect against DNA damage.

There is good laboratory evidence that *Cat's Claw* is able to decrease the amount of tumor cell enzyme (DNA polymerase) that allows the division of cancerous cells. But, the evidence in sick people who take *Cat's Claw* to help them with cancer and other immune system ailments has yet to be developed.
How should you use it? The usual dose is 500mg of plant material once or twice daily.

What are the side effects, contraindications, and herb-drug interactions? No serious side effects have been reported. The use of *Cat's Claw* during pregnancy or lactation is not recommended because there is a lack of information on its toxicity. *Cat's Claw* is not recommended for children under the age of 3 years because safety data is lacking. At this time, *Cat's Claw* is contraindicated in persons who take drugs to suppress their immune systems (autoimmune diseases) and in patients who are candidates for or who are taking drugs for transplantation. *Cat's Claw* is contraindicated in persons taking anticoagulant medications. *Cat's Claw* has some blood pressure lowering effects so it should not be used in persons taking anti-hypertensive medications.

Feverfew

What is it? This is the perennial plant *Tanacetum parthenium*, common names *Feverfew* and *Bachelor's buttons*, a member of the *Asteraceae* (*Compositae*) botanical family. The active component is *parthenolide*. As early as 1649 the famous English herbalist, Culpeper, wrote that *Feverfew* was beneficial for headaches. The medicinal parts are the leaves, stems, and roots.
When should you use it? *Feverfew* has anti-inflammatory, antispasmodic, and antimigraine effects. *Feverfew* is mainly used as a preventive in migraine headaches. It prevents the release of serotonin from platelets which may be how it decreases the frequency of migraines.

How should you use it? A usual dose for migraine prevention is 250mg of *Feverfew* extract (which has been standardized to 0.7% *parthenolides*) 1-3 times daily depending on severity. You may need to take it daily for 2-8 weeks before any beneficial effects become evident. Do not stop taking it suddenly but rather taper over two weeks.

What are the side effects, contraindications, and herb-drug interactions? *Feverfew* has no serious side effects and can be taken long-term. *Feverfew* is contraindicated during pregnancy and lactation. If you have been taking *Feverfew* over a protracted period and wish to stop for any reason, it is best to taper over two weeks in order to prevent rebound migraine headaches which are sometimes associated with insomnia and joint pains. Allergy to *Feverfew* leaves and flowers can occur, resulting in contact dermatitis. *Feverfew* is contraindicated in persons taking anticoagulant medications.

Garlic

What is it? This is the perennial plant *Allium sativum*, common names *Garlic and Poor Man's Treacle*, a member of the *Liliaceae* botanical family. The medicinal part is the bulb (containing the cloves), either whole fresh or dried.

When should you use it? *Garlic* has been used by *Homo sapiens* as a medicinal remedy for several millennia. *Garlic* has been approved by *German Commission E* for treatment for the following disorders: arteriosclerosis (hardening of the arteries), hypertension (high blood pressure), and hypercholesterolemia (high cholesterol). However, recent medical evidence is ambivalent with regard to *garlic's* abilities to lower cholesterol. *Garlic* may be useful to treat bacterial and fungal infections. *Garlic* may be used as a cancer preventive due to its antioxidant properties, although more medical research has to be done on humans. *Garlic* has blood sugar lowering (hypoglycemic) properties. *Garlic* has the ability to protect the liver from toxins. *Garlic* possesses the ability to modulate the immune system. The active principle in *Garlic* is *allicin*, a sulfur-containing compound. *Allicin* is partially inactivated during cooking so the fresh clove is preferred for its health benefits. Another sulfur-containing compound *ajoene* may play a role in the prevention and treatment of cancer.

How should you use it? The label on *Garlic* preparations states the amount of *allicin* it contains. The recommended dosage of *Garlic* is 500mg twice daily. Wakunaga (the makers of Kyolic) make an *Aged Garlic Extract* which is odor-free and palatable as well as a liquid garlic preparation. You may contact Wakunaga at 800-421-2998 or info@wakunaga.com. You may prefer the fresh cloves of *Garlic*. Eat one or two cloves twice daily. When you peel your fresh garlic cloves, chop or crush them, then let them set for 15 minutes before cooking. That way you'll maximize *Garlic's* anti-cancer properties.

What are the side effects, contraindications, and herb-drug interactions? *Garlic* should not be used during anticoagulant therapy (such as *warfarin* [*Coumadin*], *clopidogrel* [*Plavix*], *aspirin*, and other blood thinners) due to decreased platelet stickiness (aggregation). *Garlic* should be discontinued at least 2 weeks prior to elective surgery. *Garlic* should not be used prior to labor and delivery for the same reason. *Garlic* may lessen the ability of certain medications to lower blood pressure (antihypertensives) such as: *diltiazem* (*Cardizem*), *nicardipine* (*Cardene*) and *verapamil* (*Calan*). *Garlic* may interact with certain protease-inhibiting drugs which are used to treat HIV/AIDS and drugs which suppress the immune system (such as *cyclosporine* [*Sandimmune*]). *Garlic* may interact with antidiabetes drugs including *insulin*, *glipizide* (*Glucotrol*), *rosiglitazone* (*Avandia*) and *chlorpropamide* (*Diabinese*). *Garlic* may reduce the drug effects of oral contraceptives.

Using *Garlic* during lactation may improve nursing by increasing the breastfeeding times. But, some infants may be sensitive to *Garlic* which may result in colic in the newborn. There have been no adverse reports on the use of *Garlic* during pregnancy. However, it is wise to discontinue *Garlic* one month prior to delivery so that your ability to clot will not be affected.

Side effects of *Garlic* include bad breath (halitosis) which can be (almost completely) eliminated by choosing a "deodorized" preparation. However, the more "deodorized" the *Garlic* pill, the less active *allicin* it contains. Other side effects may be abdominal discomfort with bloating, nausea, vomiting, and diarrhea. Allergy to *Garlic* does occur.

Ginkgo biloba

What is it? *Ginkgo biloba* is a dioecious tree (male and female flowers are on separate trees) which generally lives for hundreds of years. The tree is 20 years old before it is ready to reproduce. *Ginkgo biloba* first appeared on the earth about 200 million years ago, making it our planet's oldest living tree. *Ginkgo biloba* is the only species belonging to the *Ginkgoaceae* botanical family. The medicinal part is the leaves. The active components are *flavonoid glycosides* and *ginkgolides*, sometimes called *ginkgoflavongycosides*.

When should you use it? *Ginkgo biloba* has been shown to increase blood flow to the cerebral cortex, the thinking part of the brain. *Ginkgo biloba* also has antioxidant and protective effects on the brain's ability to withstand decreased oxygen which may occur during normal aging. *Ginkgo biloba* has been approved by *German Commission E* to treat organic brain syndromes, dementia and pre-dementia (such as Alzheimer's disease), difficulties with memory and concentration, dizziness, and tinnitus (ringing in the ears). *Ginkgo biloba* is also used to treat poor circulation in the lower extremities (peripheral arterial occlusive disease or intermittent claudication).

Although much clinical research has validated the use of *Ginkgo biloba* to enhance memory and cognitive functioning, some well-performed studies do not show positive results on memory, learning, and concentration. A recent study did not show *Ginkgo biloba* to be more effective than placebo for treating tinnitus.

How should you use it? Take 60mg of *Ginkgo biloba* leaf extract which has been standardized to contain 24% *ginkgoflavongycosides*, 1-4 times daily depending on severity and response.

What are the side effects, contraindications, and herb-drug interactions? *Ginkgo biloba* has few serious side effects when taken at the recommended dosage. The side effects most commonly noted are nausea, heartburn or indigestion, headache, diarrhea, and allergic skin reactions.

Ginkgo biloba may interact with anti-hypertensive medications (*thiazide* diuretics such as *Hygroton* and *Esidrix*), anti-insomniac-antidepressant medication *trazodone* (*Desyrel*), and antidepressant medications of the MAO inhibitors group (such as *Nardil*, *Parnate* and *Marplan*). *Ginkgo biloba* is contraindicated in persons taking anticoagulant medications such as *warfarin* (*Coumadin*) or *clopidogrel* (*Plavix*). *Ginkgo biloba*'s antiplatelet effect may be increased (increasing the risk of excessive bleeding) when it is used with other drugs having an antiplatelet effect such as *aspirin* (and other nonsteroidal anti-inflammatory drugs [NSAIDS]), *Feverfew*, *Ginseng* and *Garlic*. If you are taking an antiplatelet drug (or drugs) it is a good idea to limit your dose of *Ginkgo biloba* to 60mg once daily. Some persons may show allergic symptoms to *Ginkgo biloba*. It is not generally used in children under the age of 12 years. *German Commission E* considers it to be safe to take during pregnancy and lactation. However, good data on safety during pregnancy and lactation are lacking.

> **Note:** Some herbalists recommend the combination of *Ginkgo biloba* together with *Hawthorn* to treat jet lag. Take one-half teaspoon of the tinctures of both herbs 3 times daily until relief. If you start using the combination before your trip you may be able to prevent jet lag entirely.

Ginseng

What is it? This is the perennial plant *Panax ginseng*, common names *Chinese* (or *Korean* or *Japanese*) *Ginseng*, a member of the *Araliaceae* botanical family. *American Ginseng* is the species *Panax quinquefolius*. *Siberian Ginseng* is *Eleutherococcus senticosus*, a different genus altogether, possessing some characteristics which are similar and some which are different from those members of the *Panax* genus. (*Eleutherococcus senticosus* is said to possess more calming action than *Panax ginseng*.) The word *Panax* is derived from the Latin word *panacea*, or cure-all. The medicinal part is the dried main and lateral roots, which are said to resemble a human body. The pharmacologically active chemicals are called *ginsenosides*, of which there are at least 25 different ones.

When should you use it? *Ginseng* is an *adaptogen*, one of a group of tonic herbs including *Siberian Ginseng*, all the *Panax* species, *Rhodiola rosea* and *Ashwagandha* (*Withania somnifera*, containing the active principle *withanolides*, known as *Indian*

Ginseng used in Ayurvedic medicine). Adaptogens enhance the body's ability to cope with stress by their modulating effects on the adrenal gland. Stress elicits certain hormonal responses which may not be unhealthy. The unhealthy part is the way some of us react to those signals. Our individual reactivity to stress is one of the causes of many of the chronic diseases so prevalent in our times.

Ginseng has been used for thousands of years to enhance libido and improve sexual functioning. Now there is clinical research showing that *Ginseng* may correct erectile dysfunction, decrease premature ejaculation, and increase libido. *Ginsenosides*, the active components in *Ginseng*, have been shown in laboratory research to increase the release of nitric oxide which acts to dilate the corpus cavernosum of the penis, thereby enhancing erections.

In addition to its stress-balancing and sexual functioning effects, *Ginseng* increases energy, vitality, physical stamina, athletic performance, and mental functioning. *Ginseng* also has antioxidant and liver-protecting effects. It tends to lower blood glucose and to lower total cholesterol while increasing HDL cholesterol as well. There is some research showing that *Ginseng* may have anti-cancer activity.

> **Note:** *Withania somnifera* (*Ashwagandha*) is an herb with adaptogenic properties, relieving stress similar to *Ginseng*. Its sexual enhancing powers are also similar to *Ginseng*. It may be safely used to stimulate libido in both men and women and to enhance sexual performance in men. Although *Ashwagandha* has energizing actions, it is also used to treat anxiety and insomnia because of its sedative properties. So be careful when you first start to use this herbal remedy until you determine how it affects you.

> **Note:** *Siberian Ginseng*, commonly called *Eleuthero*, augments immunity and as such may be beneficial in preventing infection with the influenza virus (the "flu"). Take 250-500mg capsules twice daily.

> **Note:** It may be a good idea to take *Panax ginseng* during convalescence from an illness as it helps to restore physical and mental energy during

recovery. It has been shown to reduce the time to recovery from simple colds and influenza. In some studies, *Ginseng* prevented the onset of viral upper respiratory infections.

How should you use it? The daily dosage is 200mg of *Ginseng* extract standardized to 4-7% of *ginsenosides*, usually taken 100mg twice daily. *Ginseng* tea is an effective stress reducer and mid-afternoon pick-me-up. Dr. Andrew Weil recommends using *adaptogens* during convalescence from an illness, or during periods of fatigue and debility, because if used on a continuous basis, tolerance or resistance may develop. If tolerance or resistance does develop, you may stop taking *Ginseng* for about 2 weeks and then start again for a 3-month cycle.

What are the side effects, contraindications, and herb-drug interactions? *Ginseng* should not be used with anticoagulants (such as *warfarin* [*Coumadin*], *aspirin* and other *NSAIDs*), MAO inhibitors (such as *Nardil, Parnate* and *Marplan*). In addition, *Ginseng* should not be used with *estrogen, steroids, digoxin* and *insulin* (or other drugs that lower blood sugar, such as *glipizide* [*Glucotrol*], *rosiglitazone* [*Avandia*] and *chlorpropamide* [*Diabinese*]). *Ginseng* should be used cautiously in persons who have heart disease (cardiovascular disease) or diabetes. If you or your family member has either of those conditions, it is best to seek the advice of your health care professional before taking *Ginseng* supplements.

Ginseng is generally not recommended for use during pregnancy or lactation. (A report that *Ginseng* causes an increase in the male characteristics of the newborn [neonatal androgenization] was discredited.) However, *Ginseng* is used during pregnancy in China as well as in Germany as the *German Commission E* monograph does not prohibit its use. My recommendation is that *Ginseng* should not be used during pregnancy and lactation until we have more data on its safety under these conditions. There is some, albeit unproven, suspicion that *Ginseng* may have some estrogenic properties.

Prolonged high doses of *Ginseng* may produce the *Ginseng Abuse Syndrome* which consists of headaches, nervousness, insomnia, high blood pressure, and vomiting.

> **Note:** You may want to try *Altovis*, a combination herbal remedy for fatigue

manufactured by Berkeley, the same company that makes *Avlimil* (please refer to **Chapter 21: Herbal Remedies for Women's Health**). The active ingredients in *Altovis* include: *Green tea* (containing 100mg of *caffeine* in each tablet), *Cordyceps*, *Eleutherococcus senticosus*, *Panax ginseng*, *vinpocetine* and (*octacosanol*). Take one tablet daily. You may order at 1-800-ALTOVIS.

Note: Make sure to buy a reputable brand of *Ginseng* because the quality of the remedy is not uniform between different brands. You may check the brands that deliver the proper amount of *Ginseng* at ComsumerLab.com.

Green Tea

What is it? This is the evergreen shrub *Camellia sinensis*, or *Thea sinensis*, common name *Tea*, a member of the *Camelliaceae* botanical family. The medicinal part is the dried leaves. The 3 kinds of tea, *Green*, *Oolong* and *Black*, all come from the same plant. The difference lies in the processing after harvesting the leaves. *Green tea* is made when tea leaves are heated immediately after harvesting. This tends to decrease any chemical changes. A short delay until heating produces *Oolong tea* (which is slightly fermented) and a longer delay until heating (fermented) gives *black tea*. Of the three teas, *Green tea* has the most *flavonoid* antioxidants but all three have impressive amounts.

When should you use it? One of the active chemical components in *Green tea* is *polyphenols* which are classified as *flavonoids*. *Polyphenols* possess potent antioxidant effects. This probably explains some of *Green tea*'s anticancer activity. However, *Green tea* exerts an action on cancerous tumors that goes beyond its antioxidant function. It actually decreases new blood vessels growing in tumors, thereby shutting down their blood supply and slowing their growth rate. *Green tea* shows anticancer activity against most cancers along the entire digestive tract as well as those that are estrogen-dependent, such as breast cancer. In one study, *Green tea* drinkers who smoked had less damage to their DNA (a precursor

to cancer) than smokers who didn't drink *Green tea*.

Other *flavonoids* in *Green tea* are *catechins* which increases the body's production of heat, thereby increasing metabolic rate. This is probably the chemical constituent that makes *Green tea* the beverage of choice in persons with obesity.

The most potent *catechin* is *epigallocatechin gallate* or *EGCG*. *EGCG* exhibits antioxidant powers up to 100 times that of Vitamins C and E.

Green tea displays antiviral, antibacterial, and antifungal activity. Drinking *Green tea* decreases your risk for heart disease and stroke, lowers total cholesterol, blocks the oxidation of LDL cholesterol, increases HDL ("good") cholesterol, and enhances your immune system. If that's not enough, *Green tea* has been proven to contribute to higher bone mineral density.

How should you use it? In order to obtain the antioxidant and other benefits from *Green tea*, you need to drink one cup 3-5 times daily, or on average 4 times daily. The recommended daily dosage of *polyphenols* is 300-400mg. Three cups has about 240-320mg of *polyphenols*.

Green tea extract (in both liquid and capsule form) has 250mg of *Green tea* standardized to contain 75% *polyphenols*. Take one or two daily.

For persons sensitive to caffeine, I recommend drinking the decaffeinated *Green tea* even though the decaffeination process decreases the *flavonoid* content by 50% (from 140mg per 100 grams of tea to 70, according to the Nutrient Data Laboratory of the United States Department of Agriculture). If you are not sensitive to caffeine, you may choose to drink regular *Green tea*, each cup of which has less than one-third the amount of caffeine compared to coffee (8-30mg/cup vs. 100-135, according to *Harvard Women's Health Watch*, October 2004).

> **Note:** *Mega Green Tea Extract* from *Life Extension* contains 725mg of powdered green tea extract (which translates into 246.5mg of *epigallocatechin gallate* (*EGCG*) and 427.75mg of other polyphenols in every capsule. *Mega Green Tea Extract* comes in lightly caffeinated or decaffeinated forms.

What are the side effects, contraindications, and herb-drug interactions? Young infants should not drink *Green tea* because it may cause anemia by interfering with iron metabolism. Drinking *Green tea* is safe during pregnancy and lactation but I do not recommend taking *Green tea* concentrated supplements. Persons with kidney failure probably should not drink tea of any type. Other than the foregoing, there are no health hazards from drinking *Green tea* or taking a *Green tea* supplement, as long as it is in line with the recommended daily dosage.

> **Note:** In the past few years *White tea* has become both popular and increasingly available. *White tea* also comes from *Camellia sinensis* like *Green tea*. *White tea* is harvested in the early spring when the leaves and buds are just beginning to emerge from winter's dormancy. The leaves of *White tea* are flash-steamed which makes it the least processed of all the kinds of tea. This may result in *White tea* containing the highest concentration of *polyphenols*. I continue to recommend *Green tea* because there is more medical research data than for *White tea*. It seems likely that both types of tea will turn out to have similar health benefits. We may find that *White tea* will be better than *Green tea* in fighting infections from bacteria, viruses, and fungi.

> **Note:** *Rooibus tea* (sometimes called *red tea*) is an herbal tea because it comes from the South African plant *Aspalathis linearis* rather than from *Camellia sinensis*. Although *Rooibus tea* does contain a high level of antioxidants (mostly *quercetin*) they are different ones and not as much as the teas derived from *Camellia sinensis*.

Hawthorn

What is it? This is the shrub or small tree *Crataegus laevigata* (or *Crataegus oxyacantha*), common name *Hawthorn, English Hawthorn*, and *Mayflower*, a member of the *Rosaceae* botanical family. The medicinal parts are the flowers, berries, and leaves. Along with many other biologically active compounds, *Hawthorn* contains *proanthocyanidins* and *flavonoids* which are potent antioxidants.

When should you use it? *Hawthorn* is indicated as a treatment for heart disease, especially congestive heart failure, and also for high blood pressure (hypertension), cardiac arrhythmias, angina, and arteriosclerosis. *Hawthorn* has been shown to improve the blood supply to the heart muscle by dilating the coronary arteries. *Hawthorn* also increases the heart muscle's force of contraction, thereby improving cardiac function. Since *Hawthorn* is clearly indicated for serious heart disease, it is imperative that you consult your health care provider whenever you want to use it.

How should you use it? The recommended dosage for *Hawthorn* is 600-900mg daily. However, some people regularly take up to 1800mg daily.

What are the side effects, contraindications, and herb-drug interactions? Some sources report that *Hawthorn* is considered safe during pregnancy and lactation. However, the *PDR for Herbal Medicines* recommends that *Hawthorn* not be taken during the first trimester of pregnancy. The same source recommends that *Hawthorn* not be given to children under the age of 12 years. *Hawthorn* may potentiate the effects of *digitalis* (*digoxin*) and certain other *cardiac glycosides*. The dosage of those prescription drugs would likely need to be lowered. *Hawthorn* should not be used with beta-blockers as it may cause an increase in blood pressure. It should not be used with antiarrhythmia drugs, or with potassium channel drugs such as *cisapride*. At lower dosages, some mild side effects may occur, such as headache and dizziness. However, at higher dosages (900-1800mg per day), heart palpitations and chest pain have been reported.

> **Note:** Some herbalists recommend the combination of *Ginkgo biloba* together with *Hawthorn* to treat jet lag. For directions please see under *Ginkgo biloba*.

Milk thistle

What is it? This is the annual or biennial plant *Silybum marianum*, common name *Milk thistle, Wild Artichoke*, a member of the *Asteraceae* (*Compositae*) botanical family. The medicinal parts are the ripe seeds. The *flavonolignan* group of compounds called *silymarin* is the main active component. It possesses antioxidant effects. *Silymarin* contains 3 different active isomers: *silibinin, silycristin* and *silydianin*.

When should you use it? *Milk thistle* is considered to be a liver tonic and detoxifier. It has been proven in animal studies to prevent penetration of liver toxins into the liver cell, thereby protecting the liver from damage. *Milk thistle* stimulates regeneration of liver cells (hepatocytes) and reverses toxic liver damage. *Milk thistle* increases the production of the antioxidant *glutathione* inside liver cells. *Milk thistle* has been proven to shorten the course of viral hepatitis. *Milk thistle* is useful to treat diseases of the liver and gallbladder, especially for chronic inflammatory liver diseases (Hepatitis C) and cirrhosis from any cause. I recommend taking *Milk thistle* as a preventive for persons who consume more alcohol than the recommended amount taken to improve cardiovascular health.

The *American Institute for Cancer Research* gave researchers at Columbia University a grant to study *Milk thistle* in children with acute lymphoblastic leukemia (ALL). The hope is that *Milk thistle* will protect the liver allowing the children with ALL to complete the entire course of chemotherapy. Studies are under way to elucidate *silibinin*'s effects on lung cancer.

How should you use it? The usual daily dose of *Milk thistle* is 200-400mg, standardized to 80% *silymarin*.

What are the side effects, contraindications, and herb-drug interactions? *Milk thistle* may decrease the effectiveness of prescribed *estrogen* and *oral contraceptives*. *Milk thistle* may potentiate the effects of anticoagulant drugs such as *warfarin* (*Coumadin*) and *clopidogrel* (*Plavix*) because it may increase the risk for bleeding. Persons who are scheduled for surgery should discontinue taking *Milk thistle* at least 2 weeks prior to surgery. When taking *Milk thistle* there may be increased side effects from these prescription drugs: the allergy drug *fexofenadine* (*Allegra*), the anti-seizure drug *phenytoin* (*Dilantin*), antifungal drugs *itraconazole* (*Sporanox*) and *ketoconazole* (*Nizoral*), and "statin" drugs to lower cholesterol such as *pravastatin* (*Pravachol*), *simvastatin* (*Zocor*) and *atorvastatin* (*Lipitor*). *Milk thistle* may increase the sedative effects of *alprazolam* (*Xanax*), *diazepam* (*Valium*) and *lorazepam* (*Ativan*).

Note: Despite the above list of herb-drug interactions and precautions, Dr. Andrew Weil's *Self-Healing Newsletter* states that *Milk thistle*'s interactions are more theoretical than real and haven't been found in recent clinical studies.

Milk thistle is considered to be particularly safe and may be taken for long periods, perhaps indefinitely. No health hazards or side effects (except for a mild laxative effect) at recommended dosage levels have been reported.

Milk thistle has no reported adverse effect on pregnancy and lactation but extensive data does not exist, so caution is recommended.

Note: Your liver is an amazing organ (is there an organ that isn't?). Your liver extracts waste products from your bloodstream and transforms them into metabolically inert compounds ready for excretion. Your liver detoxifies toxins and normal byproducts of metabolism. Your liver stores energy in the form of glycogen and triglycerides. Your liver stores fat-soluble vitamins A, D, E and K as well as the minerals copper and iron. Your liver manufactures cholesterol. Your liver is intimately involved in protein, fat, and carbohydrate metabolism. One of the ways you can keep your liver healthy is to ingest as few pesticides and other chemical toxins as possible. And if you drink alcohol do so only in the recommended amounts for good cardiovascular health.

Note: *Schisandra chinenis*, common name *Schizandra*, is another herbal remedy used to improve liver function during and after infection with the hepatitis virus. Take 1.5 grams everyday. There is not as much medical literature on *Schisandra* as there is on *Milk thistle*.

Note: The herbal remedy *Gynostemma pentaphylum* has been proven to reverse the effects of nonalcoholic fatty liver. It also has some value in weight loss.

Psyllium

What is it? This is the perennial "weed" *Plantago psyllium* (although some sources list the species as *Plantago ovata*) common names *Ispaghula, Plantain* and *Psyllium Husk*, a member of the *Plantaginaceae* botanical family. The medicinal part is the seeds and leaves. The seed coat contains a soluble fiber called *mucin*.

When should you use it? The seeds of *Psyllium* contain large amounts of *dietary fiber*, a volume normalizer, which exert both laxative and anti-diarrheal effects in the gastrointestinal tract, by modulating the amount of water in the stool. *Psyllium* is useful to treat both constipation and diarrhea which gives it a primary place in the treatment of irritable bowel syndrome and ulcerative colitis. *Psyllium* is used to improve glucose control in persons with diabetes mellitus type 2. *Psyllium* can also play a healthy part in a weight loss program as it tends to decrease fat intake and increase feelings of fullness. *Psyllium* lowers LDL ("bad") cholesterol and triglycerides while raising HDL ("good") cholesterol. *Psyllium* can be part of the dietary plan in persons with hemorrhoids and anal fissures. *Psyllium* is used as adjunctive treatment for hypertension (high blood pressure).

How should you use it? *Psyllium* comes in capsules (commonly but not exclusively 880mg per capsule) and powder (2gm or 6gm per teaspoon). Read and follow the directions on the label of the preparation you choose. The usual dose to treat constipation is one or two teaspoons three times daily. It is always best to start taking *Psyllium* slowly, one capsule or one teaspoon of powder daily, and work up to the recommended dosage so that your digestive tract adjusts to the increased fiber. *Metamucil* and *Fiberall* are popular brand names. It is necessary to drink one glass of fluid for every capsule or teaspoon of powder taken to prevent bowel obstruction because *Psyllium* requires water to expand properly in your digestive tract.

What are the side effects, contraindications, and herb-drug interactions? Persons who have obstructions of the bowel should not take *Psyllium*. It is necessary to drink one glass of fluid for every capsule taken to prevent bowel obstruction. Allergic symptoms have been reported with *Psyllium* although severe symptoms are rare. Discontinue taking the herb if you experience any allergic symptoms. Some persons with diabetes will need to lower their insulin dosage after taking *Psyllium*. *Psyllium* is not recommended for use during pregnancy because some *Plantago* species promote menstruation. *Psyllium* may be used during lactation as it will not affect the newborn.

Saw Palmetto

What is it? This is the evergreen palm *Serenoa repens*, also called *Sabal serrulata*, common name *Saw palmetto* or *Palmetto scrub*, a member of the *Arecaceae* botanical family. It is a native North American plant. The medicinal part is the fresh or dried berries. The chemical health promoting components are *sterols*.

When should you use it? *Saw palmetto* has been proven to be helpful in treating the urinary complaints associated with enlargement of the prostate gland (benign prostatic hypertrophy). The urinary problems that are symptomatic of benign prostatic hypertrophy and improved by *Saw palmetto* are: difficulty initiating urination, weak urinary stream, dribbling and frequent nighttime urination (nocturia). *Saw palmetto* decreases the urinary problems but probably does not decrease the enlargement of the gland, although it may reduce its progression. *Saw palmetto* interferes with the binding of dihydrotestosterone in the prostate gland, which if it does accumulate, jump-starts the enlargement process. *Saw palmetto* has been proven to be as effective as *finasteride* (*Proscar*) in reducing urinary complaints associated with prostate enlargement. However, *Proscar* lowers the PSA levels (prostate specific antigen), potentially masking a cancerous change in the prostate gland, whereas *Saw palmetto* leaves the PSA levels unchanged. This means that *Saw palmetto* allows your doctor to continue to follow your PSA levels as an indication of the presence or absence of prostate cancer.

How should you use it? The recommended dosage for *Saw palmetto* is 160mg twice daily or 320mg once daily standardized to contain at least 85% of fatty acids and 0.2% sterols. Many preparations come with the addition of *Pygeum africanum* (100mg daily) and *Urtica dioica* (*Stinging Nettle*) (100mg daily).

Pygeum and *Urtica* tend to increase *Saw palmetto's* effectiveness.

> **Note:** *Pygeum africanum* is known to improve sexual functioning in men who suffer from benign prostatic hypertrophy. Adding *Pygeum* to the antibiotic regimen in men who have chronic prostatitis has been shown to alleviate sexual dysfunction. *Pygeum* is generally safe with no herb-drug interactions. The dosage is 100-200mg daily.

What are the side effects, contraindications, and herb-drug interactions? *Saw palmetto* is contraindicated during pregnancy and lactation because of its presumed anti-estrogenic and anti-androgenic hormonal effects. In addition, it is not recommended for use in patients with hormone-dependent cancers, such as prostate cancer. Therefore, it is essential that you consult with your health care provider before beginning a course of *Saw palmetto* to make sure you do not have prostate cancer as a cause of your urinary symptoms.

Saw palmetto is considered to be non-toxic and free from significant side effects. *Saw palmetto* is not recommended for use in women; however, it is sometimes used (by health practitioners only) as a treatment for polycystic ovary syndrome.

St. John's Wort

What is it? This is the perennial shrub *Hypericum perforatum*, common name *St. John's Wort*, a member of the *Hypericaceae* botanical family. Homeopathic *Hypericum perforatum* plays a prominent role in the homeopathic healing of traumatic nerve injuries. For the herbal remedy, the medicinal parts are the fresh buds and flowers. The active components of *St. John's Wort* are *hypericin, pseudohypericin* and *hyperforin*. The name was bestowed upon the plant because it blooms with its gorgeous, bright yellow flowers around June 24th, St. John The Baptist's birthday.

When should you use it? *St. John's Wort* has been proven to be effective to treat mild to moderate depression and anxiety. The antidepressant action of *St. John's Wort* in the brain is probably due to its ability to inhibit the reuptake of the brain neuro-transmitters serotonin, dopamine, and norepinephrine, thereby increasing the brain levels of these chemicals. *St. John's Wort* has other properties, such as anti-viral, antibacterial, and anti-inflammatory, but it is usually used for its antidepressant effects in the U.S.

A research study by the *Hypericum Depression Trial Study Group*, was published in April 2002 in the *Journal of the American Medical Association*, a prominent medical journal, entitled, *Effect of Hypericum perforatum (St. John's Wort) in Major Depressive Disorder-A Randomized Controlled Trial*. This study randomly assigned 340 patients with major depression to receive either *St. John's Wort or sertraline (Zoloft)* or placebo for 8 weeks. The results of this study showed that *St. John's Wort* and *Zoloft* and placebo all performed equally well for patients with moderately severe major depression. The conclusion by the media was that *St. John's Wort* did not treat major depression. But, then in that study, neither did *Zoloft*! *St. John's Wort* has been shown by many well-designed medical studies to effectively treat mild to moderate depression. It is prescribed in Europe as the first-line drug for patients with mild to moderate depression.

How should you use it? *St. John's Wort* is standardized to 0.3% of *hypericin* (although recent evidence suggests that *hyperforin* is probably the significant mood elevator). Take one 300mg capsules 2 or 3 times daily. If there is no improvement within 4-6 weeks, you may double the dose up to 2 capsules 3 times daily. If there is no change in symptoms after 4-6 weeks at the higher dosage level, then you may consider that *St. John's Wort* is not helpful for your particular case. When discontinuing *St. John's Wort*, I believe it is safest to taper over a two-week period. Halve your dosage for the first week, and then take one-quarter for the second week. Then stop. A preparation of *St. John's Wort* that comes standardized to 3% *hyperforin* is available, called *Perika* by Nature's Way. The dose is the same as above.

What are the side effects, contraindications, and herb-drug interactions? According to the *Consumer Reports on Health* (November 2002), *St. John's Wort* may interact with the following drugs to decrease their effects to potentially ineffective levels: antibiotics *clarithromycin (Biaxin)*, and *erythromycin (E-Mycin)*; *irinotecan (Camptosar, an anticancer drug)*;

antidepressants *amitriptyline* (*Elavil*) and *nortriptyline* (*Pamelor*); *fexofenadine* (*Allegra*, for allergies); *digoxin* (*Lanoxin*, for heart failure); *theophylline* (*Theo-Dur* for asthma); beta-blockers *propranolol* (*Inderal*), *metoprolol* (*Lopressor*); calcium-channel blockers *verapamil* (*Calan*) and *felodipine* (*Plendil*); anticoagulant *warfarin* (*Coumadin*); "statin" drugs to lower cholesterol such as *pravastatin* (*Pravachol*), *simvastatin* (*Zocor*) and *atorvastatin* (*Lipitor*); cyclosporine (*Sandimmune*) for organ transplantation; *sildenafil* (*Viagra*) for impotence; and oral contraceptives.

When taking *St. John's Wort* side effects of certain drugs may be more likely: antidepressants in the SSRI group of drugs like *paroxetine* (*Paxil*), *fluoxetine* (*Prozac*), and *sertraline* (*Zoloft*); antidepressants in the MAOI group of drugs like *isocarboxazid* (*Marplan*), *phenelzine* (*Nardil*), *tranylcypromine* (*Parnate*); and anti-migraine drugs like *naratriptan* (*Amerge*) and *sumatriptan* (*Imitrex*). When *St. John's Wort* is taken with a drug in the SSRI group, it may lead to the serotonin syndrome which consists of sweating, flushing, tremors, and confusion. When *St. John's Wort* is taken with a drug in the MAOI group, it may lead to an hypertensive crisis.

The *German Commission E Monograph* reports that *St. John's Wort* is safe for use during pregnancy and lactation. Side effects of *St. John's Wort* are not common. They include mild digestive tract symptoms, allergy, sun sensitivity, and fatigue. People taking *St. John's Wort* should avoid sunlight as much as possible because an increase in sensitivity to the sun's effects (photosensitization) may occur upon exposure to ultraviolet light.

In contrast to SSRIs, sexual dysfunction is not a side effect of *St. John's Wort*. Due to *St. John's Wort*'s effects on coagulation, it should be discontinued 2 weeks prior to surgery.

> **Note:** For more information on *St. John's Wort* please visit the *National Center for Complementary and Alternative Medicine* (*NCCAM*) at http://nccam.nih.gov/health/stjohnswort/sjwataglance.htm.

Tea Tree

What is it? This is the plant *Melaleuca alternifolia*, common name *Tea Tree*, a member of the *Myrtaceae* (*Myrtle*) botanical family. The medicinal parts are the leaves and tips of branches from which the essential oils from are extracted. The active components are chemicals called *terpenes*, of which *terpineol* is probably the most active.

When should you use it? *Tea tree oil* has antiseptic, germicidal, and disinfectant properties. *Tea Tree* oil is used as a topical antibacterial, anti-fungal and anti-viral agent for infections of the skin, nails, and mouth. It is also useful to treat the pain and itching from insect bites and poison ivy.

How should you use it? Today *Tea tree oil* is found in numerous products that treat acne, skin infections (Athlete's foot, head lice), skin rashes (poison ivy), nail fungi, cold sores, canker sores, and gingivitis. It is applied externally directly onto the skin or nail or mucus membranes. It is found as an ingredient in toothpaste, mouthwash, soap, antiseptic cream, body lotion, deodorant, shaving gel, shampoo, conditioner, foot spray, and foot powder. I recommend that you purchase 100% *Tea tree oil* manufactured by *Thursday Plantation* (made by Nature's Plus) in a 50 ml bottle. Apply once or twice daily to the affected area. The bottle is made from amber glass so the *Tea tree oil* is protected from exposure to light which may cause it to become unstable. *Life Extension* makes a toothpaste that contains *Tea tree oil*.

What are the side effects, contraindications, and herb-drug interactions? *Tea tree oil* is not to be taken internally as it can cause confusion and coma. No side effects or herb-drub interactions are reported when used in the recommended manner.

> **Note:** Please do not confuse *Tea tree oil* with *Tea oil* which is used for cooking and therefore taken internally. *Tea oil* is made from the seeds of the tea plant, *Camellia sinensis*.

Tea Tree oil is not recommended for use during pregnancy and lactation. Some persons with sensitive skin may be allergic to *Tea tree oil*.

Other herbs have similar actions to *Tea tree oil* (except that only *Tea tree oil* has antifungal properties). *Calendula officinalis* (*marigold*) has anti-inflammatory properties as well as antibacterial and antiviral. It is found as an eye wash, gargle, soap, and skin ointment. *Calendula* accelerates healing of the skin which makes it a popular ointment to treat diaper rash and superficial skin wounds. *Calendula* products are often prescribed for children with sensitive skin. *Calendula* may be an ingredient in skin moisturizers and massage oils. No side effects are reported other than sensitization (contact dermatitis) after frequent use.

The juice of the succulent plant *Aloe vera* possesses the same properties as *Calendula*. *Aloe vera* is often used externally to treat sunburns and skin rashes. It is never used internally. *Aloe vera* is often an ingredient in sunscreens and skin moisturizers.

Chamomile (*Matricaria recutita*) is also useful to treat minor wounds and diaper rash. *Chamomile* possesses most of the actions as *Calendula* and *Aloe vera*. Remember that only *Tea tree oil* has antifungal properties. *Chamomile* is sometimes an ingredient in skin moisturizers. *Chamomilla* is the homeopathic remedy made from the same plant.

> **Note:** To combat toenail fungus use 100% *Tea tree oil*. At bedtime, soak a cotton ball in *Tea tree oil* tape it (use paper tape) to the infected nail and leave it on all night. It's a good idea to put a sock on that foot because *Tea tree oil* tends to stain the bed sheets otherwise.

Valerian

What is it? This is the plant *Valeriana officinalis*, common name *Valerian*, a member of the *Valerianaceae* botanical family. The medicinal parts are the dried roots, rhizomes (underground stems) and stolons (underground horizontal stems).

When should you use it? *Valerian* has 3 specific calming actions in the body: sedation, decrease of anxiety, and muscle relaxation. *Valerian* is used to decrease nervousness, anxiety, restlessness, and insomnia. Hippocrates wrote about using *Valerian* to treat insomnia. The chemical *valerenic acid* found in *Valerian* is the component that increases the available amount of the brain neurotransmitter *gamma-aminobutyric acid* (*GABA*). *GABA* is our body's natural sedative. In addition, *Valerian* contains a high amount of *glutamine*, an amino acid that is converted to *GABA*.

How should you use it? Take 150-300mg of *Valerian* during the day but you may take 400-900mg ½-1 hour before bedtime. Other safe herbal remedies for insomnia include: *Passionflower* (*Passiflora incarnata*), *Skullcap* (*Scutellaria baicalensis*), *Hops* (*Humulus lupu-*

lus), *Chamomile* (*Matricaria recutita*) and *Lemon Balm* (*Melissa officinalis*). These are often combined with *Valerian* to treat anxiety and insomnia. *Herbal Sleep* manufactured by Vitamin Research Products (1-800-877-2447 or www.vrp.com) contains: *L-theanine*, *Hops*, *Lemon Balm*, *Passionflower* and *Valerian* root extract. The dosage is 2-3 capsules one hour before bedtime. If you are experiencing insomnia, you may wish to experiment with *Chamomile*, *Passionflower* and *Lemon Balm* teas along with Valerian capsules at bedtime. I also recommend *Lavender* (*Lavandula angustifolia*) as aromatherapy oil in your bath or applied to your pillow.

What are the side effects, contraindications, and herb-drug interactions? *Valerian* may increase the effectiveness as well as the dangerous side effects of certain sedatives such as *alprazolam* (*Xanax*), *diazepam* (*Valium*) and *lorazepam* (*Ativan*). *Valerian* may increase the effects of: *fexofenadine* (*Allegra* or allergies); antifungal drugs such as *itraconazole* (*Sporanox*) and *ketoconazole* (*Nizoral*); and "statin" drugs to lower cholesterol such as *pravastatin* (*Pravachol*), *simvastatin* (*Zocor*) and *atorvastatin* (*Lipitor*). *Valerian* should not be taken with alcohol. *Valerian* at the higher dosage level may impair driving ability. *Valerian* is not used during pregnancy and lactation. It is considered to be safe for long-term use. Rare side effects of headache and sleeplessness have been reported with long-term use.

> **Note:** *Melatonin* is a hormone produced by the pineal gland in the brain. It is involved in the regulation of the sleep cycle in humans. *Melatonin* supplements may be effective for some sleep disorders, especially to decrease the time it takes to fall asleep. Some people get nightmares when taking *melatonin*. The long-term safety of melatonin is unknown and because it is a hormone, I do not recommend its use other than for short periods to alleviate jet lag. Take 2.5mg of *melatonin* as a dissolvable tablet under your tongue at bedtime for one to three nights. Remember that *Ginkgo biloba* together with *Hawthorn* also treats jet lag. *Melatonin* has also been used to decrease the frequency of migraine headaches.

Guidelines for Consulting Your Health Care Provider

You should consult your health care provider if:
- the patient doesn't look right or act right (trust your instincts!)
- the patient is getting worse instead of better over the course of the illness
- the patient is having trouble breathing or complaining of chest pains or there is mental confusion or lethargy or irritability
- the patient develops allergic symptoms (hives, itchy or watery eyes, runny nose, scratchy throat, asthma, shortness of breath) after taking an herbal remedy
- after beginning a herbal remedy the patient experiences *new onset* of any serious symptoms such as:
    paralysis, weakness, tingling, inability to focus or concentrate, blurred or double vision or blindness, slurred speech, severe headaches, seizures, irritability, dizziness, disorientation, memory loss, anxiety, depression, insomnia, blackouts, fainting, or the person complains of not feeling like himself
- the patient is taking *ANY* prescription medication
- the patient is pregnant or breastfeeding
- the patient has any serious disease which may become life-threatening, such as:
    autism, cancer, HIV and AIDS, arthritis, multiple sclerosis, coronary artery disease, heart attack (myocardial infarction), blood dyscrasia, cancer (of any type), congestive heart failure, diabetes mellitus, obesity, thyroid disorders, high blood pressure (hypertension), stroke, seizures, acute and chronic kidney (renal) failure, schizophrenia, bipolar disorder, borderline personality disorder, eating disorders, fibromyalgia, chronic fatigue syndrome, Crohn's disease, ulcerative colitis, celiac disease, mental deficiency disorders, chromosomal disorders, infertility, frequent miscarriages, polyneuropathy, cystic fibrosis [Adapted from *The Merck Manual* at www.merck.com]

Note: Do not delude yourself into believing that herbal remedies somehow are not medicines. They are. You must disclose the herbal medicines you or your family member is taking to your health care provider.

Note: Do not discontinue taking any pharmaceutical medication that has been prescribed by your health care provider unless you or your family member is under the supervision of a physician.

Note: Do not take any herbal remedy without first consulting a health care provider if you or your family member is pregnant or breastfeeding. In addition, it is a good idea to check with your health care provider if your family member is either very young or very old because herbal remedies given injudiciously may overwhelm the body's defenses in those age groups.

Note: Self-care for persons who already had/have cancer is not a sound practice in any case. Do not take any herbal supplement to prevent or treat cancer or augment your immune system without first consulting with your health care provider especially if you or your family member is taking a prescription medication to treat cancer or its complications or is pregnant or breastfeeding.

Note: The most important thing to understand about using *homeopathy, herbal remedies, and nutritional supplements* for the treatment of cancer is that these must not be given during chemotherapy or radiation therapy. This is because the effects of *homeopathy, herbal remedies, and nutritional supplements* may actually go against the action of chemotherapy or radiation therapy. For this reason *homeopathy, herbal remedies, and nutritional supplements* are taken after the chemotherapy or radiation therapy sessions are finished, or during the respite between sessions.

Note: *Urtica dioica* (*Stinging Nettle*) is an herbal remedy that may be helpful to treat hay fever during the allergy season. The dose is 400-600mg capsules twice daily of the freeze-dried herb.

Note: *Butterbur* (*Petasites hybridus*) is an herbal remedy that may be helpful to treat hay fever as well as the migraine headaches that often accompany seasonal allergies. *Butterbur*, in some studies, has been shown to be as effective as the prescription medications *Allegra* and *Zyrtec* in treating seasonal allergies. *Petadolex* is the brand that has been used in medical research. The dosage is 50mg three times daily.

Note: *Artemisinin*, an extract from the dried leaves of the plant *Artemisia annua*, common name *Sweet wormwood*, or *Qinghao* in Chinese, is used to treat malaria. It acts quickly and effectively even against drug-resistant strains of malaria. There are no significant side effects. It is usually taken together with *lumifantrine* as the drug *Coartem*.

Putting It All Together

If you are considering using an herbal remedy, it is a good idea to familiarize yourself with **Chapter 19: Introduction to Herbal Medicine**.

Then, after you have decided to use an herbal remedy to prevent or treat a certain ailment, it makes good sense to investigate the homeopathic remedy indicated for that ailment as well. That's because homeopathic remedies are safe, have no side effects, and can be used together with herbal remedies and Western pharmaceutical medicines without concern. You may read about your sick person's homeopathic remedies in **Chapters 3-18**. And you may want to better understand homeopathy by reading **Chapter 2: Basic Homeopathy**.

Whenever you have decided to go ahead with herbal remedies, it is a good idea to consider giving the sick person's homeopathic constitutional remedy as well (please refer to **Chapter 9: Homeopathic Remedies for Constitutional Problems in Infants, Children, and Adolescents** or to **Chapter 18: Homeopathic Constitutional Remedie**s if you are dealing with an adult; or **Chapter 13: Homeopathy for Elderly Persons** if you are dealing with an elderly person).

People who are taking an herbal remedy will likely require all the vitamins and minerals necessary to repair and replenish tissues (please refer to **Chapter 23: Vitamins and Minerals**) as well as a general antioxidant supplement (please refer to **Chapter 24: Antioxidant Phytochemicals**).

People who are taking an herbal remedy may also benefit from certain nutritional supplements, depending on the particular ailment. After reading **Chapter 22: Introduction to Nutritional Supplements**, you may read about your sick person's specific nutritional remedies in **Chapters 23-31**.

Chapter 21

Herbal Remedies for Women's Health

Herbal Remedies for Women's Health in General

Ailment/Disorder/Symptom	Herbal Remedy
Menopause, hot flashes	*Black Cohosh*
Premenstrual syndrome	*Chasteberry*
Urinary tract infection	*Cranberry*
Menstrual complaints	*Dong quai*
Breast tenderness, eczema, ADD/ADHD	*Evening Primrose Oil*
Nausea of pregnancy and indigestion	*Ginger*
Phytoestrogens	*Soy*
Natural progesterone	*Wild Yam*

Guidelines for Consulting Your Health Care Provider
Putting It All Together

Herbal Remedies for Women's Health in General

The average female today is entering puberty by the age of 10 years. She is marking the transition from girlhood to womanhood with her first menstrual period (menarche) by the age of 12 years. And on average, she is transitioning from menstrual cycles to menopause between the ages of 50-52 years, although perimenopausal symptoms may often begin ten years earlier.

The passages of a woman's life could be and should be healthy ones. None of these transitions in themselves should be considered an illness or a disease and this includes menstruation, pregnancy, childbirth, and breastfeeding. In order to *prevent* the complications all too commonly seen during these life passages (such as osteoporosis, breast and reproductive tract cancers) it is essential that you pay attention to the **good health practices**:

>—no smoking, moderate alcohol, nutritionally healthy diet, adequate daily physical exercise, adequate sleep, time for daily relaxation techniques, seeking humor and love in everyday life, engaging in activities for intellectual stimulation, doing things for other people, and participating in preventive health testing.

But, sometimes the pathway through these life passages is strewn with such discomfort that one's quality of life markedly diminishes. The healthy way to treat disabling symptoms is to combine the three essential natural alternatives, homeopathy, herbal remedies, and nutritional supplements.

For most ailments, I recommend using homeopathic remedies first (since there are no side effects and they have a good chance to be effective) then instituting the appropriate nutritional supplements (to augment the homeopathic remedies), and then, only if needed, begin the recommended herbal remedies. In this manner, most of the time, you will find yourself using herbal remedies only when homeopathic remedies have not given you the relief you seek.

This chapter and **Chapter 20: Herbs You Need to Know** presents herbal remedies that have an established safety record so that they lend themselves to self-care. However, you will still need to carefully check side effects, contraindications, and herb-drug interactions before beginning to take any herbal remedy.

If you or your family member is pregnant, breastfeeding, or is very young or very old, you will need to take even more stringent precautions. By reading this chapter carefully you yourself should make sure that the herbal remedy you have selected is not contraindicated for pregnant or lactating females, infants, or elderly persons. Then you should check with your health care provider before taking any herbal remedy.

Ever since the report from the *Women's Health Initiative Trial* concerning the increased risk of certain diseases when taking hormone replacement therapy (*HRT*; combined estrogen and progesterone, or *Prempro*) during the menopausal years was published in 2002, women have been searching for safe and effective alternatives. The results from that study proved that taking *HRT* increases your risk for developing coronary heart disease, stroke, thromboembolism (blood clots), Alzheimer's disease, and invasive breast cancer. *HRT* decreases your risk for hip fracture and does not change your risk for developing colon cancer.

A good source of accurate information on menopause is The North American Menopause Society at www.menopause.org, a non-profit organization devoted to healthy menopause. You can read their journal, *Menopause*, online. A good book source on menopause is *The Truth About Hormone Replacement Therapy: How to Break Free from the Medical Myths of Menopause*, written by women medical authors of the National Women's Health Network (Prima Publishing, 2002).

The two-volume set, *Women's Health* by Burton Goldberg and the editors of the magazine *Alternative Medicine* (www.alternativemedicine.com) gives you a thorough understanding of 17 common health problems that afflict women particularly. *Women's Health* emphasizes prevention of these maladies by recommending lifestyle changes, homeopathy, herbal medicines, and nutritional supplements. Unfortunately, *Women's Health* also tends to recommend additional alternative therapies which you may ignore as they are usually unnecessary for optimal health.

Another well-respected source of medical information (if you want to learn more about your body from a respected source) is *The New Harvard Guide to Women's Health* by Carlson, Eisenstat and Ziporyn.

The herbal remedies for women's health discussed below are those most commonly used by me in my clinical practice of alternative medicine. I have not included certain herbs (such as *Red Clover* [*Trifolium pratense*]) because so far there is no good medical evidence that they are helpful for menopausal symptoms.

> **Note:** Some new but preliminary evidence points to *Red Clover* having a beneficial effect on bones in post-menopausal women.

When using herbal remedies for self-care of any and all ailments you must pay strict attention to the **Guidelines for Consulting Your Health Care Provider** at the end of this chapter. You may want to refer to the last section **Putting It All Together** for ideas on how to integrate the essential natural alternatives, homeopathy, herbal remedies, and nutritional supplements.

Black Cohosh

What is it? This is the perennial woodland plant *Cimicifuga racemosa*, common name *Black cohosh*, a member of the *buttercup* or *Ranunculaceae* botanical family. The medicinal parts are the fresh and dried roots and rhizomes (underground stems). When *Cimicifuga racemosa* is prepared as the homeopathic remedy (abbreviated as *Cimic*), it is most commonly used to treat menstrual cramps and headaches associated with menstruation.

When should you use it? The active plant chemicals in the herbal remedy *Black Cohosh* are *triterpene glycosides*. *Black Cohosh* has estrogen-like effects, although the exact mechanism of action has not been elucidated. But, it appears likely that *Black Cohosh* does not have direct estrogenic effects. This means that *Black Cohosh* won't increase your risk for breast cancer. Nonetheless, until more evidence on the safety of *Black Cohosh* is obtained, it is best not to use it in women who have or had breast cancer. *Black Cohosh* has been proven effective to decrease

menopausal symptoms, most specifically hot flashes, night sweats, vaginal dryness, irritability, mood swings, and insomnia. It is also used to treat premenstrual symptoms (PMS) such as irritability and mood swings. *Black Cohosh* has also been helpful in some cases of painful menstrual periods (dysmenorrhea).

> **Note:** A large NIH study did not find any benefit from taking *Black Cohosh* over placebo on the number of hot flashes and night sweats.

How should you use it? The dose of *Black Cohosh* is 40mg daily (although recently 80mg has been suggested to counter severe cases of hot flashes). It is not recommended for use longer than six months because the long-term effect on the uterine lining (endometrium) is unknown. One of the theoretical effects may be an increase in the uterine lining (endometrial hyperplasia) which may increase the risk for uterine cancer, although this remains unproven.

One of the most reliable and popular brands of *Black Cohosh* is *Remifemin* (from *GlaxoSmithKline*) containing 20mg of *Black Cohosh*. Take 2 tablets daily. *Remifemin* is standardized to contain 5% (2mg) *triterpene glycosides*.

There are many complex herbal preparations containing *Black Cohosh* as one of the ingredients. Another product is *Menopause Plus Formula* from *Emerita*, containing *Black Cohosh* (80mg in 2 tablets) along with *Red Clover* (*Trifolium pratense*), *Siberian Ginseng* (*Eleutherococcus senticosus*), *Dandelion* (*Taraxacum officinale*), *Alfalfa* (*Medicago sativa*) and *Chasteberry* (*Vitex agnus-castus*).

> **Note:** *Avlimil* is an herbal remedy for addressing the symptoms of Female Sexual Dysfunction, that includes *Black Cohosh* (calling it by its old name, *Actaea racemosa*), along with *Sage leaf* (*Salvia officinalis*), *Red raspberry leaf* (*Rubus idaeus*) and *isoflavones* (see *Soy* below) from *Kudzu root* extract (*Pueraria montana*) and *Red clover* extract (*Trifolium pratense*), with *Capsicum* pepper (*Capsicum annuum*), *Licorice* root (*Glycyrrhiza glabra*), *Bayberry* fruit (*Morella cerifera*), *Damiana* leaf (*Turnera diffusa*), *Valeriana* root (*Valeriana officinalis*) and *Ginger* root (*Zingiber officinale*)

(see *Ginger* below). The proprietary blend of *Avlimil* makes it specially formulated to improve libido and sexual response in the female. Take one tablet every day. Pregnant women (and women who may become pregnant) and lactating women should not take *Avlimil*.

Note: *Rhodiola rosea* may enhance libido for both men and women. Other herbal remedies that are used to increase libido in women are *Ashwagandha* (*Withania somnifera*), *Eleuthero* (*Eleutherococcus snticosus*) and *Catuaba* (*Erythroxylum catuaba*). Herbal remedies that may enhance libido for men are *Horny goat weed* (*Epimedium grandiflorum*), *Yohimbe* (*Pausinystalia yohimbe*) and *Ginseng* (*Panax ginseng*). *Yohimbe* may cause high blood pressure and anxiety, especially in combination with Viagra. For these reasons it is not recommended. *Horny goat weed* has a better safety profile.

Caution: As a woman, if you have low libido and are searching for help to increase your libido, do **NOT** take testosterone treatments. There are no safety data on long-term use of testosterone by women. Testosterone may even be more dangerous than estrogen in increasing your risk to develop breast cancer. Libido is such a complex phenomenon, embracing psychological as well as physiological pathways, that it is imperative that you seek the advice of your health care provider to rule-out certain common diseases causing low libido, such as hypothyroidism, depression, and diabetes.

The herb *Eurycoma longifolia*, common name *Malaysian Ginseng*, from Southeast Asia, has been used for centuries to increase libido in both men and women. Side effects have not been reported. However, due to scanty data, please do not take *Eurycoma* during pregnancy or lactation. Make sure you take *Eurycoma* supplements made from the root of the plant only.

In addition, you may want to try the homeopathic personal lubricant formulas for women manufactured by Sen-suaorganics, such as *Libido Formula*. The Sensuaorganics topical homeopathic products are available for men as well as for women, and they come in different flavors. Call Sensuaorganics at 1-800-983-1993.

What are the side effects, contraindications, and herb-drug interactions? *Black cohosh* probably does not stimulate estrogen-receptor-positive breast cancer cells and it may actually increase the anti-tumor effects of *tamoxifen*. However, because at this time *Black Cohosh*'s effects on breast cancer cells has not been well studied, it is not advisable for women with breast cancer (in self or first-degree relatives) to take it. This warning is also pertinent for other estrogen-sensitive cancers, such as ovarian and uterine. Research studies are being conducted to better delineate the effects of *Black Cohosh* in patients taking *tamoxifen* to prevent recurrence in breast cancer.

The side effects of *Black Cohosh* at the recommended dosage level are none to minimal. Some mild gastrointestinal discomfort, headaches, dizziness, weight gain, and leg cramps have been reported. *Black Cohosh* is contraindicated during pregnancy (as it may increase the risk for miscarriage) and lactation. *Black Cohosh* in higher than recommended dosages may increase the effects of medications used to treat high blood pressure, thereby possibly causing dangerously low blood pressure. No drug interactions have been reported with *Black Cohosh*.

Note: For more information from the *National Center for Complementary and Alternative Medicine* (*NCCAM*) please visit http://nccam.nih.gov/health/blackcohosh/.

Note: *Black Cohosh* may increase the risk to develop inflammation of the liver. More studies need to be done to elucidate the connection. Do not take *Black Cohosh* if you have liver disease.

Chasteberry

What is it? This is the plant *Vitex agnus-castus*, common name *Chasteberry* and *Chaste Tree*, a member of the *Verbenaceae* botanical family. The medicinal parts are the dried ripe berries.

When should you use it? *Chasteberry* is primarily used to treat premenstrual syndrome (PMS), relieving such symptoms as headache, bloating, anger, irritability, mood swings, and breast tenderness. *Chasteberry* is also used to treat menstrual irregularities, especially during perimenopause, or as a result of endometriosis. *Chasteberry* probably has some beneficial effect on hot flashes, but it is not as consistent as *Black Cohosh*. It may help to increase libido and decrease depression during menopause. Dr. Andrew Weil recommends *Chasteberry* to help treat endometriosis as it may restore hormonal balance to the female reproductive system. Some people recommend *Chasteberry* to increase fertility in women who are having difficulty conceiving, especially if they have a hormone imbalance in the progesterone phase (second half) of the menstrual cycle. However, the recommendation is to take *Chasteberry* for three cycles to restore hormonal balance while you are not trying to conceive because you do not want to become pregnant while taking *Chasteberry*.

FertilityBlend for Women is a preparation that may help infertile women conceive. It combines *Chasteberry* with the amino acid *L-arginine* (improves circulation to the uterus) along with *Green tea*, Vitamins B6, B12, folic acid, Vitamin E, iron, magnesium, zinc and selenium. More information about *FertilityBlend* is available at www.fertilityblend.com. *FertilityBlend for Men* consists of *L-carnitine, ferulic acid* (the antioxidant component of *Dong quai* [please see below] which is said to improve sperm quality), along with the same vitamins and minerals present in *FertilityBlend for Women*.

How should you use it? Different preparations of *Chasteberry* contain between 40 and 200mg per day. I recommend *Chasteberry* 200mg daily for the treatment of PMS symptoms and for menstrual regulation. In treating PMS, *Chasteberry* is used throughout the cycle.

What are the side effects, contraindications, and herb-drug interactions? *Chasteberry* has not been shown to be safe for use during pregnancy or lactation. There are reports in the literature that recommend *Chasteberry* during breastfeeding, but other reports have shown it to inhibit milk flow. Until the effects are definitely known do not use *Chasteberry* during lactation.

The *German Commission E Monograph* does not report any herb-drub interactions with *Chasteberry*. No significant side effects have been reported other than rare allergic rash.

Cranberry

What is it? This is the herbal remedy *Vaccinium macrocarpon*, common name *Cranberry*, a member of the *Ericaceae* botanical family. The berries are the parts of the plant that are used to make the herbal remedy.

When should you use it? *Cranberry* possesses anti-bacterial, anti-cancer, and antioxidant activity. It is used to prevent recurrent urinary tract infections. However, the medical evidence for the treatment of urinary tract infections is less convincing. In my own clinical experience with my patients, it is worthwhile trying it for treatment as well as prevention. The mode of action is probably that *Cranberry* contains an anti-adherence factor that make bacteria (specifically *E. Coli*, but others as well) unable to adhere to the wall of the urinary tract, thereby preventing infection. *Cranberry* is also useful to prevent formation of dental plaque and to prevent recurrence of infection with the bacteria that causes stomach ulcers, *Helicobacter pylori*.

How should you use it? *Cranberry* juice is usually diluted with other juices to make it less tart and more palatable, but this decreases its effectiveness and adds often unwanted calories. The best way to take *Cranberry* is to take *CranAction* manufactured by Solaray. This contains 200mg of *Cranberry* in each chewable tablet. The adult dose is one up to 4 times daily. Children take half the dose. For prevention, if you are prone to recurrent urinary tract infections, I recommend that you take one tablet every day.

What are the side effects, contraindications, and herb-drug interactions? There are no serious side effects with taking *Cranberry* as a nutritional supplement. However, pregnant and lactating women should drink *cranberry* juice rather than take the nutritional supplement until more information becomes available. For more information please visit http://nccam.nih.gov/health/cranberry/.

Dong quai

What is it? This is the perennial herbaceous plant *Angelica sinensis*, common name *Dong quai* and *Chinese Angelica root*, a member of the *Apiaceae* (*Umbelliferae*, or *parsley*) botanical family. The medicinal part is the root.

When should you use it? *Dong quai* has been used for centuries in China as a tonic for women, often called the "*Female Ginseng*." *Dong quai* is the main herb used to treat menstrual complaints, such as: menstrual cramps (dysmenorrhea), amenorrhea (cessation of menstrual cycles), oligomenorrhea (infrequent menstrual cycles) and menstrual blood flow problems (either too heavy and/or for too long). The antioxidant present in *Dong quai* is *ferulic acid* which may improve sperm quality.

How should you use it? Take *Dong quai* 200mg three times daily of an extract that is standardized to contain 1% *ligustilide*, the probably active component. Some popular brands contain 500mg to take once daily.

What are the side effects, contraindications, and herb-drug interactions? *Dong quai* may interact with anticoagulant prescription medications (*warfarin* or *Coumarin*) and *aspirin*. Due to this ability of *Dong quai* to increase bleeding, it is not recommended for use during the menstrual blood flow. It is not recommended for use during pregnancy and lactation. The only side effects of note are that it may increase your sensitivity to sunlight and it may increase blood sugar.

Evening Primrose Oil

What is it? This is the biennial plant *Oenothera biennis*, common name *Evening Primrose Oil*, a member of the *Onagraceae* botanical family. The plant flowers in the second year. The medicinal part is the ripe seeds. These contain the important essential fatty acids, linoleic acid (LA) and gamma-linolenic acid (GLA; an omega-6-fatty acid) as well as others. In the body, LA is converted to GLA. GLA is important in the body's production of the class of hormones called *prostaglandins*, specifically *prostaglandin E*. The GLA in *Evening Primrose Oil* functions as a natural anti-inflammatory agent in the body. It is essential for normal neural tube development in the fetus and it is found in breast milk. Omega-6-fatty acids function in the body to decrease the formation of atherosclerotic plaques in arteries and supplementing with GLA may decrease total cholesterol.

When should you use it? *Evening Primrose Oil* is used to treat symptoms of menopause and PMS. However, the data is not convincing that *Evening Primrose Oil* is beneficial in these conditions. *Evening Primrose Oil* has been shown to be helpful in treating breast tenderness during the menstrual cycle. Although research has not shown consistent benefit, some clinicians prescribe *Evening Primrose Oil* for children with Attention Deficit/Hyperactivity Disorder (ADD/ADHD) because of its high content of GLA. Some clinicians recommend using *Evening Primrose Oil* to relieve eczema and neurodermatitis. In addition, it has been used to relieve symptoms of polyneuropathy especially in diabetic patients. *Evening Primrose Oil* has also been useful to thicken hair growth on the scalp, especially after menopause-induced hair thinning.

How should you use it? *Evening Primrose Oil* is taken in 500mg capsules that contain 9% GLA and 91% LA. Take 1-3 capsules daily. Using *Evening Primrose Oil* for menopause-induced hair loss may take 6-8 weeks for noticeable change. *Black Currant Oil* at the same dosage may have the same effect.

What are the side effects, contraindications, and herb-drug interactions? *Evening Primrose Oil* should not be used in persons who have had seizures (convulsions, epilepsy) because it may lower the seizure threshold, precipitating seizures. Persons with schizophrenia and patients taking *phenothiazine* drugs should not take *Evening Primrose Oil*. Side effects have not been reported. *Evening Primrose Oil* is considered safe for use during pregnancy and lactation and it may help to decrease breast pain during breastfeeding, although this has not been proven.

Ginger

What is it? This is the plant *Zingiber officinale*, common name *Ginger*, a member of the *Zingiberaceae* botanical family. The medicinal part is the fresh root, the underground rhizome.

When should you use it? *Ginger* is well studied as an effective aid to treat nausea and indigestion from many causes, such as motion sickness, morning sickness, chemotherapy, and surgery. *Ginger* also has anti-inflammatory actions and is now being studied in osteoarthritis, migraine, autoimmune diseases, and for the treatment of ovarian cancer. The anti-nausea effects of *Ginger* are probably due to its soothing action on the digestive tract.

How should you use it? *Ginger* is widely available as a tea, spice, fresh root, powder, capsules, syrup, and as candied (crystallized) *Ginger*, where you bite off a piece and chew, as you need it to control symptoms. The daily dose of *Ginger* root powder to prevent or treat motion sickness, morning sickness, indigestion, and to ease the pains of arthritis is usually 1-2 grams daily taken as 500mg 2-4 times daily.

What are the side effects, contraindications, and herb-drug interactions? There is controversy concerning the safety of *Ginger* during pregnancy because high doses have been used in Chinese Traditional Medicine to promote menstruation. Clinical data derived from the use of *Ginger* in pregnant women for thousands of years tell us *Ginger* is safe for use during pregnancy in recommended doses only. Data is insufficient to recommend *Ginger* during breastfeeding. *Ginger* inhibits clotting so persons who are taking anticoagulants should not use it. *Ginger* should not be used in persons who suffer from gallstones. No side effects at recommended dosages are reported. At high doses *Ginger* can sometimes cause a burning feeling in the stomach. If it does, you may have to take your *Ginger* along with some food.

> **Note:** *QueasEase* made by Pacific BioLogic is a chewable herbal remedy containing *Ginger* in conjunction with 11 other herbs, according to the tenets of Traditional Chinese Medicine. *QueasEase* is indicated for the prevention and treatment of motion sickness but not for morning sickness because it may not be safe for pregnant women. Follow the directions on the label.

> **Note:** Other herbal remedies helpful for indigestion are: *Peppermint* (*Mentha piperita*), *Fennel seed* (*Foeniculum vulgare*), *Chamomile* (*Matricaria chamomilla*) and *lemon balm* (*Melissa officinalis*). These herbal remedies are also helpful for colicky pains in infancy. They are present in *Calma Bebi* herbal tea. *Gripe water* is another remedy worthy to try in cases of infant colic. There are many formulations available, but most have *Fennel seed* or *Dill seed oil* or *Ginger* and some have *sodium bicarbonate*.

Soy

What is it? Soybeans, *Glycine max*, are technically not herbs but rather legumes or beans, eaten as a healthy food and marketed as nutritional supplements. However, *soy* belongs in this section because of its profound effects on the health of women.

When should you use it? *Soy* contains *phytoestrogens*, chemicals that function in the body like estrogen, but which are not actually estrogen. The *phytoestrogens* found in *soy* have both weak estrogen-like and anti-estrogen-like effects in the body. The *phytoestrogens* found in *soy* are called *isoflavones*. *Soy isoflavones* come in 3 types: *daidzen*, *genistein* and *glycitein*. *Soy isoflavones* also function as antioxidants and may possess anti-cancer activity. *Soy isoflavones* have been used to treat menopausal symptoms and to prevent osteoporosis in both men and women. People in countries where more *soy* foods are eaten have decreased numbers of breast, lung, and prostate cancers and leukemia. They also have a lower rate of cardiovascular diseases, possibly due to *soy*'s cholesterol lowering effects.

In countries, like Japan, where *soy* foods constitute the dominant protein in the daily diet, breast cancer occurs much less frequently compared to America. One of the reasons may be that *soy* is consumed early on in a female child's life and continues through the breast-tissue development years. It is likely that benefits accrue to young boys as well.

How should you use it? I strongly urge you to consume *soy* foods (like tofu, tempeh, edamame, *soy* nuts, *soy* burgers, *soy* milk, *soy* cheese and textured *soy* protein) rather than *soy* supplements because the estrogen-like effects of very high doses of *soy* *isoflavones* have not yet been well studied. We just don't know enough about *soy* supplements' abilities to initiate or advance breast and/or prostate cancer. *Soy* foods are considered beneficial and healthy even when consumed as much as 1-2 times daily, but no more than 25 grams of *soy* protein daily.

> **Note:** The National Institute of Environmental Health Sciences (at www.niehs.nih.gov) reported that when mice are fed a diet high in *genistein*, they have menstrual and fertility problems. When *genistein* is given to newborn mice, their ovaries become abnormal. Although mice and humans are not the same, these results are so chilling that they make me very cautious about *soy* protein supplements, at least until this is studied in humans. But, 1-2 servings of *soy* foods (as distinct from *soy* supplements) have been proven healthy in both laboratory animals and humans. This same study has made me reluctant to endorse *soy*-based formulas for infants as either supplemental feeding or as complete replacement for breast milk or cow's milk.

> **Note:** *Soy* flour contains no gluten and is high in protein and fiber.

What are the side effects, contraindications, and herb-drug interactions? *Soy* supplements are contraindicated during pregnancy and lactation due to insufficient medical data on safety. However, *soy* foods (as distinct from *soy* supplements) are considered safe and healthy to eat 2-4 times per week during pregnancy and lactation. No drug interactions have been reported with *soy* *isoflavone* supplements. *Soy* supplements for persons who currently have or in the past have had breast cancer are not recommended. *Soy* foods for these people are considered safe to eat no more than 2 times weekly.

> **Note:** There are some doctors who do not allow any *soy* foods and *soy* supplements for women with breast cancer who are taking tamoxifen to prevent recurrences because of the possible increased risk for cancers of the liver and uterus. However, Dr. Andrew Weil believes the evidence for this is inadequate to completely proscribe *soy* foods for this subpopulation of women on tamoxifen.

> **Note:** Since *soy* foods contain naturally occurring *goitrogens* (chemicals that interfere with thyroid hormone production), it is a good idea to limit your intake if you or your family member is being treated for hypothyroidism (thyroid hormone deficiency). In this case, you should probably not ingest more than one serving of *soy* foods per day. In addition, you should not eat *soy* foods within 3 hours of taking your thyroid hormone replacement medicine.

> **Note:** Take a look around at all the different *soy* milks that are available. You need to be extra vigilant if you want to control the amount of added sugar in *soy* milk. You may choose *soy* milk (fortified with calcium and Vitamin D) sweetened with the sugar-substitute *Splenda* (*sucralose*), unsweetened, or sugar sweetened and flavored. Please be sure to buy *soy* milk with added *calcium carbonate* and remember to always shake the carton before pouring because *calcium carbonate* tends to settle on the bottom.

Wild Yam

What is it? This is the perennial vine plant *Dioscorea villosa*, common name *Wild Yam*, a member of the *Dioscoreaceae* botanical family. The medicinal parts are the root and rhizome.

When should you use it? *Wild Yam* contains certain chemicals which are precursors for the hormone progesterone, produced by your ovaries along with estrogen. *Wild Yam* is used to manufacture *natural progesterone* which is identical to the progesterone in the female body. During perimenopause and menopause, both estrogen and progesterone become deficient and contribute to symptoms, like hot flashes, depression, low libido, sleeplessness, irregular bleeding, and more severe PMS. A woman who has her uterus intact and takes estrogen as a prescription medication needs to supplement with progesterone as well so as not to increase her risk for uterine cancer (endometrial cancer). *Wild Yam* becomes a natural alternative to synthetic progesterone, but only when it is used in the manufacturing process. *Wild Yam* is not converted to progesterone inside the human body, so topical products containing *Wild Yam* may not contain any progesterone. The product has to contain *USP progesterone* or *natural progesterone* to be active in your body.

How should you use it? One of the ways to take *natural progesterone* made from *Wild Yam* is to spray it onto your skin 2-3 times daily in a product like *TransMist* by Health Freedom Nutrition. Each spray contains 6mg of *USP progesterone*. Use a total of 1-5 sprays per day, depending on severity of symptoms. Visit www.hfn-usa.com for more information.

Emerita makes the popular *Pro-Gest Body Cream* in tubes and single-use packets. Massage a packet containing ¼ teaspoon of cream (20mg of *USP progesterone*) into the skin twice daily for the 2 weeks prior to menstruation or, for women no longer menstruating, for 3 weeks out of every month. Some women may need ½ teaspoon to control symptoms.

> **Note:** Emerita also makes a water-based *personal lubricant* with *Aloe vera, Calendula, Chamomile, ginseng, Black walnut* and *Vitamin E* designed for menopausal women who want to alleviate vaginal dryness.

There are many other brands containing *USP progesterone* (or *natural progesterone*) for transdermal (topical) use. Men sometimes use *natural progesterone* (e.g., *Adam's Equalizer*) to increase libido because progesterone is a precursor of testosterone in the body.

> **Note:** Hormone replacement therapy (*HRT*) for a woman who still has her uterus usually involves taking both estrogen for relief of menopausal symptoms and progesterone to help prevent uterine cancer. The form of progesterone that is the closest fit to the natu-

rally occurring hormone is *Prometrium* 200mg capsules. *Prometrium* contains *micronized natural progesterone* made from *Wild Yam*.

> **Note:** *FemGest* progesterone cream made by Home Health contains progesterone "from natural sources" but does not contain *USP progesterone* from *Wild Yam*.

What are the side effects, contraindications, and herb-drug interactions? Too much *natural progesterone* may cause depression and mood swings as well as abdominal discomfort, bloating, and breast tenderness. But, *natural progesterone* supplementation is considered safe for long-term use. It is safe for use during pregnancy and may actually help to maintain the pregnancy. Discontinue use at least 2-3 weeks before expected delivery. *Natural progesterone* may be used during breastfeeding.

Guidelines for Consulting Your Health Care Provider

You should consult your health care provider if:
- the patient doesn't look right or act right (trust your instincts!)
- the patient is getting worse instead of better over the course of the illness
- the patient is having trouble breathing or complaining of chest pains or there is mental confusion or lethargy or irritability
- the patient develops allergic symptoms (hives, itchy or watery eyes, runny nose, scratchy throat, asthma, shortness of breath) after taking an herbal remedy
- after beginning a herbal remedy the patient experiences *new onset* of any serious symptoms such as: paralysis, weakness, tingling, inability to focus or concentrate, blurred or double vision or blindness, slurred speech, severe headaches, seizures, irritability, dizziness, disorientation, memory loss, anxiety, depression, insomnia, blackouts, fainting, or the person complains of not feeling like himself

- the patient is taking *ANY* prescription medication
- the patient is pregnant or breastfeeding
- the patient has any serious disease which may become life-threatening, such as:

autism, cancer, HIV and AIDS, arthritis, multiple sclerosis, coronary artery disease, heart attack (myocardial infarction), blood dyscrasia, cancer (of any type), congestive heart failure, diabetes mellitus, obesity, thyroid disorders, high blood pressure (hypertension), stroke, seizures, acute and chronic kidney (renal) failure, schizophrenia, bipolar disorder, borderline personality disorder, eating disorders, fibromyalgia, chronic fatigue syndrome, Crohn's disease, ulcerative colitis, celiac disease, mental deficiency disorders, chromosomal disorders, infertility, frequent miscarriages, polyneuropathy, cystic fibrosis   [Adapted from *The Merck Manual* at www.merck.com]

Note: Do not delude yourself into believing that herbal remedies somehow are not medicines. They are. You must disclose the herbal medicines you or your family member is taking to your health care provider.

Note: Do not discontinue taking any pharmaceutical medication which has been prescribed by your health care provider unless you or your family member is under the supervision of a physician.

Note: Do not take any herbal remedy without first consulting a health care provider if you or your family member is pregnant or breastfeeding. In addition, it is a good idea to check with your health care provider if your family member is either very young or very old because herbal remedies given injudiciously may overwhelm the body's defenses in those age groups.

Caution: If you are searching for an alternative treatment for infertility, the safest path is to try homeopathic remedies that are safe without any side effects. No herbal remedy is completely safe in the first few days and weeks of pregnancy—when you are still wondering if you might be pregnant.

Note: If you suffer from bloating at the onset of your menstrual cycle, you may want to try the herbal remedy *parsley* (*Petroselinum crispum*) for its diuretic properties. *Parsley* contains the diuretic chemical *apiole* which acts by stimulating the kidneys to excrete urine. Do not use *parsley* if you are pregnant because it stimulates uterine contractions too.

Putting It All Together

If you are considering using an herbal remedy, it is a good idea to familiarize yourself with **Chapter 19: Introduction to Herbal Medicine**.

Then, after you have decided to use an herbal remedy to prevent or treat a certain ailment, it makes good sense to investigate the homeopathic remedy indicated for that ailment as well. That's because homeopathic remedies are safe, have no side effects, and can be used together with herbal remedies and Western pharmaceutical medicines without concern. You may read about homeopathic remedies for women's reproductive tract health in **Chapter 10: Homeopathic Remedies for Disorders of Menstruation, Fertility, Pregnancy, Labor, Childbirth, Lactation, and Menopause**. And you may want to better understand homeopathy by reading **Chapter 2: Basic Homeopathy**.

Whenever you have decided to go ahead with an herbal supplement, you may want to consider giving the sick person's homeopathic constitutional remedy as well (please refer to **Chapter 18: Homeopathic Constitutional Remedies** if you are dealing with an adult; or **Chapter 13: Homeopathy for Elderly Persons** if you are dealing with an elderly person).

Women who are taking a herbal remedy for reproductive tract health will likely require all the vitamins and minerals necessary to repair and replenish tissues, especially *folic acid, iron, calcium* and *magnesium* (please refer to **Chapter 23: Vitamins and Minerals**) as well as a general antioxidant supplement (please refer to **Chapter 24: Antioxidant Phytochemicals**). Reproductive tract health, like the health of other body systems, may be dependent upon *omega-3 fatty acids* (please refer to **Chapter 31: Oils and Fats**). In addition, it is a good idea to incorporate *probiotics* (please refer to **Chapter 30: Prebiotics and Probiotics**) into your daily supplements because your may find your reproductive tract problems to be sensitive to enhanced gastrointestinal health.

Weight gain during menopause is a very nearly universal phenomenon in our culture. If you or your family member has gained to an unhealthy body weight, you may want to read **Chapter 26: Nutritional Supplements for Healthy Weight Control** for a consideration of appropriate nutritional supplements. Other medical problems can be tackled by reading **Chapters 25-31**.

PART THREE

Nutritional Supplements

Chapter 22

Introduction to Nutritional Supplements

Understanding Nutritional Supplements: Vitamins, Minerals, Antioxidants, and Phytonutrients

What are nutritional supplements?

Nutritional supplements refer to vitamins, minerals, antioxidants and all the wondrous substances one derives from plants, called phytonutrients, as well as many other substances used as foods. Phytonutrients or phytochemicals refer to the thousands of chemicals found in plants that help them survive. They are structured to interact with our own chemistries because humans and plants are interconnected on this planet. Phytonutrients are protective chemicals both for the plants that make them and for the animals that eat those plants.

Antioxidants refer to any substance (certain vitamins and minerals, certain phytochemicals) that renders free radicals harmless in the body. Free radicals are produced in the course of normal cellular metabolism (sometimes called oxidative metabolism). When unchecked, free radicals have been implicated in the development of cancer, cardiovascular disease, stroke, arthritis, diabetes, and other chronic conditions.

What are essential nutrients?

"Essential nutrients" are those nutritional chemicals that are not made inside our bodies although they are required, or "essential" in order to create the energy that allows us to live. "Essential nutrients" include: water; certain minerals like calcium, potassium, phosphorus, magnesium, sodium and chloride; trace minerals like chromium, copper, iron, selenium, zinc and others; essential amino acids derived from proteins; essential fatty acids from fats; and certain vitamins like C, B, A, D, E and K.

When should we use nutritional supplements?

Nutritional supplements are used to promote health, prevent disease, and also to treat certain chronic conditions. They are now considered indispensable to a healthy lifestyle because diet alone is no longer able to satisfactorily promote health. Why is this true?

First, it is almost impossible to get the amounts of nutrients we need from diet alone if we want to protect ourselves from certain diseases of modern life, such as heart disease, hypertension, stroke, cancer, diabetes, arthritis, osteoporosis, and others, as well as to correct the effects of pollution on our bodies.

> **Note:** Chronic ailments, like heart disease, hypertension, stroke, cancer, diabetes, arthritis, osteoporosis, and many others may be linked to inflammatory proteins that may be produced in the body as a consequence of chronic stress. If you wish to combine proven stress-relieving techniques with homeopathy, herbal remedies, and nutritional supplements, it is a good idea to purchase Harvard Medical School's *Guide to Relieving Stress* available at www.health.harvard.edu.

Second, our foodstuffs have been altered and their nutrient content diluted by modern growing techniques and the use of fertilizers and pesticides. This, taken together with modern storage methods, means that we sometimes run into oranges that have no Vitamin C or tomatoes with little or no *lycopene*.

Vitamins and minerals are essential in cellular metabolism because they act as coenzymes, or enzyme cofactors, thereby having a central part to play in the work of all our living cells. Vitamin and mineral coenzymes allow enzymes to do their work of converting foodstuff into energy and then detoxifying and eliminating the end-results of these reactions. Vitamins and minerals are essential for our survival on this planet.

The colorful diet

It is axiomatic that Americans do not eat enough fruits and vegetables on a daily basis to stay healthy and prevent chronic diseases, such as cancer, cardiovascular disease, hypertension, diabetes, arthritis, and many other "lifestyle" diseases so prevalent in our times.

The *Food Pyramid*, a fatally flawed creation of the U.S. Department of Agriculture, still recommends that we eat 5 portions of fruits and vegetables. However, the *American Institute for Cancer Research* (www.aicr.org) has studied the deficiencies in the American diet and now recommends that every one of us eat 10 portions of fruits and vegetables daily, essentially doubling the recommendation. The increases in the fruit and vegetable portions should be offset by decreases in the number of portions of carbohydrates and starches in the daily diet.

The *American Institute for Cancer Research* and the *National Cancer Institute* recommend that people should eat at least one portion of every color fruit and vegetable daily because each color contains different phytochemicals and antioxidants. The more deeply colored the fruit and vegetable, the greater the amounts of phytochemicals, vitamins, and minerals they contain.

The colorful diet includes fruits and vegetables of the following groups:

Greens: green leafy vegetables such as spinach, Romaine lettuce, collard greens, kale, beet greens, escarole, mustard greens, Swiss chard and turnip greens, green grapes, and the cruciferous vegetables: broccoli, cabbage and Brussels spouts;

Reds: watermelon, tomatoes, red grapes, pomegranates;

Whites: the cruciferous vegetable cauliflower, garlic, white onions, and leeks;

Yellow-oranges: carrots, butternut squash, sweet potatoes, peaches, apricots, pumpkins, cantaloupe, mangoes, lemons;

Blue-purples: blueberries, blackberries, purple grapes, plums, eggplants.

Note: Grapefruits and grapefruit juice contain a chemical that interferes with the metabolism of certain commonly prescribed pharmaceuticals. The result is to potentiate their actions in the body which may result in toxic side effects. Do not eat grapefruits or drink grapefruit juice if you are taking any of the following drugs: *astemizole* (*Hismanal, an antihistamine*); cholesterol-lowering drugs such as *Zocar* and *Lipitor* ("statins"); estrogens, caffeine, *saquinavir* (*Invirase*, for HIV infection); immunosuppressants *cyclosporine* (*Sandimmune*) and *tacrolimus* (*Prograf*); *alprazolam* (*Xanax*) and *triazolam* (*Halcion*); calcium channel blockers *felodipine* (*Plendil*), *nifedipine* (*Adalat, Procardia*), *nimodipine* (*Nimotop*), and *verapamil* (*Calan, Isoptin, Verlan*); *cisapride* (*Propusid*); and *cilostazol* (*Pletal*).

Should you get your phytonutrients from foods or supplements?

In theory, the healthier choice would be to eat your phytonutrients from foods rather than from supplements because the natural plant actually contains hundreds of chemicals all acting together in a natural balance. Supplements cannot achieve this profuse variety and wondrous balance. Supplement manufacturers take one of the plant's chemicals, purify and concentrate it, and make it into tablets or capsules.

Research has sometimes shown that choosing one antioxidant phytochemical and taking it as a supplement may not protect us from disease the way eating the natural vegetables do. But, other research shows that certain antioxidant phytochemicals in the form of nutritional supplements do the job we want them to do.

The same reasons we no longer rely on our food to supply us with the vitamins and minerals we need to cope with the health dangers of our modern, active, polluted, stressful lives apply to this situation.

Yes, you should strive to obtain your daily dose of phytonutrients from the five colors but you probably should also take certain nutritional supplements, especially at the very least, a daily multivitamin-multimineral supplement and calcium supplement, depending on your individual health and circumstances.

Putting good health practices and nutritional supplements together

It is not possible to compensate for an unhealthy diet and lifestyle by taking vitamins, minerals, and other nutritional supplements, even in megadoses.

In order for you and your family members to derive benefit from the **essential alternative health** practices such as nutritional supplements, it is an absolute requirement that you adhere to the **good health practices**:

—no smoking, moderate alcohol, nutritionally healthy diet, adequate daily physical exercise, adequate sleep, time for daily relaxation techniques, seeking humor and love in everyday life, engaging in activities for intellectual stimulation, doing things for other people, and participating in preventive health testing.

The alphabet soup of recommendations for vitamins and minerals

More than 60 years ago the U.S. government published the **Recommended Dietary Allowances** **(RDAs)** of vitamins and minerals. The goal of **RDAs** was to prevent vitamin deficiency diseases. But we've learned so much in those intervening years. We now want to recommend levels of vitamins and minerals that would *prevent* many of the killer diseases and *promote* long-term health.

To that end, in early 2003, the Food and Nutrition Board of the Institute of Medicine published new nutritional standards, called the **Dietary Reference Intakes (DRIs)**. **DRIs** vary by gender and by the different stages and situations of life (infancy, childhood, adolescent, adult, pregnancy, lactation, 60 years of age and older).

But, when not enough information was known about a certain vitamin or mineral the **Adequate Intake (AI)** value was used. In addition, they created the **Upper Intake Levels (ULs)** which is the highest amount of vitamins or minerals that would do no harm in the human body. The **UL** is designed to prevent excessive intake of vitamins and minerals.

This alphabet soup has not made understanding which vitamins and minerals to take and in what amounts any easier. But it has led us to more meaningful recommendations and puts us on the road towards individualizing prescriptions for vitamins and minerals to fit gender and life cycle stage.

> **Note:** Most of the **DRIs** and **ULs** in this book are excerpted from the bimonthly newsletter (now defunct), *The Dietary Supplement*, Issue No. 13, 2002, written and published by Paul R. Thomas. If you are interested in specific **DRIs** or **ULs**, you can find them in *Understanding Nutrition*, 9th Ed., by Whitney and Rolfes. This reference book may be available in your library.

Should you buy organic foods and produce?

More and more people are coming over to the organic side by buying organic fruits and vegetables. Buying organic has become an integral part of our concern with our own health as well as the health of the world we live in.

"USDA Organic" certified produce are fruits, vegetables, and grains that have been grown with none or only very small amounts of chemical fertilizers, no synthetic pesticides (although some natural pesticides are allowed), no sewage sludge, no fumigants, no chemical additives, no taste enhancers, no food colorings, no irradiation, and no genetically modified seeds.

Meat and poultry that are "certified USDA organic" come from animals that have free access to the outdoors (free range) and eat only pesticide-free, hormone-free and antibiotic-free feeds. In addition, the feed must be 100% "certified organic." "Organic" eggs and dairy products come from "organically" raised chicken and cows, respectively.

The words "all natural" on the label mean that the food contains no artificial ingredients. "All natural" does not have anything to do with "organic."

The "USDA Organic" label means that not only is there a decreased level of toxins (pesticide residues) that might otherwise come with your food, but also an increased level of nutrients are contained in that food. Eating "organic" fruits and vegetables may likely give you increased amounts of vitamins, minerals, and phytochemicals including antioxidants. This has not yet been proven conclusively by medical research, but some studies have been done which show that organically grown fruits and vegetables contain more Vitamin C, iron and other minerals, *lycopene*, and other phytonutrients than those grown with pesticides. Such studies have sometimes revealed tomatoes without detectable *lycopene* coming to market! Or oranges without detectable Vitamin C! And there is good medical data that show a decrease in chemicals from pesticides in urine of children whose diets are based on organic produce.

Another good reason to buy "organic" is the taste test. Organic fruits and vegetables taste better, fresher, fuller and they taste this way longer than their non-organically grown cousins. These results are found consistently in taste tests of organic versus conventional produce.

Yet another reason is that organic produce do not contain genetically modified organisms (GMOs) that have invaded most of our crops over the last decade. No one knows what the long-term effect of GMOs will have on human health and there are prominent medical researchers on both sides of the controversy.

> **Note:** Some of the successes behind the rapid growth of GMOs in our food supply are that we do have hardier wheat, corn, and soy and this has led to a global "green revolution" as people are better able to feed themselves. The solution to the GMO controversy will probably be a compromise so that we don't throw out the baby with the bath water.

> **Note:** The commonest genetically modified foods are corn and corn products, soy and soy products, cottonseed oil, and canola oil. For more information take a look at www.greenpeace.org.

A good way to begin to buy organic produce

You may want to test the "organic" waters for yourself and your family by beginning to buy "organic" those fruits and vegetables that have been proven to be most contaminated with pesticides. Pesticide levels are determined by the *Environmental Working Group*, a nonprofit research organization devoted to improving our environment.

The fruits most contaminated with pesticides are: cherries, nectarines, strawberries, red raspberries, apples, peaches, and pears; imported grapes and imported cantaloupe. The vegetables most contaminated with pesticides are: bell and hot peppers, spinach, potatoes, and celery.

The least contaminated fruits are: banana, kiwi, mango, papaya and pineapple. The least contaminated vegetables are: asparagus, avocado, broccoli, cauliflower, corn, onion and peas.

> **Note:** The list of the "dirty dozen" fruits and vegetables changes every few months. You can check the current list provided by the *Environmental Working Group* at www.ewg.org.

You may decide to start your family's organic odyssey by buying organic milk (brand name *Horizon* at www.horizonorganic.com) because it is produced from free-range cows fed pesticide-free feeds without the addition of antibiotics or growth hormones. *Horizon* also produces organic cheese. Organic milk and dairy products cost more than their nonorganic counterparts, but they are well worth it in health benefits. You do not want your developing children to ingest any additional hormones, especially genetically engineered bovine growth hormone. *Earthbound Farm* (www.ebfarm.com) sells organic salads, fruits, and vegetables. Many companies sell organic baby foods.

> **Note:** Organic eggs are not the same as "designer" eggs. The nutritional value of "designer" eggs varies by the kind of diet that is fed to the hens. Some "designer" eggs claim to contain increased levels of *omega-3 fatty acids* or

antioxidants or have lower saturated fat content. There are two potential problems: 1) these claims may not be justified, and 2) the changes in these levels may be insignificantly small.

Here are a few useful websites for more information about organic products: www.organicgardening.com, www.horizonorganic.com, www.localharvest.org, www.naturespath.com, www.organicconsumers.org, www.stonyfield.com, www.organicvalley.com, www.theorganicreport.org, www.wholefoodsmarket.com, www.allorganiclinks.com, www.eatwellguide.org, www.ams.usda.gov/nop, www.rodaleinstitute.org, www.ofrf.org, www.organicfqhresearch.org and www.soilassociation.org

You may want more information on topics like pesticide exposure in the foods you eat and in your drinking water. I recommend that you start reading *Environmental Nutrition: The Newsletter of Food, Nutrition, and Health.* You may contact them about subscription costs at 1-800-829-5384 or www.environmentalnutrition.com. Another reliable source of information on our environment is *E Magazine: The Environmental Magazine* published by Earth Action Network, Inc. You may visit them online at www.emagazine.com (203-854-5559).

> **Remember:** Organic farming is helping to save our planet from poisoning our food and water. Another way to help save our planet is to get involved with recycling of household garbage (usually glass, newspaper, plastic and aluminum cans). If you want more information on recycling, please visit *Grassroots Recycling Network* at www.grrn.org (706-613-7121) and the *National Recycling Coalition* at www.nrc-recycle.org (202-347-0450).

> **Note:** Another way to get involved with eating healthier is to buy locally grown produce. This may turn out to be of equal importance as buying "organic" because freshness in fruits and vegetables has been linked to increased levels of all phytonutrients.

Should you buy bottled water?

Bottled water is marketed in ever-increasing choices. You can buy spring water, mineral water, flavored water, carbonated water, oxygenated water, and even water fortified with various vitamins. The problem is that the bottled water industry is not regulated by the *Environmental Protection Agency* (*EPA*) like your public water supply is. Rather, bottled water is regulated by the *Food and Drug Administration* (*FDA*). The *FDA* does not require that companies publish records of the results of laboratory tests of their products. And these test results are known to vary as widely as the varieties of bottled waters. It all means that bottled waters are not always what they seem, or even wha you wish them to be, safe and free from contaminants.

Instead of bottled water, you may opt for a filter system. Filter systems include (from least to most expensive): the pour-through-pitcher system (only filters a few quarts of water at a time); the faucet-mounted filter; the reverse osmosis filter mounted under the sink; and the "point-of-entry" filter system which is connected at the place in the pipe where your water meter meets the main water line (the best option for well water).

My own advice: purchase a good water filter system for your tap water or a pour-through-pitcher system for your drinking water that will remove impurities (lead, mercury, and chlorine), improve the sometimes chemical taste, and filter out some microorganisms (*Giardia*, *Cryptosporidium*). *Pur* pour-through-pitchers remove the chemical pesticide *atrazine* but not *alachlor*. The *Brita* faucet-mounted filter removes both.

> **Note:** I do not recommend distilled water because it contains no minerals whatsoever which can be unhealthy.

Detoxification the gentle way

Homeopathy is the only gentle and yet effective way to achieve detoxification from environmental poisons, such as pesticides, herbicides, insecticides, fungicides, pollutants, nicotine addiction, substances of abuse, alcohol addiction, and prescription pharmaceuticals.

> **Note:** Please do not consider other methods of detoxification, such as fasting, purging, chelation or colonic irrigation. These methods are likely to be harmful, dangerous, and invasive. They surely are unnatural and they all come with side effects. Homeopathic detoxification does not.

For detoxification purposes, you may want to consider the homeopathic combination remedy called *Ubichinon Compositum*, which is manufactured by Heel, a homeopathic supply house.

> **Note:** You will find more information on *Ubichinon Compositum* in **Chapter 13: Homeopathy for Elderly Persons**.

> **Note:** Another homeopathic detoxification remedy is the *Detox-Kit*, also manufactured by Heel. It consists of 3 components, *Lymphomyosot*, *Berberis Homaccord* and *Nux vomica Homaccord*, each in a 50 ml bottle. *Lymphomyosot* detoxifies the lymphatic system; *Berberis*, the excretory organs, specifical-

ly the kidneys, skin, and liver; and *Nux vomica*, the digestive system and liver. Thus, the *Detox-Kit* provides for the elimination of diverse toxins from most sources. The directions for use are to put 30 drops of each of the three solutions into one quart of water and drink it during the day.

When to consult your physician

In the following chapters on nutritional supplements you will learn when to consult your homeopath or your Western medicine health care provider by paying strict attention to the **Guidelines for Consulting Your Health Care Provider**, found at the end of each of those chapters. You may want to refer to the last section **Putting It All Together** for ideas on how to integrate the essential natural alternatives, homeopathy, herbal remedies, and nutritional supplements.

> **Note:** Do not discontinue taking any pharmaceutical medication that has been prescribed by your health care provider unless you or your family member is under the supervision of a physician.

Chapter 23

Vitamins and Minerals

Vitamins and Minerals in General

Ailment/Disorder/Symptom	Nutritional Supplement
Eye health, fetal development, bones, skin, blood	*Vitamin A*
Brain health, muscles (including heart muscle) and nerves	*B Vitamins*
Antioxidant, anti-cancer, anti-ageing activity	*Vitamin C*
Bone health, anti-cancer activity	*Vitamin D*
Skin, heart, nervous and immune systems, oxidative damage repair	*Vitamin E*
Blood clotting (coagulation)	*Vitamin K*
Bone health, teeth, heart, muscles, nerves, and blood clotting	*Calcium*
Glucose metabolism regulation	*Chromium*
Thyroid gland function	*Iodine*
Red blood cell formation and function	*Iron*
Muscle contraction (including the heart muscle), nerve conduction, blood pressure and bone metabolism	*Magnesium*
Bone health	*Manganese*
Energy production and synthesis of nucleic acids, healthy blood pressure	*Potassium*
Antioxidant activity, anti-cancer activity	*Selenium*
Immune system function and glucose metabolism	*Zinc*

Guidelines for Consulting Your Health Care Provider
Putting It All Together

Vitamins and Minerals

Vitamins and Minerals in General

The multivitamin, known simply as the "multi," has been around for most of the 20th century, and is still going strong, or even stronger, as it enters the 21st century. The modern multivitamin is usually a multivitamin-multimineral supplement tablet that may contain other nutrients as well as herbal remedies, usually in very low dosage.

About one-half of all American adults take a "multi" every day for the most part because they feel their nutritional intake by way of food is inadequate to provide them with everything they need to prevent disease and promote good health. Expert nutritionists generally recommend that you and your family members take a multivitamin-multimineral supplement every day. And in addition, most would encourage you to include a calcium-magnesium supplement for teenagers on up (perhaps even young children and preteens), for both men and women, including pregnant and breast-feeding women.

> **Note:** The *United States Department of Agriculture* (*USDA*) publishes data on the percent change from 1975-2004 for nutrients naturally occurring in our food. The across-the-board decreases in vitamins and minerals in our food supply is another reason we should be supplementing even a healthy diet with a daily multivitamin-multimineral.

> **Note:** Medical researchers at the Harvard School of Public Health have shown that women infected with HIV who took a multivitamin supplement had a slower progression of the virus compared with those who did not. This study is an example of the powerful effect of multivitamins.

Regular use of multivitamin-multimineral supplements over a period of a decade or more has been associated with a significantly decreased risk for cancer of the colon. The important element in pre-vention is *long-term* use of a multivitamin-multimineral supplement. It is likely that future research will show the same results for the prevention of other cancers as well.

But, what if you haven't yet started yourself (or started a family member) taking a multivitamin-multimineral supplement? It's not too late. Get started by choosing a daily multivitamin-multimineral supplement from a reputable manufacturer. Read all the ingredients on the label and compare different brands. Compare prices too. And choose a formulation that fits your gender and stage in life: infant, child, adolescent, young active man or woman, sports active, pregnant or lactating woman, menopausal, elderly.

Before you buy a supplement, look for the *USP mark* on the label for quality assurance. If you want to buy a non-*USP* labeled supplement, please check first with ConsumerLab.com. They performed product reviews of many vitamin and mineral supplements. You can read the results at www. ConsumerLab.com or in their book, ConsumerLab. com's *Guide to Buying Vitamins and Supplements, What's Really in the Bottle?*

Adult men and women differ in their vitamin and mineral requirements. Children need a multivitamin-multimineral supplement specifically designed for that age, while seniors need one that suits that stage in life. Adult men and post-menopausal women do not require iron in their daily supplements as they are likely to get enough from their diets alone. They do not experience on-going blood loss like premenopausal women do during their monthly menstrual cycles. Elderly persons require a larger daily dose of Vitamin B12 because age tends to decrease the amount of stomach acid which in turn would impede absorption of that vitamin.

Women who are pregnant or breastfeeding should take a prenatal vitamin every day so that their levels of iron and folic acid are adequate. If at all possible, start taking your prenatal vitamin six months to one year before conception so that you may ensure a healthy level of iron and folic acid to prevent neural tube malformations.

Keep away from some multivitamin-multimineral supplements which are specially formulated with herbs. The herbs are there in insufficient dosage to be helpful. Never take herbs willy-nilly.

Herbs (in contrast to homeopathic remedies) are medicines and they can interact with the prescription medications you may be taking. Herbs are included in some multivitamin-multimineral supplements because the manufacturer hopes you will be duped into thinking that a better supplement is one with a longer list of ingredients. Not necessarily true.

> **Note:** An exception to this is the multi-vitamin-multimineral-plus nutritional supplement *Life Extension Mix* manufactured by Life Extension. It is a comprehensive supplement, containing veg-etable-fruit complexes for antioxidants, enzymes, amino acids, vitamins, and minerals. The problem: you have to take 9 tablets, or 14 capsules, or three scoops of powder for your daily dose. And even then you will need to take additional calcium! *Life Extension Mix* is not appropriate for men and post-menopausal women because it contains 18mg of iron.

> **Note:** *Environmental Nutrition* (June 2004) printed their *Top Picks* for general multis. They listed: *Centrum Advanced Formula, CVS Spectravite, Geritol Complete, GNC Solo Day, One-A-Day Maximum, One-A-Day Men's Health, Tie Aid Central-Vite* and *Vitamin World ABC Plus.* Here are their *Top Picks* for Ages 50+: *Centrum Silver, AARP Alphabet II, DVS Spectravite Senior, Kirkland Signature Mature Adults Daily Multi, One-A-Day Today* and *Vitamin World ABC Plus Senior.*

> **Note:** Read more about "multis" in the *Harvard Health Letter*, September 2006 at www.health.harvard.edu.

Steer clear of pricey chelated and colloidal minerals because there is no scientific evidence to support the claim that they are better absorbed or utilized in any different manner inside the body than their plainer counterparts. In fact, the opposite may be true in some cases. In addition, there is no medical evi-

dence that slow-release (or time-release) vitamins or minerals are more effective than non-time-release. The one major exception is *niacin* (please see below) because the slow-release form of high dose *niacin* (*Niaspan*) decreases the disturbing (but not harmful) side effect of skin flushing.

The controversy over natural versus synthetic vitamins is inflamed by manufacturers who want to sell you the more expensive product. Very little research has been done on the question of superiority of natural versus synthetic vitamins. The prevailing opinion is that synthetic vitamins are considered to act inside the body the same as natural ones, except for Vitamin E. Minerals are always natural because they are chemical elements that cannot be synthesized.

Supplements designed for infants do not contain the full complement of vitamins nor any minerals, except for iron. The vitamins in breast milk, except for Vitamin D, are usually adequate to maximize infant growth. Infant formulas are fortified with Vitamin D (as well as many other vitamins and minerals). Most pediatricians recommend that infants take a vitamin-mineral supplement containing Vitamins A, C and D along with iron and fluoride (unless the water supply has sufficient fluoride). I recommend that the B Vitamins be added as well to help with the rapid, critical brain growth in infancy.

The complex issues of infant feeding, breast milk versus formulas, when to start solids, which solids to start, which vitamin-mineral supplements to give, are important matters that require special attention. The chapter on *Life Cycle Nutrition: Infancy, Childhood, and Adolescence* in *Understanding Nutrition*, 9th Ed., by Whitney and Rolfes is a reliable, but technical, place to start. (You may be able to borrow the book from your local library.) The American Academy of Pediatrics at www.aap.org is another good source of information on the special nutritional needs of infants and young children.

> **Note:** For a basic understanding of Dietary Reference Intakes (DRIs) and Upper Intake Levels (ULs), please refer to **Chapter 22: Introduction to Nutritional Supplements.**

Note: Most of the DRIs and ULs in this book are excerpted from the bimonthly newsletter (now defunct), *The Dietary Supplement*, Issue No. 13, 2002, written and published by Paul R. Thomas. If you are interested in specific Dietary Reference Intakes (DRIs) or Upper Intake Levels (ULs), you can find them in *Understanding Nutrition*, 9th Ed., by Whitney and Rolfes.

Note: Harvard Medical School's *The Smart Guide to Vitamins and Minerals*, available at www.health.harvard.edu is a good resource for understanding the basics.

Vitamins are so called because they are vital to life, meaning essential not only for health but for survival. They function as coenzymes in the myriad of chemical, enzymatic reactions throughout metabolism. There are 2 basic kinds: water-soluble (Vitamins B and C) and fat-soluble (Vitamins A, D, E and K). Water-soluble vitamins are not stored in the body. Fat-soluble vitamins are stored in fatty tissue until needed for metabolic processes. Both water- and fat-soluble vitamins should not be consumed above the Upper Intake Levels (ULs) which is the highest amount of vitamins or minerals that would do no harm in the human body.

It is important to steam or microwave vegetables so that the water-soluble vitamins are preserved. Otherwise, if cooked in water, the water-soluble vitamins are leached into the water. But, if you do cook your vegetables in water, don't throw that vitamin-rich water away. Drink it or use it to make soups.

When using nutritional supplements for self-care of any and all ailments you must pay strict attention to the **Guidelines for Consulting Your Health Care Provider** at the end of this chapter. You may want to refer to the last section **Putting It All Together** for ideas on how to integrate the essential natural alternatives, homeopathy, herbal remedies, and nutritional supplements.

Vitamins

Vitamin A (retinol, retinal, retinoic acid)

Vitamin A is a fat-soluble vitamin (along with Vitamins D, E and K) which means that bile is necessary for its absorption from the intestines, and that unused amounts are stored in the liver and fat (adipose) tissue. Vitamin A is composed of 3 different chemicals (retinol, retinal and retinoic acid), each of which is essential for its own set of chemical reactions. The precursor to Vitamin A in the body is *beta-carotene*, a member of the *carotenoid* family of powerful plant antioxidants. *Beta-carotene* is water-soluble, is non-toxic, and does not accumulate in tissues.

Vitamin A is necessary for healthy vision, skin, blood, bone, and reproduction, as well as fetal development, and protein synthesis. Vitamin A deficiency results in night blindness (from lack of pigment in the retina), total blindness (from destruction of the cornea), growth retardation, susceptibility to infections, cancers, and death. Topical forms of retinoic acid are used to treat acne and psoriasis.

Children in developing countries are particularly vulnerable to Vitamin A deficiency. When children eat diets low in Vitamin A, they tend to have a higher mortality rate from infectious diseases such as measles. Hypervitaminosis A (Vitamin A toxicity) results from excess Vitamin A ingestion. Excess *beta-carotene* ingestion just turns the skin yellow-orange but does not cause toxicity because the body converts only as much *beta-carotene* as it requires into Vitamin A. If either too much (more than 10,000 IU/day) or too little Vitamin A is ingested during pregnancy birth defects may result. Ingesting high levels of Vitamin A (from retinol, not from *beta-carotene*) is associated with an increased rate of bone fractures from osteoporosis in both men and women.

Food sources: fish, fish oils, liver, eggs, dark leafy vegetables, orange and yellow fruits and vegetables. Retinol, retinal, and retinoic acid are found in animal sources; *beta-carotene* is found in plant sources.

DRI for men 3,000 IU (900 micrograms) and **DRI** for women 2,300 IU/day (700 micrograms), 2,500

IU/day during pregnancy, and 4,300 IU/day during lactation.

UL: for Vitamin A (from retinol) is 10,000 IU/day. Choose a multivitamin preparation that contains no more than 3,000-5,000 IU (or at most 1,500 micrograms) of Vitamin A. If your multivitamin supplies Vitamin A from *beta-carotene*, no more than 10,000 IU should be ingested on a daily basis. Most prenatal vitamins include 5,000 IU Vitamin A per tablet and a proportion is derived from *beta-carotene*.

The popular multivitamin-multimineral brands *Centrum* and *Centrum Silver* both contain 3,500 IU of Vitamin A with 29% as *beta-carotene*.

> **Note:** Vitamin A and Vitamin E are still listed on labels in IU (International Units), an old way of measuring amounts of vitamins.

The B Vitamins

There are nine B Vitamins: thiamin (Vitamin B1), riboflavin (Vitamin B2), niacin or nicotinamide (Vitamin B3), pantothenic acid (Vitamin B5), pyridoxine (Vitamin B6), cobalamin (Vitamin B12), folic acid or folate or folacin, biotin, and choline.

All the B Vitamins are water-soluble which means that they dissolve in water rather than fat and are not stored in the body. Each of the B Vitamins is involved in energy production in the body, either producing energy from carbohydrates (sugar and starches), or from fats and proteins. The entire B family is necessary for healthy function of your brain, muscles (including heart muscle) and nerves. Members of the B family often work together.

> **Note:** A natural way to get your daily dose of the entire complex of B Vitamins is by taking *Brewer's Yeast*. I recommend the brand *Lewis Laboratories; 100% Pure Premium Imported Brewer's Yeast* because it tastes good. Acceptable taste has been the problem with other brands. You can add it to foods and soups (after cooking because B Vitamins are destroyed by heat) to enhance flavor and increase nutritional value. *Brewer's Yeast* not only contains B Vitamins, but many other vitamins and minerals as well as 18 amino acids. It is a very nutritious

food. But remember that *Brewer's Yeast* contains about 120 calories in 2 tablespoons (one serving size).

Thiamin (Vitamin B1)

Thiamin or Vitamin B1 is essential to energy production in the body by its presence as a coenzyme in the conversion of glucose and amino acids into energy. Thiamin is present on nerve cell membranes. Thiamin deficiency disease is called *beriberi*, affecting nerves and muscles, and usually occurring as a result of alcoholism. Relative thiamin deficiency is probably present in at-risk populations, such as alcohol abusers, homeless persons, and pregnant and lactating women.

> **Note:** *Benfotiamine* is a close chemical cousin of thiamin but since it is fat-soluble it penetrates into certain cellular places where thiamin does not. *Benfotiamine* functions as an enzyme cofactor. It increases the activity of transketolase, a critical enzyme in glucose metabolism. *Benfotiamine* is being investigated as an agent that may be useful to boost metabolism and prevent complications from diabetes.

Food sources: whole grains, legumes, nuts and seeds, and pork. In contrast, refined foods contain little, if any, thiamin.

DRI for men 1.2mg/day. **DRI** for women 1.1mg/day, 1.4mg/day during pregnancy and lactation.
UL: has not been established.

Riboflavin (Vitamin B2)

Riboflavin or Vitamin B2 is essential as a coenzyme for chemical reactions that convert foodstuffs into energy. Deficiency of riboflavin causes cracking at the corners of the mouth, sensitivity to light and other eye and skin symptoms. Among people who suffer from migraine headaches, those who take 400mg of riboflavin daily have fewer and less severe episodes This effect is compounded when magnesium (400-800mg/day) is added.

Food sources: whole grains, dairy products, dark green leafy vegetables.

DRI for men 1.3mg/day. DRI for women 1.1mg/day, 1.4mg/day during pregnancy and 1.6mg/day during lactation.
UL: has not been established.

Niacin (nicotinamide, Vitamin B3)

Niacin can be produced in the body by converting the amino acid, tryptophan into niacin. Recommended amounts for niacin is given in mg NE/day or "niacin equivalents." One NE is either 1mg of niacin present in food or 60mg of tryptophan present in food which is then converted to 1mg of niacin in the body.

Niacin is an essential coenzyme for more than 50 chemical reactions which convert glucose and fat into energy. Niacin deficiency disease is called *pellagra* which produces a constellation of symptoms called "the four Ds": diarrhea, dermatitis, dementia (with depression), and death.

Food sources: meat, fish, poultry, whole grains, green leafy vegetables, legumes, eggs, milk, nuts and seeds.

DRI for men 16mg NE /day. DRI for women 14mg NE/day, 18mg NE/day during pregnancy and 17mg NE/day during lactation. Sometimes you can experience an uncomfortable "niacin flush" (a painful flushing of the skin with sweating and tingling) when niacin is ingested in higher than recommended dosages. High-dose niacin is used in Western medicine to treat high triglycerides in the blood, a condition that may have harmful effects on the cardiovascular system, similar to high cholesterol. There are newer pharmaceutical preparations (such as *Niaspan*) that slow-release niacin into the blood to prevent "niacin flush." Niacin in doses of 500-1,500mg daily can raise HDL ("good") cholesterol by as much as 35% and lower triglycerides by as much as 50%. You must be under your doctor's care when taking high-dose niacin or *Niaspan*. Your doctor will need to monitor your liver function when taking high-dose niacin to lower triglycerides.
UL: 35mg/day of niacin.

Pantothenic acid (Vitamin B5)

Pantothenic acid is a coenzyme for many of the enzymes in carbohydrate metabolism, helping to convert foodstuff to energy. It is also involved in the synthesis of steroid hormones in the body. Pantothenic acid deficiency is rare because it so widespread in foods.

Food sources: milk, meats, eggs, whole grains, legumes, many vegetables.

DRI for men and women 5mg/day. DRI 6mg/day during pregnancy and 7mg/day during lactation. Toxicity from overdosage has not been reported.
UL: has not been established.

Pyridoxine (Vitamin B6)

Pyridoxine or Vitamin B6 functions as coenzyme PLP (pyridoxal phosphate) in amino acid metabolism. PLP allows the body to manufacture certain amino acids that are not necessary to get from our food (non-essential amino acids). Pyridoxine converts the amino acid tryptophan into serotonin, the brain chemical (neurotransmitter) that controls mood and depression, eating, sleeping, and other survival functions. Pyridoxine is necessary for proper functioning of the immune system. Pyridoxine deficiency causes depression and confusion.

Food sources: meats, fish, poultry, legumes (including soy), bananas.

DRI for men and women 1.3mg/day. DRI for men older than 50 years 1.7mg/day, for women older than 50 years 1.5mg/day. DRI 1.9mg/day during pregnancy and 2.0mg/day during lactation.
UL: 100mg/day. Some practitioners recommend high doses of Vitamin B6 to treat various nerve dysfunction diseases (carpal tunnel syndrome, polyneuropathy) for which it is sometimes beneficial. However, it is worthwhile to keep in mind that prolonged use of high doses of Vitamin B6 have been known to be toxic, causing signs of nerve damage such as numbness and muscle weakness.

Vitamin B12 (cobalamin, cyanocobalamin)

Vitamin B12 has cobalt in its chemical formula. Vitamin B12 and folate (folic acid) are intertwined and interdependent in chemical reactions inside the body. Both have to do with synthesis of DNA and RNA, thus with the creation of all new cells in the body. Vitamin B12 is required to maintain the protective sheath around nerve fibers (called myelin) so it is an essential nutrient for a healthy nervous system.

In the stomach, under acid conditions, Vitamin B12 is released from food, and binds with "intrinsic factor" in order for Vitamin B12 to be absorbed into the bloodstream. Vitamin B12 deficiency can result from poor absorption due to lack of stomach acidity or lack of "intrinsic factor." These situations are more common in elderly people. When Vitamin B12 deficiency is caused by a lack of "intrinsic factor" it is called pernicious anemia (which is anemia coupled with irreversible peripheral polyneuropathy).

> **Note:** Since medicines for heartburn block the formation of stomach acid, persons taking drugs like *Nexium*, *Tagament* and *Prilosec* may develop Vitamin B12 deficiency after prolonged use. Chronic indigestion with or without gastroesophageal reflux (GERD) is sometimes called "acid indigestion" (a synonym for heartburn). The medical establishment's treatment of the whole issue of "acid indigestion" is based on a false premise. Antacids, Histamine H2-receptor blockers (H2-blockers), and Proton Pump Inhibitors (PPIs) all treat "acid indigestion" as though the cause is *too much acid* in the stomach, whereas the real situation is, in 90% of cases, exactly the opposite, *too little acid* in the stomach. It is a good idea to stay away from those drugs, especially on a chronic basis. If you want to read more about this, I recommend the book, *Why Stomach Acid Is Good for You* by Jonathan Wright and Lane Lenard, published by M. Evans and Company, 2001. A safe and effective way to treat "acid indigestion" and GERD is with homeopathy, herbal remedies, and nutritional supplements.

The other cause of Vitamin B12 deficiency is inadequate intake of the vitamin in the diet which tends to occur in people who do not eat animal products. Vegetarians who do not eat dairy or eggs (called vegans) are especially vulnerable to Vitamin B12 deficiency. Vegans and vegetarians should take multivitamin supplements containing Vitamin B12. Symptoms of Vitamin B12 deficiency include memory loss (dementia can occur in the most severe form), inability to concentrate, and confusion.

A low level of Vitamin B12 in the blood often predicts a high level of the amino acid homocysteine, which is associated with coronary artery disease (atherosclerosis or hardening of the arteries of the heart).

Food sources: only in animal products: milk, cheese, meats, eggs, poultry, fish, shellfish.

DRI for men and women 2.4 microgram/day. **DRI** 2.6 microgram/day during pregnancy and 2.8 microgram/day during lactation. Toxicity from overdosage has not been reported. It is essential to supplement pregnant and lactating women with Vitamin B12 if they do not eat animal products. **UL:** has not been established.

Folic acid **(folate, folacin, pteroylglutamic acid)**
Vitamin B12 and folate (folic acid) are intertwined and interdependent in chemical reactions inside the body. Folic acid becomes the active coenzyme only with the help of Vitamin B12. Both have to do with synthesis of DNA and RNA, thus with the creation of all new cells in the body. Folic acid is also involved in the transfer of single carbon atoms during metabolism of amino acids.

Folic acid deficiency during early pregnancy can result in devastating neural tube defects in the developing fetus. It is likely that folic acid deficiency in the pregnant woman may predispose to cleft lip and palate in the fetus as well. Folic acid supplements ideally should be started 6 months to one year *before conception* and taken throughout pregnancy and lactation. In fact, all women of childbearing age are urged to take 800 micrograms of folic acid every day because so many pregnancies are unplanned.

> **Note:** Fetal neural tube defects include spina bifida (when the two sides of the vertebral column does not fuse together thereby exposing the spinal column) and anencephaly (when the brain is underdeveloped). These errors in embryonic development cause the fetus and newborn to suffer neurological

damage and sometimes death. The incidence of these defects is cut by half when 400-800 microgram of folic acid is taken by the pregnant woman.

Folic acid, at levels of 800 micrograms daily, protects against cardiovascular disease, some cancers (colon, breast, cervical), stroke, dementia, and depression. Low levels of Vitamins B6, B12, and folate are associated with high levels of the amino acid homocysteine. High levels of homocysteine are a risk factor for heart disease, stroke, Alzheimer's disease, and certain cancers. Low levels of folic acid are also associated with depression and supplementation with folic acid may actually increase the effectiveness of certain antidepressant medications. Folic acid is essential for the body's manufacture of the chemical *S-adenosylmethionine* (*SAMe*). Among other things, SAMe is involved in mood and depression.

Food sources: legumes, green leafy vegetables, artichoke, asparagus, seeds, whole grains, brewer's yeast.

DRI for men and women 400 microgram/day. **DRI** 800 microgram/day during pregnancy and 800 microgram/day during lactation. Many doctors are now recommending 1,000 microgram/day during pregnancy and lactation as well as for the older population at risk for cardiovascular disease, cancer, stroke, and dementia.
UL: 1,000mg/day.

> **Note:** Some doctors have started to recommend 800 micrograms/day of folic acid for all their patients on the strength of results of a medical research study. Folic acid given at doses of 800 micrograms daily slowed the decline in cognitive functioning and improved memory in an aging population.

> **Note:** If folic acid is given to Vitamin B12 deficient people, it can correct the anemia part of pernicious anemia while masking the ongoing Vitamin B12 deficiency, allowing the irreversible peripheral polyneuropathy to develop. If you or your family member has anemia, it's a good idea to have laboratory tests not

only for iron, but for folic acid and Vitamin B12 as well.

Biotin

Biotin is a B Vitamin that acts as a coenzyme in chemical reactions in energy and fat metabolism. Biotin deficiency is exceedingly rare. It can occur in persons who consistently eat raw egg white because it contains a protein (avidin) which binds to biotin in the intestines, preventing absorption. Biotin is important for hair and nail health.

Food sources: nuts, meats, egg yolk, legumes, whole grains.

DRI for men and women 30 microgram/day. **DRI** 30 microgram/day during pregnancy and 35 microgram/day during lactation. Toxicity from overdosage has not been reported.
UL: has not been established. Recently, some researchers have recommended 300-500 microgram/day, an amount that is difficult to obtain even taking a B Complex 100 supplement (containing 100 micrograms of biotin). You may need an additional stand-alone biotin nutritional supplement to treat hair loss or peeling nails.

Choline

Choline is required to make acetylcholine, the neurotransmitter chemical that causes muscular action, and *lecithin*, a component of all cells. Choline is necessary for normal brain formation during fetal life. After birth, choline is essential for memory function. Choline is called a "conditionally essential nutrient" because the body is able to synthesize it from the amino acid methionine. But synthesis is not enough, so ingestion of choline is required in order for the body to sustain the chemical reactions that involve choline.

Food sources: milk, eggs, peanuts, wheat germ, beef. Breast milk is a good source of choline for infants.

DRI for men 550mg/day, for women 425mg/day. **DRI** 450mg/day during pregnancy and 550mg/day during lactation. Toxicity from overdosage has not been reported.
UL: 3,500mg/day.

Note: *Inositol* functions together with *choline* and is necessary for the production of *lecithin*. *Inositol* is a component of cell membranes. *Inositol* has been used to treat depression and panic disorders. It is being investigated for its anti-tumor activity as well.

Vitamin C (Ascorbic Acid)

About thirty years ago, the Nobel laureate chemist Dr. Linus Pauling, first popularized taking large doses (megadoses) of Vitamin C to foreshorten the course of the common cold. His book, *Vitamin C and the Common Cold* was revolutionary for that time. He coined the term, "orthomolecular medicine" to mean using nutrition to treat disease.

Vitamin C is involved in at least 300 chemical reactions in the body, more than any other vitamin, functioning as a cofactor in many chemical reactions and as the body's most important antioxidant. Antioxidants prevent damage to cells and DNA and if damage does occur, they repair it.

Since Vitamin C prevents DNA damage, it is considered to possess anticancer activity as well as anti-aging properties. In addition, Vitamin C protects against cardiovascular disease, and is essential for the synthesis of collagen and for the proper functioning of the immune system. It is essential for the proper functioning of every organ in the human body. Vitamin C acts together with Vitamin E to protect against oxidative damage in cells.

The Vitamin C deficiency disease is called *scurvy*. The symptoms include bleeding gums, tendency towards infections, dryness of eyes and mouth, weakness, depression, anemia, muscle pains, non-healing wounds, and diarrhea, and in severe cases coma and death.

Vitamin C is water-soluble. It is sometimes buffered (most commonly with calcium ascorbate) since the reduced acid form may digest more easily. Some manufacturers offer Vitamin C with acerola cherries or rose hips, two highly concentrated sources of the vitamin. Some add citrus *flavonoids* (naturally occurring with the vitamin), which may help in the absorption of Vitamin C. However, the benefits of acerola, rose hips, and flavonoids have not been proven and these preparations tend to be more expensive than when the ingredient is Vitamin C simply as ascorbic acid. A popular version of Vitamin C is Ester C whose claim (by the manufacturer) is that it maintains higher blood and tissue levels for a longer time. It contains calcium ascorbate, *quercetin*, rutin and proanthocyanidins.

Note: The concentration of Vitamin C is highest in fresh oranges. However, if you can't squeeze your own juice from fresh oranges, then you may want to choose frozen orange juice concentrate with a higher concentration of Vitamin C over orange juice in cartons.

Remember: Oxidation of Vitamin C occurs readily once you allow air to come in contact with the cut fruit or the juice. Oxidation decreases the antioxidant power of Vitamin C.

<u>Food sources:</u> citrus fruits and cruciferous vegetables such as kale, cauliflower, brussels sprouts, cabbage and broccoli as well as green leafy vegetables and peppers of all colors.

DRI for men 90mg /day. **DRI** for women 75mg/day, 85mg/day during pregnancy and 120mg/day during lactation. As little as 10mg/day prevent scurvy.
UL: 2,000mg/day. Today, many alternative health practitioners recommend 1000-4000mg/day for adults, doubling that dose when trying to prevent or foreshorten a viral upper respiratory infection. Megadoses of Vitamin C are not toxic but diarrhea can result.

Vitamin D (calciferol)

Vitamin D is a fat-soluble vitamin. This means it is stored in body fat. Vitamin D can be produced in your skin, in the presence of sunlight (ultraviolet B radiation), so it is technically not an essential nutrient. About 90% of our Vitamin D comes from sunlight, depending on many factors, especially geographic location and skin color (the darker your skin color, the more sunlight you need to form Vitamin D). At least 10 percent of our Vitamin D has to come from foods and supplements. Many people wear sunscreen whenever they are exposed to sunlight, which blocks UVB, thereby interfering with the skin production of Vitamin D.

Vitamin D plays its most important role in the formation of bone, the prevention of bone loss, and the slowing of degenerative joint disease (osteoarthritis) as well as lowering the risk for rheumatoid arthritis. Vitamin D maximizes the body's absorption of calcium. Vitamin D deficiency is called *rickets* in children and *osteomalacia* in adults. Osteomalacia causes bone pain and muscle weakness.

Vitamin D tends to decrease blood pressure by lowering the kidney hormone rennin. Taking Vitamin D supplements has been proven to lower your risk for coronary artery disease. Vitamin D may also have a role in lowering the risk of multiple sclerosis and the prevention of schizophrenia. Vitamin D also affects muscle function. Periodontal disease is associated with a low level of Vitamin D. Low levels of Vitamin D are associated with Type 1 and Type 2 diabetes mellitus.

Vitamin D also plays a prominent role in preventing cancer by inhibiting cell proliferation. Deaths from skin cancer are higher in sunny parts of the globe, but deaths from colon, prostate, breast, and ovarian cancers are lower. This lower death rate for these particular cancers has been shown to be related to the protective effects of Vitamin D. People who have surgery to remove their primary cancers during the summer months have a much reduced likelihood of metastases five years later compared to those who have surgery during the winter months.

A large excess of Vitamin D over a long period of time (from supplements) may cause toxicity from calcium imbalance. Vitamin D toxicity does not occur as a result of exposure to sun. It is much more likely to have a deficiency of Vitamin D rather than an excess.

> **Note:** Due to the risk of serious skin cancer (melanoma), many health conscious people slather on sunscreen whenever they go outdoors. As it turns out, this may not be a good idea. Now some medical researchers are saying it's probably healthier to expose our skin to a limited amount (around 15 minutes) of sun every few days (before applying sun block) in order to get the benefits of

Vitamin D. Remember that 90% of Vitamin D is manufactured by our skin. But under no circumstances should you expose the skin to sunburn. Sunburn is the trigger, many years later, associated with the development of melanoma.

> **Note:** UVB sunlight is too weak during the winter months for people who live in the northeast to get enough Vitamin D via their skin. And these same northern latitudes show higher cancer rates for many common cancers, including breast, colon, and prostate. The implication here is that Vitamin D supplementation may help to prevent some cancers.

Food sources: milk, eggs, fish.

> **Note:** Vitamin D is not present in plant-based foods but Vitamin D-fortified soy milk is available.

DRI for men and women (and for pregnancy and lactation) is 5 microgram/day (200 IU), aged younger than 50 years, 10 microgram/day (400 IU) for men and women aged 51-70, and 15 microgram/day (600 IU) for men and women older than 70 years. But these recommendations are based on getting most of your Vitamin D from sunlight. The older you are, the more difficult it is for your skin to manufacture Vitamin D from sunlight, so more and more doctors and researchers, like Dr. Walter Willett, Chairperson of the Nutrition department of Harvard's School of Public Health and Dr. Andrew Weil are now recommending 800-1,000 IU/day after age 50. It is likely, for those over 50, that in order to reach that level of Vitamin D intake every day, you will need to take a supplement. You should know the amount of Vitamin D contained in your multivitamin-multimineral supplement and then you must add the remainder in supplement form to achieve the new recommended intake at least 800-1,000 IU/day. Find a Vitamin D supplement that does not contain Vitamin A. You will find Vitamin D together with calcium in many preparations.
UL: 50-60 microgram/day (2,000-2,500 IU).

Vitamin E (tocopherols and tocotrienols)

Vitamin E is another fat-soluble vitamin. The Vitamin E family, a mixture of 8 different chemicals, consists of tocopherols and tocotrienols, and there are four different forms (alpha, beta, gamma, and delta) in each group. Alpha-tocopherol is the form that is mainly active in the human body. All chemicals in nature are found in two forms called d- (for dextro) and l- (for levo) isomers. Alpha-tocopherol is active inside your body only in the d- form.

> **Note:** Synthetic Vitamin E is a combination of d- and l- isomers of alpha-tocopherol, making it less physiologically active inside your body. It is important that you purchase Vitamin E supplements containing natural d-alpha-tocopherol. This is not a worrisome factor in the other vitamins when synthetic ingredients are indistinguishable in the body from natural.

Recent studies have also recognized a role for gamma-tocopherol, the form found in corn and soybeans. Taking a supplement with mixed tocopherols (alpha, beta, and gamma) may be preferred to taking only alpha-tocopherol alone.

Vitamin E has powerful antioxidant activity, being the most important antioxidant of the lipids (fats) in your body. As an antioxidant, it functions as a single-electron oxidant scavenger. Vitamin E protects cell membranes and lipoproteins (like LDL and HDL, parts of your total cholesterol) from oxidative damage. Considering that cell membranes are present in every cell of every organ, it is evident that Vitamin E performs widespread antioxidant actions throughout the body. It has been proven to protect your skin, heart, nervous and immune systems against oxidative damage.

In addition to its general antioxidant healthful effects in the body, Vitamin E has been proven to lower the risk of cancer (breast, colon, prostate), and it may protect against Alzheimer's disease. However, it probably does not lower the risk of heart disease, and this may be true in both healthy and unhealthy people.

> **Note:** A recent medical research report from the Cleveland Clinic found that Vitamin E was not successful in decreasing deaths from cardiovascular disease

among persons who already had heart disease. However, it is uncertain at this time whether Vitamin E would protect if you start supplementation when you do not yet have heart disease. Some researchers believe that the study results might have been positive if the study subjects had taken mixed tocopherols in their supplement instead of only the alpha form.

> **Note:** Another study, called a meta-analysis, done by researchers at Johns Hopkins University School of Medicine, pooled together results from 19 research studies (about 135,000 subjects). The unexpected results showed a small *increase* in dying from cardiovascular disease for those persons using Vitamin E supplements at more than 400 IU daily, compared to those who took less. The difficulty with this approach is that most of the studies in the analysis included older people who were chronically ill with Alzheimer's disease, cancer, heart disease, and kidney failure. These people would have a higher risk of death independent of their Vitamin E supplements. This study did not help us to understand the effects of Vitamin E on younger, healthy people.

My prudent recommendation until more data become available is to keep the Vitamin E dosage level at around 200-400 IU daily (or 80mg of mixed tocopherols and tocotrienols daily).

To put this in perspective, the Institute of Medicine (IOM) still says that according to its review of the overall scientific literature, 1,500 IU of Vitamin E is safe.

Also, it's important to remember that studies that use the synthetic alpha-tocopherol form of Vitamin E may not show beneficial effects.

> **Note:** Another study from the Women's Health Study published in the *Journal of the American Medical Association* (July 6, 2005) on almost 20,000 healthy women

aged 45 and older showed no effect of Vitamin E 600 IU daily on the commonest cancers in women (breast, lung, and colon), non fatal heart attacks, and non fatal strokes. However, there were fewer cardiovascular deaths in the Vitamin E treated group, especially among women 65 years and older. It appears that Vitamin E may not be a panacea against heart disease, but in modest doses, it remains a heart healthy antioxidant vitamin, more especially for older women.

Vitamin C is another powerful antioxidant, acting in the water-soluble part of the cell's interior. Vitamin C complements the actions of Vitamin E that is active in the fatty part of cells, the cell membrane. For this reason, Vitamin E is called a lipophilic antioxidant. In addition, Vitamin C acts to regenerate the active form of Vitamin E.

Medical research has proven that there is a neuroprotective effect after chemotherapy when Vitamin E supplementation is used. It may have some protective power against Alzheimer's disease. Vitamin E has anti-cancer activity as well. Supplementation with Vitamin E decreases the risk for skin cancer.

It is also a naturally occurring anticoagulant in your body, acting to decrease the stickiness and clumping (aggregation) of platelets. This causes a delay in the clotting mechanism of blood.

The trace mineral selenium (please see under **Minerals**, in this chapter) acts together with Vitamin E in your body to enhance the protective effects against cardiovascular disease and cancer (especially prostate).

Vitamin E deficiency is rare, causing a type of anemia called hemolytic anemia, which occurs when the cell membrane surrounding red blood cells can no longer function. Vitamin E toxicity is also rare. Very high levels of Vitamin E may counteract the action of Vitamin K, causing bleeding.

Food sources: polyunsaturated vegetable oils (olive), whole grains, wheat germ, egg yolks, nuts (almonds) and seeds (sunflower), legumes. Food sources contain different levels of Vitamin E family components. For example, alpha-tocopherol is found mainly in *olive oil*, nuts, and seeds whereas gamma-tocopherol is mainly in corn and soybeans.

DRI for men and women 15mg/day (or 22 IU/day), for pregnant women 15mg/day (or 22 IU/day), and for lactating women 19mg/day (or 30 IU/day).
UL: 1,200 IU/day. Vitamin E supplements come in 200 IU, 400 IU, and 1,000 IU capsules. The daily dose necessary to achieve the protective effects of Vitamin E is 200-400 IU/day. Vitamin E should be stopped at least two weeks before surgery so that coagulation of the blood is normalized. Do not take Vitamin E supplements without talking with your homeopath or physician if you or your family member is taking aspirin or *Warfarin* (*Coumadin*), or other anti-coagulant therapy. Vitamin E, *Garlic* and *Ginkgo biloba* have similar effects on the coagulation system, so be sure to consult your homeopath or physician before taking these together.

Ointments containing Vitamin E protect the skin against sun damage, thereby contributing to anti-aging of the skin. After the skin has been damaged (by any mechanism causing inflammation), Vitamin E supplementation enhances repair mechanisms. In addition, rubbing Vitamin E oil or ointment into a wound has been shown to decrease the formation of scar tissue thereby resulting in a smoother cosmetic effect. Vitamin E supplementation decreases the time of healing of a skin wound after a burn or surgical procedure.

Vitamin K (phylloquinone, menaquinone, menadione)

Vitamin K is a fat-soluble vitamin because it is stored in body fat. Vitamin K is a combination of three substances: K1 (phylloquinone), K2 (menaquinone), and K3 (menadione). Vitamin K can be manufactured to some extent in your intestines by the bacteria naturally present there, so it (like Vitamin D) is technically not an essential nutrient.

Vitamin K's primary action in the body is to activate the complex processes of coagulation of the blood. Newborn babies have a sterile intestinal tract making them vulnerable to bleeding from Vitamin K deficiency (called *hemorrhagic disease of the newborn*). All newborn babies receive an injection of

Vitamin K in the delivery room. Symptoms of Vitamin K deficiency in adults are easy bruising and bleeding.

 Note: Hemorrhaging in a hemophiliac is not due to Vitamin K deficiency.

Vitamin K is also necessary for bone health, helping calcium and Vitamin D to prevent osteoporosis. Vitamin K has been proven to reduce fractures in post-menopausal women.

 Vitamin K is also important in bone formation because it is essential in the production of osteocalcin, the bone-forming protein. It has been shown to help prevent hip fractures. Vitamin K supplements help to increase bone mineral density. But vitamin K supplements are not given to persons who are taking anticoagulant drugs.

 Broad-spectrum antibiotics may annihilate the intestinal bacteria thereby causing an inadvertent Vitamin K deficiency. Persons who suffer from Crohn's disease, ulcerative colitis, or liver disease may be deficient in Vitamin K.

Food sources: dark leafy green vegetables (kale, spinach, collard greens), cruciferous vegetables, milk. People taking anticoagulants like *Warfarin* (*Coumadin*) should be careful when eating leafy green vegetables to test their blood coagulation to make sure it remains in the range dictated by your physician.

DRI for men 120 microgram/day, for women, and pregnant and lactating women, 90 microgram/day. It is likely that these levels will be increased as more research results become available.

UL: has not been established.

Minerals

All the minerals in your body are essential for metabolic processes. They fall into two groups, major minerals and trace minerals. The only difference between the two groups is that major minerals are found in the body in larger amounts than trace minerals. Major minerals include: calcium, magnesium, phosphorus, sulfur, and the electrolytes chloride, potassium, and sodium. Trace minerals include: chromium, copper, fluoride, iodine, iron, manganese, molybdenum, selenium and zinc.

 Five other minerals belonging to the trace group are also essential for a healthy body, but we do not have enough information on them to provide specific recommendations. These five are: arsenic (yes, the poison, all depending on amounts), boron, nickel, silicon and vanadium.

 Minerals are chemical elements. That means that they carry electron charge and tend to form chemical compounds in your body. Calcium tends to bind with phosphorus, for example, to form *calcium phosphate*, an important part of your bones. Sodium tends to bind with chloride to form sodium chloride, salt, an important part of every cell in your body as well as the fluid that baths every cell. The list of chemical compounds containing minerals working inside your cells is not endless, but close to it!

Calcium

Calcium is the most abundant mineral in your body. Calcium is essential for the health of our bones, teeth, heart, muscles, nerve, and coagulation (blood clotting) mechanism. Calcium together with Vitamin D protects against osteoporosis. Calcium together with magnesium prevents painful muscle cramps and may dampen premenstrual symptoms. Calcium is essential for your heart to beat normally. The American Cancer Society's research showed that people taking calcium supplements had a lower incidence of colorectal cancer. It is hypothesized that calcium might inhibit the formation of polyps, the precancerous stage of colon cancer. And there is preliminary evidence that people who have higher daily calcium intakes gain less weight over time. Among people who are on calorie-restricted diets, the group losing the most weight was consuming the most dairy calcium per day.

 Osteoporosis affects about 10 million Americans, 20% of them men. Men do not have the fast fall-off in bone mass that women do around age 55 or 60, but by age 70, men and women are losing bone mass at the same rate. Peak bone mass is achieved during middle to late adolescence, by the early 20s at the latest. This is why it is crucial that young boys and girls get their daily recommended intake of calcium, preferably by a mix of calcium-rich foods and supplements.

Note: Recent medical research showed that the fracture rate among women aged 70 and over (all of whom had had previous fractures) was the same in those taking calcium supplements and those not taking them. This means that you must get your daily calcium early on in life in order to affect peak bone mass.

The blood level of calcium has to remain in a fairly narrow range so that normal muscle contraction can take place. The blood level of calcium is maintained by either calling forth calcium from the bones or by dumping excess calcium into the bones. The hormones from your thyroid gland that balance calcium in the blood are parathormone and calcitonin.

Food sources: dairy products, calcium-fortified orange juice, soy milk and tofu, kale, broccoli, bok choy, collard greens, turnip greens, mustard greens, beans (legumes), raw parsley, raw watercress, raw and cooked spinach, dried figs, the bones in canned sardines, mackerel and salmon, raw oysters.

Note: Although caffeine does not interfere with the absorption of calcium to any great degree, it does increase its excretion into urine. *Green tea* is a healthier drink than coffee.

DRI for boys and girls aged 9-18, 1,300mg/day; for men and women younger than 50, 1,000mg/day; for men and women older than 50, 1,200mg/day; and 1,000mg/day for pregnant and lactating women. **UL:** 2,500mg/day.

Note: Dr. Andrew Weil has lowered his recommendations for supplemental calcium based on medical evidence that showed a link with prostate cancer in men who took more than 600mg/day. He advises men over the age of 19 to take no supplemental calcium.

Since the body has difficulty absorbing more than 600mg of calcium at a time, it is wise to take your calcium supplement at two different times during the day, morning and evening, or morning and lunchtime.

Calcium supplements should come together with Vitamin D (800 IU/day) and magnesium (400mg/day). Some preparations include zinc, copper, manganese and boron, all important trace minerals for bone health. I often recommend *Caltrate 600-D Plus* (in the purple package).

Calcium and cholesterol sometimes combine with proteins inside arterial walls, resulting in plaque, which in turn causes arteriosclerosis. Calcium supplements do not contribute to this process. In fact, calcium supplements may actually lower the risk for heart disease.

Calcium carbonate is cheaper than calcium citrate (Citracal) but not as well absorbed. Coral calcium is not recommended. It has not been proven to possess any superior health benefits over calcium carbonate or calcium citrate. Calcium carbonate needs to be taken with food because it requires stomach acid for absorption. Calcium citrate does not require stomach acid for absorption so it may be taken with or without food. Some calcium preparations from unrefined oyster shells have been found to be contaminated with lead.

I do not recommend ingesting calcium from animal sources (bone meal) because of the possibility, albeit remote, of bovine spongioform encephalitis (BSE, or "mad cow" disease). Although the FDA does not allow supplement manufacturers to import cow products from countries that have BSE, it is safer to forego those products altogether.

Note: BSE is caused by a class of proteins called prions. Prions "jump ship" from infected cows to humans causing a lethal, degenerative disease of the brain, which is similar in both species. (The same disease exists in sheep as "Scrapie.") There have been a handful of cases found in cattle in North America, including 3 proven cases in U.S.A., which suggests that we need to re-examine our testing methods. Japan tests every slaughtered cow whereas the U.S. tests only a small fraction of them (1%).

Note: If you are concerned about BSE and want to protect against the development of the human form of it (variant Creutzfeldt-Jakob disease or vCJD) in the future (as much as possible), you may want to consider eating kosher meats. Kosher meats differ from non-kosher in several slaughtering practices. Kosher meats come from young animals only and BSE tends to occur in the older population of animals. "Downer" animals are not considered kosher. Most cattle are killed by injecting pressurized air into the animal's brain, thereby raising the possibility of brain tissue ending up in other organs. Kosher animals are killed by a knife cutting the carotid arteries in the neck. And every kosher animal's organs are examined for signs of illness and the animal is rejected as not kosher if they are found. These differences may make kosher meat safer than non-kosher, although this is still theoretical.

And: A safe practice in buying both kosher and non-kosher meats is to avoid eating any of the specialty items that are manufactured by "automatic meat recovery" (like hot dogs, sausage, and ground meat) because they would tend to have more chance to contain nervous tissue than muscle cuts. Also avoid bone-in steaks and choose boneless steaks instead.

Remember: Weight-bearing exercises like weight training (strength training) are a vitally important part of bone health. You should aim for 30-60 minutes 3-4 times/week of weight-bearing exercises. Exercises to improve balance and flexibility are also recommended because these will help you to avoid falling and perhaps breaking your bones. If you have entered menopause, please ask your doctor about bone density screening (dual energy X-ray absorptiometry, or DEXA scan).

Note: Persons taking calcium-channel blockers to decrease blood pressure need the same amount of daily calcium.

Note: Contrary to public opinion, peo-ple with kidney stones should *not* lower their intake of calcium. Instead, they require lower amounts of protein (50 gms/day) and salt (2,400mg/day) in their daily diets. If you or a family member suffers from kidney stones, I strongly recommend that you seek the advice of a registered nutritionist so that you may benefit from the latest in medical knowledge in this field.

Note: *Phosphoric acid* in colas (but not in other carbonated drinks) interferes with the absorption of calcium from foods. This is a good reason to stay away from drinking colas.

Note: Copper is also involved in bone formation. Copper is essential for the laying down of collagen and forming cross links between the strands. Once laid down, they are then mineralized into bone.

Chromium

Chromium is an essential trace mineral working along with insulin and acting to promote a steady state of glucose in the blood. A deficiency of chromium leads to a diabetes-like condition with impaired glucose tolerance.

Chromium picolinate supplementation (200 microgram/day) has been used (without convincing medical evidence) to increase lean body mass and decrease body fat. Chromium picolinate may be beneficial to weight loss (unproven), but it must be used with diet and exercise to be effective.

Laboratory studies in animals have revealed that very high amounts of chromium picolinate may damage DNA which in turn may lead to the development of cancer. The long-term safety of chromium picolinate supplements has not been evaluated.

Chromium is a component of *Glucose Tolerance Factor (GTF)*, a complex compound regulating insulin activity in your body. *GTF* chromium supplements (1000 micrograms/day) are used to improve insulin sensitivity. Since this form of chromium increases the body's sensitivity to insulin, it may delay the onset of frank diabetes in obese people with prediabetes. For persons with hypoglycemia who want to stabilize blood glucose, the daily chromium supplement dose is 120-240 microgram/day.

Food sources: whole grains, nuts, meats, vegetable oils, mushrooms, tea, wine, beer, brewer's yeast, cheese.

DRI: for men younger than 50 years, 35 micrograms/day; for women younger than 50, 25 micrograms/day; for men older than 50, 30 micrograms/day; for women older than 50, 20 micrograms/day; for pregnant women, 30 micrograms/day; for breastfeeding women, 45 micrograms/day.

UL: has not been established. Liver toxicity may occur at intake levels of 1200-2400 microgram/day.

> **Note:** Taking Chromium picolinate at levels of 1000 microgram/day has been shown to decrease heart arrhythmias in people prone to them.

Iodine

Iodine is present in foods and converted to iodide (an ion) for use in the body. Iodide is essential for the manufacture of thyroid gland hormones (triiodothyronine and thyroxin). Thyroid hormones regulate your metabolic rate by controlling the amount of oxygen used by every cell in your body. Thyroid hormones are essential for growth and reproduction. A complete deficiency of thyroid hormones is incompatible with life. Iodine deficiency causes the thyroid gland in your neck to become larger, causing a goiter, or if it occurs during pregnancy, the newborn infant may be born with cretinism, a severe form of mental retardation. The World Health Organization estimates that as of 2001 as many as 50 million children had been born into the world at risk for inadequate maternal iodine intake.

Food sources: iodized table salt, seafood, kelp, seaweeds, and vegetables grown in iodine-rich soils.

DRI for men and women 150 microgram/day; for pregnant women 220 microgram/day; for breast-feeding women 290 microgram/day.

UL: 1,100 microgram/day.

> **Note:** Potassium iodide protects the thyroid gland from thyroid cancer after radioactive iodine is released during a nuclear explosion. The dose for all adults over the age of 18 years (including pregnant and lactating women) is one 130mg tablet of potassium iodide once every 24 hours during exposure to radioactive iodine. The dose for children 3-18 years, is one-half tablet; for children 1 month to 3 years, one-quarter tablet; for neonates from birth to one month of age, one-eighth tablet. Potassium iodide tablets by *Life Extension* contain 99mg of iodine and 31mg of potassium in each 130mg tablet. Contact information for *Life Extension* is 1-800-544-4440 and www.lef.org. Persons with allergy to iodine or iodide should not take potassium iodide supplements.

> **Note:** Persons with thyroid cancer will need to follow a low iodine diet. This means that your multivitamin-multimineral supplement tablet must be iodine-free. In addition, you will need to learn how to avoid iodine-rich foods like iodized table salt, seafood, kelp, and seaweeds.

Iron

Iron is an essential trace mineral, involved in the cellular processes that transport oxygen and electrons. Iron is essential for the synthesis of hemoglobin, the protein in red blood cells that carries oxygen and releases it into cells. Iron deficiency may cause learning impairment and anemia, and if it occurs during pregnancy, it may cause low birth weight and preterm delivery. Iron is also part of myoglobin, a protein in muscle cells.

The World Health Organization estimates that approximately 25% of the world's population is at risk for iron deficiency and anemia. Iron deficiency manifests as fatigue and apathy along with anemia.

It is the most prevalent nutritional disorder in the world. However, iron overload disorders (hemochromatosis, a genetic disorder and hemosiderosis, an iron storage disorder) are common in this country. Iron overload is a cause of cirrhosis of the liver with consequent liver failure, and congestive heart failure.

Menstruating females are at risk for iron deficiency because they lose the iron in the red blood cells that are shed with the uterine lining every month. Growing infants and children and menstruating females generally require iron supplementation. Post-menopausal females and grown men, assuming no active bleeding, do not require iron supplements because the iron in red blood cells is recycled rather than lost. They can obtain the iron they require from food sources alone. In fact, grown men and postmenopausal women should take a multivitamin-multimineral supplement that does not contain any iron or no more than 5mg. The popular multivitamin-multimineral brand *Centrum Silver* does not contain any iron.

Restless legs syndrome is an overwhelming compulsion to move your legs, especially when resting or sitting down. It is worse from midnight to 2 a.m., and is a common cause of disturbed sleep and insomnia. Restless legs syndrome has been associated with low iron levels. If you or a family member has restless legs syndrome, please have your ferritin level checked. Ferritin is the protein that carries iron in the blood. If your ferritin level is low, you should take iron supplements in the form of ferrous sulfate.

Food sources: red meats, poultry, fish, eggs, beans (especially lentils), dried fruits (especially raisins), green vegetables.

DRI for men and postmenopausal women 8mg/day; menstruating women 18mg/day; pregnant women 27mg/day; breastfeeding women 9mg/day.
UL: 45mg/day. The iron in supplements is usually ferrous sulfate or ferrous gluconate. Abdominal symptoms such as bloating, constipation, and black stools may occur as a side effect of iron supplementation.
> **Remember:** Iron poisoning can occur when infants and young children ingest iron-containing multivitamin-multi-mineral supplements. These should be stored in childproof containers.

Magnesium

Magnesium is an essential mineral working inside your body in over 300 metabolic reactions. Magnesium is involved in the production of biologic energy inside the mitochondria, specialized energy factory organelles present in every cell. Magnesium is responsible for electrical stabilization of cell membranes and is an integral factor in muscle contraction (including the heart muscle), nerve conduction, normalization of blood pressure, and bone metabolism. Magnesium and calcium often work together inside the body, either synergistically (with each other) or antagonistically (against each other). This magnesium-calcium interaction is apparent in muscle contraction (including the heart), regulation of blood pressure, blood coagulation and bone metabolism.

Magnesium deficiency is associated with insulin resistance, a fundamental part of type 2 diabetes mellitus and the metabolic syndrome. Magnesium prevents and treats a serious disease of women in labor, called pre-eclampsia, as well as migraine headaches, muscle cramps, and fibromyalgia. Magnesium together with calcium is used to prevent and treat premenstrual syndrome (PMS). The amount of magnesium necessary to treat these disorders is 400-800mg/day (or more).

There are several magnesium compounds available in supplements: magnesium oxide, taurate, chloride, sulfate, citrate and glycinate. The more bioavailable forms are magnesium citrate, chloride, or glycinate, but the differences are small.

Food sources: beans, nuts and seeds (especially almonds and cashews), green leafy vegetables, avocado, whole grains, seafood, chocolate, cocoa.

DRI for men 420mg/day; for women 320mg/day; for pregnant women 350mg/day; for breastfeeding women 320mg/day.
UL: 350mg/day. Too much magnesium (usually more than 400mg/day in a supplement) can cause diarrhea. Do not use magnesium supplements in persons who suffer from kidney failure without the

advice of a physician. Some practitioners use as much as 2,500mg/day of magnesium to treat high blood pressure.

Manganese

Manganese is an essential trace mineral. Manganese, like magnesium, is involved in the production of biologic energy inside the mitochondria, specialized organelles present in every cell. Manganese has a role in the growth and development of bone.

Food sources: nuts, green leafy vegetables, whole grains, tea.

DRI for men 2.3mg/day; for women 1.8mg/day; for pregnant women 2.0mg/day; for breastfeeding women 2.6mg/day.
UL: 11mg/day.

Potassium

Potassium, an element whose chemical symbol is K, is an essential mineral, crucial to the transmission of nerve impulses that result in muscle contraction. Potassium is an integral part of the production of energy and the synthesis of nucleic acids (like DNA). Potassium, together with sodium and chloride, maintains fluid and electrolyte balance throughout your body. People who eat a potassium-rich diet have been shown to have lower rates of high blood pressure, strokes, kidney stones, and osteoporosis.

Potassium deficiency, usually a side effect of the prolonged use of diuretics or the abuse of laxatives, may also result from vomiting, diarrhea, and dehydration. When taking a diuretic, most people will take a potassium supplement (prescribed by a doctor), most often potassium chloride, in order to prevent muscle weakness and confusion. Potassium citrate, gluconate, and bicarbonate are also used.

Potassium supplements should be taken *only under the supervision of a physician* because potassium in large amounts may cause fatal heart rhythms (arrhythmia). Most people obtain their daily potas-

sium from healthy eating rather than supplements. Only a small amount is usually included in most daily multivitamin-multimineral supplements, due to the fear of overdosage. So it is up to us to eat potassium-rich foods to protect against high blood pressure, strokes, kidney stones, and osteoporosis.

Food sources: meats, dairy products, vegetables (especially green leafy (spinach with 450mg in 1/2 cup cooked), sweet potatoes (540mg in 1/2 cup cooked), and white potatoes, (940mg in 1/2 cup cooked), tomato paste and puree), fruits (citrus and especially bananas with 490mg in 1/2 cup raw and kiwifruits, cantaloupe and honeydew melons), avocado, whole grains, beans, fish, nuts.

DRI: New guidelines recommend at least 4,700mg/day for men and women.
   Note: Potassium iodide and potassium iodate are compounds that protect the thyroid gland from thyroid cancer after radioactive iodine is released during a nuclear explosion.

Selenium

Selenium is an essential trace mineral. Oxidation reactions in your body produce energy but their metabolic by-products are toxic forms (free radicals) of oxygen, sulfur, nitrogen, and other elements. Selenium is involved in defending cells against the ravages of free radicals. Selenium is an antioxidant mineral, helping enzymes to protect cells from oxidative damage.

Low levels of selenium have been associated with an increased risk for some cancers, especially cancer of the prostate. The commonly used dosage for cancer prevention is 200 micrograms/day. This underscores selenium's basic role in immune system health. Selenium plays a role in moderating the virulence of viruses. Together with Vitamins C and E, selenium protects your skin from damage due to sun exposure, commonly called aging. Selenium is also an important part of heart health.

The thyroid gland contains the highest concentration of selenium than any other organ in the body because selenium functions as a coenzyme in the production of thyroid hormones. If you suffer from hypothyroidism, you may want to take 200 micrograms of selenium every day.

Food sources: seafood, meats, whole grains, Brazil nuts. Eating only 2 Brazil nuts daily deliver 200 micrograms of selenium.

DRI for men and women 55 microgram/day; for pregnant women 60 microgram/day; for breastfeeding women 70 microgram/day.
UL: 400 microgram/day.

> **Note:** Daily amounts of selenium over one milligram are toxic to hair, nails, and the nervous system. The safe daily amount is around 200 microgram/day. Be sure to count up the selenium in your daily multivitamin-multimineral supplement along with the amount in your selenium supplement. If you are taking selenium supplements, it is wise not to eat Brazil nuts as one ounce of these contain 544 micrograms. No other food has this high concentration of selenium.

Zinc

Zinc is an essential trace mineral. Zinc is the metal cofactor for more than 100 enzymes in your body. Zinc protects cells against free radicals by stabilizing cell membranes. Zinc promotes healthy immune function and healthy sperm production. Zinc regulates the activity of genes by interacting with DNA to direct the manufacture of proteins in your body. Zinc and copper are the two metal coenzymes for the antioxidant enzyme, *superoxide dismutase* (*SOD*). It is involved in glucose metabolism by regulating the storage and release of insulin. Zinc has been shown to protect retinal tissue from age-related macular degeneration. It is necessary for wound healing.

Signs of zinc deficiency include impotence, infertility, growth retardation, sexual development retardation, delay in wound healing, and hair, skin, and eye problems. Vegetarians tend to absorb less zinc than meat-eaters because of the interference of phytates found in whole grains and legumes.

Zinc lozenges decreases the duration and sever-

ity of the common cold (if taken in the first 24 hours), probably by preventing the virus from attaching to cells and from replicating itself. Zinc lozenges help to relieve sore throat, cough, congestion, and hoarseness. It is believed that the lozenge form of zinc is effective because the zinc comes into direct contact with the virus.

> **Note:** Zinc gluconate as the homeopathic remedy *zincum gluconicum* is made into a nasal gel called *Zicam Cold Remedy*. It may reduce the length and severity of a cold if taken within the first 24 hours after onset. But the FDA has begun to investigate *Zicam nasal gels* for reports that they may cause ansomia, the loss of the sense of smell. At this point, until more information is available, I recommend limited use of *Zicam Cold Remedy*, using one day's worth only within the first 24 hours after onset of the cold and then stopping.

Zinc supplements are available as the following compounds: zinc gluconate, oxide, picolinate, citrate, as well as others.

Food sources: meats, fish, oysters, poultry, eggs, nuts, whole grains, beans, wheat germ, dairy products.

DRI for men 11mg/day; for women 8mg/day; for pregnant women 11mg/day; for breastfeeding women 12mg/day. A dosage of 30mg of zinc picolinate supplements daily may be effective in curing warts while 15mg daily is used for children, teens, and adults with behavior problems associated with ADD/ADHD.
UL: 40mg/day.

> **Note:** Both too low and too high levels of zinc cause immune system malfunctioning. Taking more than 150mg of zinc daily can interfere with the absorption of copper. Copper is a trace mineral that is also involved in immune system health. And high doses of zinc may promote prostate cancer.

> **Note:** Medical research has shown that people with age-related macular degeneration (AMD) should take 80mg of zinc

oxide along with 500mg of Vitamin C, 400 IU of Vitamin E, 15mg of Vitamin A, and 2mg of cupric oxide (a form of copper). It is also a good idea to take between 6 and 20mg of *lutein*, the antioxidant present in high concentration in the macula of the retina.

Guidelines for Consulting Your Health Care Provider

You should consult your health care provider if:
- the patient doesn't look right or act right (trust your instincts!)
- the patient is getting worse instead of better over the course of the illness
- the patient is having trouble breathing or complaining of chest pains or there is mental confusion or lethargy or irritability
- the patient develops allergic symptoms (hives, itchy or watery eyes, runny nose, scratchy throat, asthma, shortness of breath) after taking a nutritional supplement
- after beginning a nutritional supplement the patient experiences *new onset* of any serious symptoms such as:

  paralysis, weakness, tingling, inability to focus or concentrate, blurred or double vision or blindness, slurred speech, severe headaches, seizures, irritability, dizziness, disorientation, memory loss, anxiety, depression, insomnia, blackouts, fainting, or the person complains of not feeling like himself

- the patient is taking *ANY* prescription medication
- the patient is pregnant or breastfeeding
- the patient has any serious, chronic disease which may have complications and become life-threatening, such as:

  autism, cancer, HIV and AIDS, arthritis, multiple sclerosis, coronary artery disease, heart attack (myocardial infarction), blood dyscrasia, cancer (of any type), congestive heart failure, diabetes mellitus, obesity, thyroid disorders,

high blood pressure (hypertension), stroke, seizures, acute and chronic kidney (renal) failure, schizophrenia, bipolar disorder, borderline personality disorder, eating disorders, fibromyalgia, chronic fatigue syndrome, Crohn's disease, ulcerative colitis, celiac disease, mental deficiency disorders, chromosomal disorders, infertility, frequent miscarriages, polyneuropathy, cystic fibrosis   [Adapted from *The Merck Manual* at www.merck.com]

Note: Do not discontinue taking any pharmaceutical medication that has been prescribed by your health care provider unless you or your family member is under the supervision of a physician.

Note: Do not take any nutritional supplement, including vitamins and minerals without first consulting your health care provider if you or your family member is pregnant or breastfeeding.

Women who are pregnant and breastfeeding have special needs for vitamins and minerals. These needs are usually met by taking a prenatal vitamin. It is a good idea to start taking your prenatal vitamin six months to one year before conception to ensure that you have healthy levels of folic acid and iron in your body.

In addition, it is a good idea to check with your health care provider if your family member is either very young or very old because nutritional supplements, including some vitamins and minerals, given injudiciously may overwhelm the body's defenses in those age groups.

Putting It All Together

Most people interested in promoting good health will take a multivitamin-multimineral supplement every day (and extra calcium with Vitamin D as well). If you are considering using vitamin and mineral nutritional supplements for yourself or your family members, it is a good idea to familiarize yourself with **Chapter 22: Introduction to Nutritional Supplements**. It makes good sense to understand the role of *antioxidants* from **Chapter 24: Antioxidant Phytochemicals: Natural Anti-aging Remedies**; *omega-3 fatty acids* from **Chapter 31: Oils and Fats** and *probiotics* from **Chapter 30: Prebiotics and Probiotics**.

Then, after you have decided to use vitamin or mineral nutritional supplements to prevent or treat a certain ailment, it makes good sense to investigate the homeopathic remedy indicated for that ailment as well. Homeopathic remedies are safe, have no side effects, and can be used together with herbal remedies and Western pharmaceutical medicines without unwanted interactions. You may read about your sick person's homeopathic remedies in **Chapters 3-18**. And you may want to better understand homeopathy by reading **Chapter 2: Basic Homeopathy**.

Whenever you have decided to go ahead with vitamin or mineral nutritional supplements, it is a good idea to consider giving the sick person's homeopathic constitutional remedy as well (please refer to **Chapter 9: Homeopathic Remedies for Constitutional Problems in Infants, Children, and Adolescents** or to **Chapter 18: Homeopathic Constitutional Remedies** if you are dealing with an adult; or **Chapter 13: Homeopathy for Elderly Persons** if you are dealing with an elderly person).

People who are taking vitamin or mineral nutritional supplements may also benefit from certain specific nutritional supplements, depending on the particular ailment. You may read about your sick person's specific nutritional remedies in **Chapters 25-31**.

Chapter 24

Antioxidant Phytochemicals: Natural Anti-Aging Remedies

Antioxidants and Anti-Aging in General

Ailment/Disorder/Symptom	Nutritional Supplement
Antioxidant and anti-aging activity	*Alpha-lipoic Acid*
Anti-inflammatory activity	*Carotenoids*
Heart function, anti-cancer activity	*Beta-carotene*
Eye function	*Lutein* and *zeaxanthin*
Prostate cancer prevention	*Lycopene*
Blood clotting	*Polyphenols*
Heart, cholesterol, blood vessel function	*Flavonoids*
Cardiovascular system	*Anthocyanins* and *proanthocyanidins*
Heart and blood pressure, anti-cancer and anti-inflammatory activity	*Quercetin*
Immune system	*Glutathione*
Metabolic detoxification	*Isothiocyanates*
Anti-cancer and antioxidant activity	*Sulphoraphane*
Phytoestrogens	*Lignans*
Anti-cancer, anti-inflammatory and anti-aging activity	*Resveratrol*

Guidelines for Consulting Your Health Care Provider
Putting It All Together

Antioxidants and Anti-Aging in General

What are antioxidants?

Antioxidant phytochemicals are chemical substances, grouped into families, found in fruits and vegetables, part of the plant kingdom's elaborate scheme for survival. All forms of antioxidants (phytochemicals as well as certain vitamins and minerals) act inside your body to counter the effects of oxidation. Oxidation is the process—indispensable to life—by which we convert food into energy, using oxygen. But, in doing so, these chemical reactions cause damage to cells. The damage is cumulative, occurring every minute of every day of every year of your life.

The cause of the damage is free radicals. Free radicals are produced as a by-product of oxidation. Free radicals are molecules which contain an unpaired electron, an unstable state in nature. This unpaired electron casts about to "steal" an electron from another chemical molecule in order to become stable. This in turn produces a free radical. Thus, a chain reaction is generated, one molecule becoming stable at the expense of the next. This chain reaction damages vital cellular processes as well as the structure and function of DNA. It is the basis of aging.

Antioxidants prevent the destabilization of molecules that oxidation creates. Antioxidants "squelch" free radicals and block the damage that potentially would occur. How do they do it? They donate electrons to free radicals to stabilize them without becoming free radicals themselves. (Another example of how nature's solutions are simple yet elegant.)

The damage done by free radicals is one of the mechanisms that accelerates the aging process. And potentiating aging is not the only result of unchecked free radicals. The damage they cause is considered to be the underlying problem in the generation of many chronic diseases, from cardiovascular disease to arthritis, from diabetes to cancer. The damage is sometimes to the cell membrane, sometimes to the mitochondria where metabolic processes are being carried out, and sometimes to DNA itself, causing mutations and perhaps cancer.

> **Note:** Mitochondria are organelles present in the cytoplasm (outside the nucleus) of every cell. They actually generate energy for cells' life processes. Mitochondria are responsible for generating the energy molecule ATP (adenosine triphosphate). Thus they are the energy powerhouses, the factories where oxidation takes place, basic to life as we know it. It is hypothesized that aging and degenerative diseases occur as mitochondria become less efficient. Certain antioxidants maintain healthy mitochondrial function.

> **Note:** Some researchers believe that oxidative damage is synonymous with aging. Aging is seen as the inexorable consequence of cellular damage over a long period of time. And so *antioxidants* are often called *anti-aging chemicals*.

Anti-aging magic bullets

Since youthfulness is so highly prized in our society, it is no wonder that we are bombarded with nutritional supplements that supposedly reverse aging or even prevent it altogether. Those claims will unlikely be upheld when examined by medical research.

Human growth hormone (HGH) is one of those unabashedly advertised supplements that claim to fight the symptoms of aging. I believe you should stay away from any and all nutritional supplements that purport to increase your levels of *HGH*. The reason is that taking *HGH* itself (synthetic *HGH*, by injection) or oral supplements that increase your own levels of *HGH*, come with too high a price to pay for youthful energy levels or good looks. Medical researchers are concerned that taking *HGH* supplements may increase your risk for cancer, joint pains, diabetes, and even premature death!

However, you may wish to take *HGH* in the form of a homeopathic remedy to enhance the function of your own *HGH*, rather than taking it as a nutritional supplement. If this is the case, then I recommend that you seek the services of a homeopath not because homeopathic *HGH* is not safe, but rather changing *HGH* inside your body in any way should not be done without proper medical supervision.

Another reputed anti-aging nutritional supplement is *dehydroepiandrosterone* (DHEA). It is naturally found inside your body as the main steroid precursor for the manufacture of the sex hormones estrogen and testosterone in both men and women. Taking *DHEA* tends to build muscle mass and increases endurance. Some believe that *DHEA* supplements increase libido and energy levels, and enhance the functioning of the immune system, hence the widespread belief that *DHEA* is an anti-aging supplement.

However, when you take *DHEA*, you cannot control where it is used inside your body. In women it could increase your levels of testosterone, making you prone to testosterone-related side effects, such as acne, male-pattern baldness, and facial hair. Or it could increase your levels of estrogen, inadvertently increasing your risk for estrogen-related cancers. In men it could increase levels of estrogen, which might have drastic effects on breast size and sperm counts. Or it could increase levels of testosterone, which might affect aggression and mood. The point is that when you take *DHEA* supplements, you do not know what might happen to you. For this reason, I strongly recommend that you stay far away from *DHEA* supplements.

> **Note:** Performance-enhancing supplements are sometimes used to increase muscle mass, strength, and endurance. Anabolic steroids (also called androgenic steroids) and prohormones such as androstenedione have not only been banned by all major sports organizations but they are controlled substances so using them is illegal. This is because using them is associated with serious side effects such as testicular atrophy and irreversible breast enlargement in males, and masculinization in females.

> **Note:** The supplement *dehydroepiandrosterone* (*DHEA*) is exempt to being classified as a controlled substance despite its being a steroid hormone. It is banned by the Olympics and many other sports organizations. *DHEA* 's exemption is based on its reputed anti-aging and weight redistribution actions. There has never been any convincing evidence as to *DHEA* 's anti-aging prowess, but in a very small study, *DHEA* decreased

abdominal fat in elderly men and women. Abdominal fat wreaks metabolic havoc with insulin causing insulin resistance, which makes people prone to diabetes. But, until more is known about *DHEA* and its long-term effects on both men and women, it is still prudent to refrain from taking it as a supplement.

A Natural Anti-Aging Remedy
There is one combination of nutritional supplements that, although still unproven, has the theoretical (and some claim, the actual) benefit of augmenting cellular health. The combination appears to be safe in the recommended amounts. This combination is *L-carnitine* 500mg twice daily (or *acetyl-L-carnitine*) along with *alpha-lipoic acid* 200 twice daily (please see below). You may buy these 2 supplements separately or together as *Weil Juvenon*. Take one capsule of *Weil Juvenon* (1-800-269-3981) twice daily with meals. Each capsule contains 500mg of *acetyl-L-carnitine* and 200mg of *alpha-lipoic acid*. Please do not take this combination if you have bipolar disease or seizures (epilepsy).

Mitochondrial Energy Optimizer manufactured by Life Extension (1-800-544-4440) contains *acetyl-l-carnitine, carnosine, R-lipoic acid, benfotiamine, Vitamin B1, Rhodiola rosea, luteolin* and *Sodzyme* (for *superoxide dismutase*). Take 4 capsules daily.

> **Note:** With normal aging comes the inevitable decline in antioxidant enzyme levels of *superoxide dismutase* (*SOD*). When *SOD* is taken as a supplement (coupled to *gliadin* for better absorption) it is possible to decrease disease-provoking inflamamtory compounds.

> **Note:** Another approach to increasing longevity is calorie restriction. The results of animal studies revealed that lifespan increases when calories are restricted. A healthy way to restrict calories is to choose low-calorie snacks. Celery is a low-calorie vegetable suitable for snacking because of its satisfying crunch that contains a compound 3-

n-butylphthalide that helps to regulate blood pressure.

Note: Physical activity is another potent anti-aging remedy. A recent Swedish study followed persons over the age of 65 for 12 years. The results showed that those persons who exercised as little as at least once a week lived longer than those who did not. And it appears that more frequent physical activity (5-7 times/week) is associated with even longer lifespans.

How is the action of antioxidants measured?
Antioxidant activity is measured by the ORAC test, the oxygen radical absorbance capacity. Foods are tested and their ORAC score determines whether or not the term antioxidant may be applied to that food. Fruits with the highest amounts of antioxidant activity as measured by the ORAC test are: blueberries, pomegranates, purple grapes, and cranberries, followed by apples, bananas, oranges, and grapefruits. Vegetables with the highest amounts are garlic, broccoli, and tomatoes, followed closely by onions, green peppers, spinach, and carrots.

Note: The United States Department of Agriculture ranked blueberries highest among 100 different foods in antioxidant activity. Blueberries are a wonder in the fiber category too, 2 grams of fiber in 1/2 cup. And they are low-calorie too, with only 40 calories in 1/2 cup.

Eat fresh foods or take supplements?
The best way to get your antioxidant phytochemicals is to eat a variety of fruits and vegetables making up the "colorful diet" (see below) every day. This is what nature intended us to do. This is the way we survived and flourished on this planet for many thousands, possibly millions, of years. Whole foods furnish healthier antioxidant compounds than do the isolated supplements. The interaction between the myriad of antioxidant compounds is probably important for health.

The American Institute of Cancer Research urges Americans to eat at least 5 fruit portions and 5 vegetable portions every single day. This recom-mendation will probably be increased as we discover more about the substances that protect us against cancer. We should also add legumes, whole grains, and nuts every day in order to get superior antioxidant benefits from foods. Since so many of us do not achieve this goal, you may wish to consider taking antioxidant phytochemical supplements along with your multivitamin-multimineral supplement.

One of the ways you might choose to augment the green leafy vegetables in your daily diet is by taking a supplement called *wheat grass*. You will find *wheat grass* from several manufacturers. It contains minimally processed green leafy vegetables, offering a rich mix of nutrients including vitamins, minerals, essential amino acids, and antioxidants. *Barley grass* is another supplement nutritionally equivalent to *wheat grass*. They are available in tablets, powder, or pellets. The whole leaf powders, rich in fiber as well, can be added to soups and casseroles. *Wheat grass* and *barley grass* are sometimes used in a detoxification program as well as for general nutritional enhancement.

The Colorful Diet
This is the same Colorful Diet as found in **Chapter 22: Introduction to Nutritional Supplements**, with the addition of the major antioxidant phytochemical associated with each color. Since phytochemicals cause the color in plants, you can guess that the more intense color in a fruit or vegetable, the more antioxidant phytochemicals you are likely to find there. This does not mean you shouldn't eat cauliflower or garlic. These are healthy too. The main axiom: eat a variety of fruits and vegetables from every color every day.

The colorful diet includes fruits and vegetables of the following groups:
Greens: green leafy vegetables such as spinach, Romaine lettuce, collard greens, kale, beet greens, escarole, mustard greens, Swiss chard and turnip greens, green grapes, and most of the cruciferous vegetables.
> **Note:** The cruciferous vegetables include broccoli, cabbage, watercress, Brussels spouts, kale, and cauliflower. These contain a group of anticancer antioxidants called *sulforaphanes*, a member of the *isothiocyanate* antioxidant family. Possibly the most impor-

tant *isothiocyanate* in cruciferous vegetables is *indole-3 carbinol* (*I3C*). Medical research shows that it possesses potent anti-cancer and anti-angiogenesis activity.

Note: Cruciferous vegetables contain *goitrogens* (chemicals that interfere with thyroid hormone production). If you or your family member is being treated for hypothyroidism (thyroid hormone deficiency), you may want to limit the amount of cruciferous vegetables that you eat daily or adjust the amount of thyroid hormone replacement medicine that you are taking. This effect seems to be particularly problematic when cruciferous vegetables are eaten uncooked.

Note: Other foods also function as *goitrogens*, like peanuts, pine nuts, and soybeans. Eating up to one portion of soy foods every day does not seem to interfere with thyroid function, but if you or your family member suffer from hypothyroidism, do not take soy supplements.

Reds: watermelon, tomatoes, skins of red grapes, pomegranates. These contain anticancer antioxidants called *lycopene*, a member of the *carotenoid* antioxidant family. Pomegranates and many kinds of berries are high in *ellagic acid* which is an especially potent antioxidant involved in protection from cancer and heart disease.

Whites: the cruciferous vegetable cauliflower, garlic, white onions, and leeks. These contain a great variety of the antioxidant family called *flavonoids*, which help cells to survive damage.

Yellow-oranges: carrots, butternut squash, sweet potatoes, peaches, apricots, pumpkins, cantaloupe, mangoes, lemons, and sea buckthorn berry. These contain *beta-carotene, lutein* and *zeazanthin* in the *carotenoid* antioxidant family, helping to lower risk for eye diseases and cancer.

Blue-purples: blueberries, elderberries, black currants, blackberries, chokeberries, purple grapes, plums, eggplants. These contain antioxidants called *anthocyanins* and *proanthocyanidins* in the *flavonoid* antioxidant family. These are especial-

ly helpful in lowering the risk for heart disease and cancer. The darker the berry, the higher the levels of antioxidants.

Remember: Vitamins A, C, and E as well as the minerals zinc and selenium function as antioxidants in your body.

When using antioxidant phytochemicals for self-care of any and all ailments you must pay strict attention to the **Guidelines for Consulting Your Health Care Provider** at the end of this chapter. You may want to refer to the last section **Putting It All Together** for ideas on how to integrate the essential natural alternatives, homeopathy, herbal remedies, and nutritional supplements.

Alpha-lipoic Acid (R-alpha-lipoic acid)

Alpha-lipoic acid (or *R-alpha-lipoic acid*) is called the "universal antioxidant" because it neutralizes free radicals throughout the entire body since it is soluble in both water and fat. It squelches many different types of free radicals, thereby reducing their concentration, as well as reconstitutes metabolically active forms of other antioxidants such as Vitamins C and E and *glutathione*.

Alpha-lipoic acid is active inside the mitochondria, the oxidation factory of the cell. It increases energy production from mitochondria. It plays a role in protecting DNA from oxidation damage. It prevents the cellular damage that occurs from high blood sugar so it may be particularly important for diabetics. It has been shown to reduce the duration of wound healing in diabetics. It is used to alleviate diabetic neuropathy.

Alpha-lipoic acid is considered an anti-aging supplement. *Alpha-lipoic acid* supplements improve the luster and texture of skin. Even though *alpha-lipoic acid* is manufactured inside your body (so it is not considered to be an essential nutrient), it may be wise to take a daily supplement after the age of 40, to augment the naturally occurring amount. The dosage is 100-300mg/day.

Note: *R-alpha-lipoic acid* occurs naturally in two forms of *lipoic acid* inside your body (the *R-alpha* and *R-dihydro* forms). Both forms scavenge free radicals. But *R-dihydro-lipoic acid* is the form that repairs oxidative damage. But, because these 2 forms readily convert to one another inside cells as they gain or lose electrons, it likely will not matter which form you take as a supplement. Since more research has been done using *R-alpha-lipoic acid*, it is a good idea to use this form.

Fruit and vegetable sources: spinach, potatoes, Brewer's yeast.

Carotenoids

The *carotenoid* antioxidant family is made up of about 500 different chemical pigments found in yellow-orange fruits and vegetables. This chemical complexity warns us that eating the whole food is likely to be superior to taking an isolated supplement. *Carotenoids* help to protect us against cumulative inflammation, probably the first step towards the development of cancer.

Beta-carotene

Beta-carotene (also known as provitamin A) is an anticancer antioxidant and has a healthy effect on the heart. However, when the Cleveland Clinic analyzed 15 studies of over 130,000 people, it was found that *beta-carotene* actually increased the risk for death from heart disease among smokers. Even though most people emphasize that the increase in deaths did not occur among nonsmokers, my recommendation is that you get your *beta-carotene* by eating yellow-orange colored fruits and vegetables rather than by taking beta-carotene supplements.

You may find that your multivitamin supplement contains 10,000 IU of Vitamin A in the *beta-carotene* form. Since the *beta-carotene* form of Vitamin A is water-soluble, non-toxic, and does not accumulate in the body, this level is acceptable. Otherwise, the Vitamin A from retinol in your multivitamin supplement should contain no more than 3,000-5,000 IU.

Fruit and vegetable sources: sweet potatoes, carrots, corn, apricots, cantaloupes, papayas, yellow squash, pumpkins.

Note: *Astaxanthin* is a *carotenoid* antioxidant that is even more potent than *beta-carotene*. It comes from the algae *Haematococcus pluvialis*.

Lutein and Zeaxanthin

Lutein and *zeaxanthin*, two *xanthophyll* compounds in the family of *carotenoid* antioxidants, protect our eyes from oxidative damage.

> **Note:** *Lutein* and *zeaxanthin* function in plants to prevent damage from too much light. This is the same function they serve in the human eye.

Lutein and *zeaxanthin* are found in concentrated amounts in the macula and lens of our eyes, up to 1,000 times greater than in any other tissue. The macula is the area in the retina that is responsible for sharp and color vision. Age-related macular degeneration (AMD), a significant cause of blindness in the older than 65 group, is lower in persons who consumed more fruits and vegetables containing *lutein* and *zeaxanthin* over a long period of time. In fact, in people who already have AMD, *lutein* and *zeaxanthin* can prevent the progression of the disease towards blindness. A diet rich in *lutein* and *zeaxanthin* also protects against cataracts. If you or a family member is at higher risk for AMD or cataracts, you may decide to take *lutein* and *zeaxanthin* supplements. The dose is 6-20mg/day.

> **Remember:** *Lutein* and *zeaxanthin* are depleted upon exposure to sunlight. This is one reason why people living in the south tend to get more cataracts.

Fruit and vegetable sources: kale, spinach, collard greens, Swiss chard, parsley, mustard greens, celery, Romaine lettuce, Brussels sprouts, broccoli, avocado.

Lycopene

Lycopene is a *carotenoid* antioxidant without being a provitamin A, that is concentrated in the prostate gland. It has been shown to decrease the risk for prostate cancer and has the ability to decrease the PSA (prostate specific antigen) levels in persons with prostate cancer. *Lycopene* also decreases the risk for heart disease. Men at particular risk for prostate cancer should consider taking *lycopene* 10-30mg/day, as well as eating a diet rich in red fruits and vegetables.

Fruit and vegetable sources: tomatoes (and tomato products), watermelon, skins of red grapes.

> **Note:** Heating tomato products (such as tomato sauce) increases the concentration of usable *lycopene*. Placing tomatoes into boiling water for one or two minutes, then easily ridding them of their skins, increases the usable *lycopene*.

> **Note:** Women who ate a daily diet with high levels of *lycopene* (about 3 medium tomatoes every day) were found by Harvard researchers to be less likely to develop heart disease.

> **Note:** *Curcumin* is another anti-inflammatory, antioxidant phytochemical that protects against prostate cancer (as well as melanoma, pancreatic cancer, and multiple myeloma). It's being used to treat Crohn's disease and liver disease from alcohol toxicity as well. *Curcumin* arrests the growth of cells that are multiplying in an out-of-control way. *Curcumin* blocks blood vessel formation (angiogenesis) in tumors. *Curcumin* is the subject of a study funded by the Cystic Fibrosis Foundation on blocking mucus in the intestinal tract in people with cystic fibrosis.

> *Curcumin* is found in the yellow spice, *turmeric* (*Curcuma longa*). It is a good idea to learn how to incorporate *turmeric* in your daily cooking recipes. *Curcumin* is available as a nutritional supplement, such as *Super Curcumin* (with *piperine* to enhance absorption) made by Life Extension. The suggested dose is 1-2 capsules of 900mg once daily with meals. Other manufactures' suggested dosages are 300-400mg three times daily. But don't take *turmeric* supplements if you are pregnant or breast-feeding (although *turmeric* used as the

spice in your food is safe for use). Take *turmeric* supplements cautiously if you are taking anticoagulants (blood-thinning drugs). Another *turmeric* product is the natural anti-inflammatory *Zyflamend* (manufactured by New Chapter) which is being used to treat all forms of arthritis and prostate cancer.

Polyphenols

Polyphenols are a large antioxidant family of naturally occurring chemicals. They consist of several kinds, like *flavanoids, catechins, isoflavones,* as well as others. *Polyphenols* help to protect arteries from oxidative damage. They play a role in increasing blood flow which in turn decreases the risk of blood clots. *Polyphenols* play a role in cell survival.

Fruit and vegetable sources: red wine, teas, grape seed extract, figs, olive oil.

> **Note:** *Rosmarinic acid* is a *polyphenol* that is present in the *Lamaiaceae* botanical family. It comes from the leaf of the culinary herb *Rosemary* (*Rosmarinus officinalis*), as well as *mint, basil, sage* and *perilla leaf*. *Rosmarinic acid* extract and *perilla leaf* extract at a dosage of 100-200mg daily are being used to treat allergy symptoms such as runny nose and nasal congestion (allergic rhinitis).

Flavonoids

Flavonoids comprise the largest group of antioxidant substances in the *polyphenol* family. The *flavonoid* antioxidant family (sometimes called *bioflavonoids*) consists of a large number of chemical compounds widely distributed in nature, occurring in fruits (especially pomegranates), vegetables, whole grains, legumes, nuts, seeds, beer, wine, tea, and cocoa (especially dark chocolate). Pomegranate juice contains more *flavonoids* than an equal amount of red wine. A good source for pomegranate juice is *POM Wonderful* which can be diluted with water or seltzer.

Chocolate is made from the cocoa bean which is

the fruit of the cocoa tree (*Theobroma cacao*). Although two-thirds of the fat in chocolate is saturated, the rest is monounsaturated. Overall, chocolate does not raise blood cholesterol. Dark chocolate contains more *flavonoids* than milk chocolate as well as less sugar. White chocolate does not contain *flavonoids* at all. For most Americans, the calories in chocolate outweigh the benefits of its *flavonoids*.

Flavonoids prevent oxidative damage to the heart and blood vessels from the metabolism of low-density lipoproteins (LDL), the form of cholesterol that contributes to clogging your arteries, especially your coronary (heart) arteries. *Grape seed extract*, a powerful antioxidant, is a good way to take your *flavonoids* as a supplement. The dose is 300mg twice daily.

Fruit and vegetable sources: fruits (especially pomegranates), vegetables, whole grains, legumes, nuts, seeds, beer, wine, tea, and cocoa (especially dark chocolate).

> **Note:** For information on *Isoflavones* please see *Soy* in **Chapter 21: Herbal Remedies for Women's Health**; and for information on *catechins* please see *Green tea* in **Chapter 20: Herbs You Need to Know**. *Isoflavones* and *catechins* belong to the *flavonoid* family of antioxidants.

> **Note:** Supplements containing *flavonoids* derived from citrus fruits like oranges and tangerines are being used to lower total cholesterol, LDL cholesterol, and triglycerides. *Nobiletin* is a *flavonoid* antioxidant derived from orange peel with anti-inflammatory activity.

Anthocyanins and *Proanthocyanidins*

Anthocyanins and *proanthocyanidins* are part of the *flavonoid* antioxidant family of chemicals. *Anthocyanins* protect the cardiovascular system against oxidative damage from free radicals. These chemicals have the ability to suppress cancer growth. They reduce inflammation naturally by decreasing COX-1 and COX-2 levels. *Anthocyanins* and *proanthocyanidins* are responsible for dark red,

blue, and purple colors in fruits and vegetables. There are more than 300 different *anthocyanins* and *proanthocyanidins*, each possessing antioxidant activity.

Fruit and vegetable sources: bilberries, blueberries, blackberries, cranberries, cherries, raspberries, strawberries, plums, red grapes, grape seed extract, beets.

> **Note:** If you want the anti-inflammatory action of *anthocyanins* from a nutritional supplement, you may try *Cherry extract*. Take 1,000mg twice daily. Dr. Andrew Weil says this is the amount you would get if you ate a pound of cherries or drank 4 cups of cherry juice.

> **Note:** The *anthocyanins* in bilberry may increase blood flow to the eyes. People who want to prevent diabetic retinopathy and macular degeneration should consider taking *bilberry* extract along with *lutein* and *zeaxanthin*.

> **Note:** Oligomeric *proanthocyanidins* (OPCs) are found in *grape seed* extract and *pine bark* extract. OPCs are particularly important for vascular health.

Quercetin

Quercetin is part of the *flavonoid* family of antioxidants. It has anticancer properties as well as helping to protect against heart disease and stroke. *Quercetin* may help to reduce allergy symptoms by its anti-inflammatory activity. It decreases the secretion of histamine from mast cells. The release of histamine is one of your body's main mechanisms to induce allergic reactions. The dosage to prevent allergy during allergy season is 500mg of *quercetin* twice daily. Children over the age of six may take *quercetin* 500mg once daily.

The herbal medicine, *olive leaf* (*Olea europaea*), contains several *flavonoids*, among them a hearty concentration of *quercetin*. *Olive leaf* extract has anti-inflammatory actions. It is being used to treat high blood pressure (hypertension), as well as the common cold, the flu (influenza virus), and herpes infections. The dose is 250-500mg of *olive leaf* extract 1-3 times daily. The extract must be standardized to contain 6-12% *oleuropein*, the main constituent with antioxidant action.

Fruit and vegetable sources: onions, wine, most vegetables. *Quercetin* is found in larger amounts in red and yellow onions compared to white onions. *Quercetin* is also found in sweet onions such as *Vidalia* and *Walla Walla*. The dose of *quercetin* taken as a nutritional supplement is 500mg twice daily.

Glutathione

Glutathione (specifically the chemical form *L-glutathione*) is a protein made up of 3 amino acids. It works together in your body with the antioxidant Vitamins C and E and the antioxidant mineral selenium. The function of *glutathione* is to regenerate vitamins C and E. The *glutathione* complex of antioxidants helps your immune system to vanquish invading organisms and to recognize foreign proteins, including cancerous cells. *Glutathione* complex also protects DNA from oxidative damage.

There is some medical evidence that *glutathione* is deficient in the brains of some people with Parkinson's disease. Some of these sick people have benefited from receiving intravenous *glutathione* in high dosages.

> **Note:** *N-acetylcysteine* (*NAC*), the sulphur-containing form of the amino acid *cysteine*, has antioxidant properties. In the body, *NAC* contributes its sulphur to renew *glutathione*'s free-radical scavenging abilities. *NAC* is also useful as a mucolytic agent for sick people with lung diseases.

Fruit and vegetable sources: brewer's yeast, garlic, avocado, walnuts, potatoes.

Isothiocyanates

The *isothiocyanate* antioxidant family is prominently found in cruciferous vegetables (broccoli, cabbage, Brussels sprouts, kohlrabi). *Isothiocyanates* help to protect the liver from doing the difficult work that the liver is programmed to do: the detoxification of

toxins that are produced as by-products of metabolism.

Fruit and vegetable sources: cruciferous vegetables (broccoli, cabbage, Brussels sprouts, kale, kohlrabi).

> **Note:** Raw cabbage, a cruciferous vegetable, contains only 17 calories per cup. Not only is it low in calories and packed with antioxidant phytochemicals but eating it requires some satisfying chewing, making it an ideal snack food. Red cabbage contains more vitamin C, *beta-carotene*, and *quercetin* than green. Cook cabbage in the microwave using very little water because *sulforaphane* and *isothiocyanates* are water-soluble. Making cabbage into sauerkraut by fermentation actually increases its *sulforaphane* and *isothiocyanate* content.

Sulphoraphane

Sulphoraphane (sometimes spelled *sulforaphane*) is part of the *isothiocyanate* antioxidant family. *Sulphoraphane* is just one of a large number of organic sulphur compounds involved in protecting your body from carcinogens. *Sulphoraphane* helps to protect your body from breast, colon, and stomach cancers.

Fruit and vegetable sources: cruciferous vegetables: broccoli, cabbage, cauliflower, mustard greens, rutabagas, kale, collard greens, and turnips; also from non-cruciferous vegetables: carrots, green onions. Broccoli sprouts contain the most concentrated amounts of *sulforaphane*.

> **Remember:** Because of possible contamination with hepatitis A virus, thoroughly cook your green onions; do not eat them raw.

> **Note:** *Brassica Tea*, made by Brassica Protection Products (www.brassicatea.com) is rich in *sulphoraphanes* extracted from broccoli. Each teabag contains 15mg of *sulphoraphane*, the same amount as one serving of broccoli, mixed together with black or *Green tea*.

Lignans

Lignans are a group of antioxidant phytochemicals that have anti-cancer properties, probably because they help to modulate the action of certain hormones, especially estrogen (phytoestrogen). *Lignans* may help to prevent breast cancer in those who have never had it. But, if you or your family member is being treated for breast cancer (or any other hormone-dependent cancer like prostate), you should avoid the *lignans* in flaxseeds. It is a good idea to follow the same recommendation if you are pregnant or lactating or if you are trying to become pregnant. *Lignans* also help to lower low-density lipoproteins (LDL), the so-called "bad" cholesterol, and in so doing, lowers your risk for heart disease.

Fruit and vegetable sources: flaxseed. Flaxseeds are available as the whole seed (providing fiber for intestinal health, a natural mild laxative), seeds ground into meal, or as sprouted flaxseeds. Flaxseed oil is also available, but it does not contain lignans. Flaxseed oil is a rich source of *omega-3 fatty acids*.

Resveratrol

Resveratrol is an antioxidant phytochemical possessing anti-cancer and anti-inflammatory properties. The anti-cancer activity of *resveratrol* is based on its abilities to block estrogen and androgens and to kill cancer cells. *Resveratrol* may increase the anti-cancer effects of Vitamin D. *Resveratrol* possesses preventive anti-cancer activity against a wide range of cancers. Recent evidence points to *resveratrol* playing a part in protecting the brain from developing Alzheimer's disease.

An exciting feature of *resveratrol* is that it has been shown to activate a longevity gene in yeast and fruit flies which in turn augments the chemical activity of a stress-response molecule. This effect on longevity has recently been shown with mice, significantly extending their lifespans when they are given *resveratrol*. Consequently, medical researchers are testing *resveratrol* on human subjects. You may consider getting your *resveratrol* in the form of nutritional supplements or the old-fashioned way, though grapes and wine.

Fruit and vegetable sources: red and purple grapes, red grape juice, red wine. *Resveratrol* is present in plants to fight fungal infections. If the grapes destined for your dessert or for your wine have been sprayed with pesticides, they will contain relatively little *resveratrol*. If you want to augment the amount of cancer-fighting *resveratrol* that you consume, is important that you choose only organic grapes and wines that are made from organic grapes.

Resveratrol as a nutritional supplement is available either alone or in combination with other antioxidants. The dose is 20mg daily of standardized *resveratrol* from organic grapes. *Longevinex* capsules contain red wine extracts with enough *resveratrol* equivalent to 5-15 glasses of red wine.

Welch Foods' research study showed that their concord grape juice increased HDL ("good") cholesterol.

Guidelines for Consulting Your Health Care Provider

You should consult your health care provider if:
- the patient doesn't look right or act right (trust your instincts!)
- the patient is getting worse instead of better over the course of the illness
- the patient is having trouble breathing or complaining of chest pains or there is mental confusion or lethargy or irritability
- the patient develops allergic symptoms (hives, itchy or watery eyes, runny nose, scratchy throat, asthma, shortness of breath) after taking a nutritional supplement
- after beginning a nutritional supplement the patient experiences *new onset* of any serious symptoms such as:

   paralysis, weakness, tingling, inability to focus or concentrate, blurred or double vision or blindness, slurred speech, severe headaches, seizures, irritability, dizziness, disorientation, memory loss, anxiety, depression, insomnia, blackouts, fainting, or the person complains of not feeling like himself

- the patient is taking *ANY* prescription medication
- the patient is pregnant or breastfeeding
- the patient has any serious, chronic disease which may have complications and become life-threatening, such as:

> autism, cancer, HIV and AIDS, arthritis, multiple sclerosis, coronary artery disease, heart attack (myocardial infarction), blood dyscrasia, cancer (of any type), congestive heart failure, diabetes mellitus, obesity, thyroid disorders, high blood pressure (hypertension), stroke, seizures, acute and chronic kidney (renal) failure, schizophrenia, bipolar disorder, borderline personality disorder, eating disorders, fibromyalgia, chronic fatigue syndrome, Crohn's disease, ulcerative colitis, celiac disease, mental deficiency disorders, chromosomal disorders, infertility, frequent miscarriages, polyneuropathy, cystic fibrosis   [Adapted from *The Merck Manual* at www.merck.com]

Note: Do not discontinue taking any pharmaceutical medication that has been prescribed by your health care provider unless you or your family member is under the supervision of a physician.

Note: Do not take any nutritional supplement, including antioxidant phytochemicals without first consulting your health care provider if you or your family member is pregnant or breastfeeding. In general, I recommend not taking any antioxidant supplement during pregnancy or breastfeeding because safety data are insufficient. A good way to get your antioxidants during pregnancy and lactation is from a healthy diet, heavy on vegetables and fruits.

In addition, it is a good idea to check with your health care provider if your family member is either very young or very old because nutritional supplements, including some antioxidant phy-

tochemicals, given injudiciously may overwhelm the body's defenses in those age groups.

Remember: You or your family member should not take supplements containing high doses of antioxidants during chemotherapy and radiation treatment for cancer. Antioxidants prevent cellular destruction by free radicals. But in the case of cancer, free radicals may be advantageous because cancerous cells would be destroyed.

During treatment for cancer you are encouraged to eat a healthy diet containing antioxidants and to continue taking your multivitamin-multimineral supplement. After treatment and during the respite between sessions, you may revert to taking your antioxidant supplement regime.

However: More and more evidence is accumulating to contradict this conventional wisdom. You may want to research this controversial issue further by reading articles from the Simone Protective Cancer Institute published in *Alternative Therapies in Health and Medicine*, January/February 2007 and March/April 2007.

Remember: If you or your family member has/had cancer, you must discuss all supplements with your oncologist.

Note: *Prolongeveity Formula* by ProVita is an herbal formula promising longevity. It includes *Ficus bengalensis* (*Banyan tree*), *Angelica keiskei* (*Ashitaba*) and *Rhodiola crenulata* along with *pantethine*, a form of *pantothenic acid*. So far, the promise is unsubstantiated.

Note: *Capsaicin* is the potent antioxidant present in hot peppers that prevents nitrites from uniting with amines to form cancerous *nitrosamines*. The amount of *capsaicin* increases as the pepper gets hotter. Jalapenos peppers are a good source of *capsaicin*.

Note: Antioxidant jucies made from *noni* (*Morinda citrifolia*), *Acai berry* (*Euterpe oleracea*), *wolfberry* and *mangosteen* are available from www.dynamic heath.com, 1-800-396-2114.

Note: Some culinary herbs have powerful antioxidant activity. The ones with the highest activity are *turmeric*, oregano, rosemary, bay leaf, coriander, sage, and dill. You can use these herbs in your cooking knowing they are not only flavorful but healthful.

Note: Please keep far away from the book *Natural Cures They Don't Want You to Know About* by Kevin Trudeau. In the University of California at Berkeley's *Wellness Letter* of November 2005 (Volume 22, Issue 2), John Swartzberg, M.D., Chairperson of the Editorial Board wrote a scathing review of this book, revealing its "empty promises, unproven assertions, and dangerous advice." "The 'natural cures' include magic juices, colonic irrigation, and other purges, bee pollen, hydrogen peroxide, enzyme pills, and a dozen other ineffective and/or harmful procedures and products." Please disregard everything Trudeau says about that long list of "natural cures" (except for enzyme pills, for which you may find more information in **Chapter 25: Heart Healthy Nutritional Supplements** and **Chapter 27: Nutritional Supplements to Prevent Cancer and Augment Your Immune System**).

Putting It All Together

If you are considering using an *antioxidant* nutritional supplement, either to forestall aging processes, optimize mitochondrial function, or for other reasons, it is a good idea to familiarize yourself with **Chapter 22: Introduction to Nutritional Supplements**. It makes good sense to understand the role of vitamin and mineral nutritional supplements from **Chapter 23: Vitamins and Minerals** and *omega-3 fatty acids* from **Chapter 31: Oils and Fats**.

Other important nutritional supplements that play a role in mitochondrial health are *Coenzyme Q10* and *L-carnitine* (please see **Chapter 25: Heart Healthy Nutritional Supplements**).

Then, after you have decided to use an *antioxidant* nutritional supplement to prevent or treat a certain ailment, it makes good sense to investigate the homeopathic remedy indicated for that ailment as well. That's because homeopathic remedies are safe, have no side effects, and can be used together with herbal remedies and Western pharmaceutical medicines without concern. You may read about your sick person's homeopathic remedies in **Chapters 3-18**. And you may want to better understand homeopathy by reading **Chapter 2: Basic Homeopathy**.

Whenever you have decided to go ahead with an *antioxidant* nutritional supplement, it is a good idea to consider giving the sick person's homeopathic constitutional remedy as well (please refer to **Chapter 9: Homeopathic Remedies for Constitutional Problems in Infants, Children, and Adolescents** or to **Chapter 18: Homeopathic Constitutional Remedies** if you are dealing with an adult; or **Chapter 13: Homeopathy for Elderly Persons** if you are dealing with an elderly person).

People who are taking an *antioxidant* nutritional supplement may also benefit from certain specific nutritional supplements, depending on the particular ailment. You may read about your sick person's specific nutritional remedies in **Chapters 25-31**.

Chapter 25

Heart Healthy Nutritional Supplements

Heart Health in General

Ailment/Disorder/Symptom	Nutritional Supplement
Heart attacks and strokes	*Alcoholic beverages*
Congestive heart failure, high blood pressure	*Amino acids*
Anti-aging activity in heart muscle	*L-carnitine*
Heart muscle contraction	*Coenzyme Q10*
Anti-inflammatory activity	*Enzymes*
Cardiovascular disease and cholesterol	*Fiber*
LDL ("bad") cholesterol lowering while raising HDL ("good") cholesterol	*Guggulipid*
Capillaries and veins, varicose veins	*Horse chestnut*
Total and LDL ("bad") cholesterol lowering	*Phytosterols*
Total and LDL cholesterol, and triglycerides lowering while raising HDL cholesterol	*Policosanol*
Total and LDL cholesterol lowering	*Red yeast rice*

Guidelines for Consulting Your Health Care Provider
Putting It All Together

Heart Health in General

Heart health refers to the health of your entire cardiovascular system, meaning your heart and your blood vessels (arteries, veins and capillaries), working together. There are many different forms of cardiovascular disease, including:

> heart attack (myocardial infarction), coronary artery disease (arteriosclerosis of the coronary arteries), angina pectoris, congestive heart failure, enlarged heart (cardiomyopathy), irregular heart beat (arrhythmias, including atrial fibrillation), diseases of the heart valves (valvular diseases), infections of the heart muscle and surrounding tissues (myocarditis, endocarditis, and pericarditis), high blood pressure (hypertension), peripheral vascular disorders (intermittent claudication), chronic venous insufficiency, blood clots in the veins (deep vein thrombosis), and varicose veins. [Adapted from *The Merck Manual* at www.merck.com]

The majority of the serious cardiovascular diseases are caused by lifestyle factors superimposed on a genetically susceptible person. The most important things you can do to prevent heart disease in yourself or a family member are stop smoking, follow a heart healthy dietary program, and exercise at least 30 minutes on most days.

> **Note:** The heart healthy dietary plan to consider is, according to Dr. Andrew Weil, the anti-inflammatory diet, which is based on the Mediterranean diet. The anti-inflammatory diet depends heavily on whole foods that grow from the earth like whole grains, fresh fruits and vegetables, with *olive oil* as your main fat source. In addition, you will need to consume foods high in *omega-3 fatty acids*, like walnuts and flaxseeds. Animal protein is at a minimum except for cold water fatty fish, again supplying *omega-3 fatty acids*. You may add *ginger* and *turmeric* to your food for their anti-inflammatory effects as well as antioxidant vitamins and minerals. You must limit your intake of processed foods, sugar and salt.

> **Note:** You may want to take a look at the dietary plans by the *American Heart Association* as well as the *American Institute for Cancer Research*. The main differences between them is the number of recommended daily portions of fruits and vegetables (5 and 10, respectively).

The *National Heart, Lung and Blood Institute* devised the *Dietary Approaches to Stop Hypertension (DASH)* eating plan, which is low in salt (sodium chloride). It is recommended for persons with high blood pressure (hypertension). The *Institute of Medicine* has lowered its recommended daily healthy salt intake from 2,400 to 1,500 milligrams per day.

> **Note:** You may take a look at the *DASH* eating plan at www.nhlbi.nih.gov/health/public/heart/hbp/dash and www.dashdiet.org.

> **Note:** The new recommendations for sodium intake are 1,200mg/day for people up to age 50, 1,300mg/day for people up to age 70, and 1,200mg/day for people over 70. One of the reasons why high blood pressure is so common today is that the average American ingests about 5,750 milligrams of salt per day (contained in one teaspoon of salt), with most of the excess coming from processed foods. Since salt is composed of 60% chlorine and 40% sodium, you would be consuming about 2,300 milligrams of sodium, about double the new recommended intake.

Kosher salt does not contain any additives (such as iodine) and has less sodium per teaspoon than table salt. Sea salt contains trace minerals (calcium and magnesium) and some brands contain less sodium per teaspoon than table salt. You may experiment with different brands for saltiness and flavor. (Please see *amino acids* below for a low-salt substitute for soy sauce and tamari.)

It is a good idea to become familiar with the Mediterranean diet to learn about its emphasis on non-animal protein sources, such as legumes, as well as healthy fats and oils.

> **Note:** Please consider using the *glycemic index* approach to eating, especially when choosing carbohydrate-containing whole foods, like grains and beans, but also for vegetables and fruits. The *glycemic index* is a way to understand what happens to food on its way to becoming glucose, the source of energy your body requires. (For more information on the *glycemic index*, please see **Chapter 26: Nutritional Supplements for Healthy Weight Control**.)

It is never too late to make these important lifestyle changes. But, it is fruitless to take heart healthy nutritional supplements without taking these steps first. These particular lifestyle changes will also help to make your heart and your immune system more resistant to the evils of chronic stress.

> **Remember:** More people die from heart disease than from any other cause. It is the leading cause of death for both men and women in the U.S.

> **Beware:** Doctors unfortunately tend to underestimate the risk for heart disease in women. And the sad part is that women do the same. All this while heart disease consistently kills more women than men every year. The *American Heart Association* has developed new guidelines to prevent fatal heart disease in women. You may visit them at www.americanheart.org.

Blood pressure measurements in the range of normal were updated in 2003 to reflect the lower cutoff point for "normal." Normal values are now less than 120/80 (previously less than 140/90). A new category, *prehypertension*, between 120/80-139/89, was added to help people become aware of their increased chances to go on to develop full-blown hypertension. If your blood pressure is in the *prehypertension* range, you have a higher chance to experience a heart attack or stroke. It is wakeup call to change those lifestyle factors that have impacted your heart health. And then you may want to choose those particular nutritional supplements that are targeted towards your heart problem.

Values for hypertension remain the same, 140/90 or higher. Persons whose blood pressure readings fall into this range need to be under the care of a physician and may require one or two prescription medications, depending on the risk level of your health problems. If you have heart disease you should discuss your choices for heart healthy nutritional supplements with your physician before you start taking anything.

Your cholesterol levels are important because the higher they are, the greater your risk for cardiovascular disease. Normal values for cholesterol levels have also been updated in 2003. The new normal level for total cholesterol is 200mg/dl or less. LDL cholesterol should be less than 130 for people without serious risks for heart disease or less than 100 if you do have risk factors. Your level of HDL cholesterol should be at least 40. HDL levels of 60 and higher are protective against heart disease. Levels of HDL below 40 indicate increased risk for heart disease.

Normal blood levels of triglycerides are less than 150mg/dl. Borderline high triglyceride levels are 150-199; high levels are 200-499; and very high triglyceride levels are 500mg/dl and higher. The first thing to do in managing high triglyceride levels is to eliminate sugar and simple carbohydrates, including alcohol from your diet.

Almost 20% of adult Americans have high blood cholesterol levels. Many are taking prescription cholesterol-lowering "statin" medications. Of course "statin" drugs may have side effects and not everyone can tolerate them. The first step in coping with elevated cholesterol levels is to provide yourself and your family with a heart healthy diet, low in total fats particularly saturated fats and negligible in *trans fats*.

While trying to buy heart healthy foods, you should avoid foods containing *trans fats*. These are fats that are formed when oils are partially hydrogenated, in the process becoming more solid and more stable for a longer shelf life. *Trans fats* are found in baked goods, like cakes, cookies, crackers, cupcakes, and some breads. New food labeling regulations by the Food and Drug Administration require *trans fats* to be listed on the Nutrition Facts label. This means that you are able to make heart healthier food choices in the supermarket by looking at both the saturated fat and *trans fat* lines on the label. You also need to scan the ingredients and if partially hydrogenated oils are used, then skip that product. Some of our most respected nutrition researchers recommend zero tolerance for *trans fats*. (For more information on *trans fats*, please see **Chapter 31: Oils and Fats**.)

A high level of the amino acid *homocysteine* is a risk factor for cardiovascular disease. High levels tend to occur in persons with diabetes and obesity. *Homocysteine* is dependent upon vitamins B6, B12, and folic acid (please see **Chapter 23: Vitamins and Minerals**) for metabolism. For persons with high levels of *homocysteine*, it is important to choose foods high in these vitamins and to consider taking heart healthy nutritional supplements as well.

Taking two baby *aspirins* (160mg) daily has become good preventive health for some men over 40 and women over 65, especially for those people with *risk factors* for cardiovascular disease (see below). This is because *aspirin* decreases the risk of cardiovascular diseases by acting as a general anti-blood clotting agent (anticoagulant) by decreasing the stickiness of platelets. If you or your family member experiences symptoms of a heart attack or stroke, whether or not he or she is taking daily preventive *aspirin*, it is a good idea to chew or crush and swallow (for faster absorption) one adult aspirin (325mg) immediately while someone else is calling 911.

Remember: If you start a regimen of taking two baby *aspirins* every day, you need to continue without forgetting. It is possible that stopping *aspirin* abruptly may cause a rebound effect, making platelets even stickier, and this may result in a new episode of heart problems or stroke. This rebound effect has been shown to be true for patients who already have heart disease. If you or your family member already has heart

disease and is considering stopping daily *aspirin* therapy in preparation for a surgical or dental procedure, please first discuss with your health care provider. It is likely that you will be advised to continue taking your daily *aspirin* tablet before most surgical operations (except for brain surgery) because *aspirin* helps to prevent blood clots (deep vein thrombosis), a potentially fatal complication of surgery.

Note: *Aspirin* is not right for everyone so you should ask your physician before you start. The side effects of *aspirin* include bleeding ulcers, hemorrhagic stroke, and allergic reactions including asthma. It may decrease kidney function in older people. Not everyone is sensitive to the anti-clotting effects of *aspirin*. These people are called *aspirin*-resistant. *Aspirin*-resistant people are much more likely to die of a heart attack than *aspirin*-sensitive people.

Note: A surprise finding in a recent study showed *aspirin* protected against cancer of the colon by decreasing the recurrence rate of polyps (precancerous growths) in the colon. This may be due to *aspirin*'s anti-inflammatory properties. This seems to be the case with breast cancer too. Women who take aspirin for heart health have a lowered risk for breast cancer.

Note: There are sex-based differences in reactivity to *aspirin* in the prevention of heart attacks and stroke. A recent study at the prestigious Brigham and Women's Hospital in Boston (called the Women's Health Study) on almost 40,000 healthy women taking 100mg of *aspirin* every other day failed to show a lower incidence of first heart attacks. But *aspirin* did decrease the risk for first heart attacks once the women were 65 years of age or older. The same study did show that those women had a lower risk for ischemic stroke (the type caused by blood clots). Unfortunately, they also had an increased incidence of hemorrhagic stroke. This study is one reason why healthy women less than 65 years of age without risk factors for heart disease need not take daily *aspirin*. This study points out why it is so important to include both genders when doing medical research.

Understanding and evaluating your personal *risk factors* is called *prospective medicine*. A full appreciation of your *risk factors* for cardiovascular disease may help you to achieve a personalized health program for lifestyle change. If you have any of the following *risk factors* you may have an increased likelihood of becoming sick with cardiovascular disease: having had any kind of heart disease or stroke; men over age 45 and women over age 50 (or in menopause); family history of having heart attacks before age 55; family history of stroke; blood pressure of 140/90; smoking; high total cholesterol or low HDL cholesterol; sedentary lifestyle with less than 30 minutes of exercise on most days; overweight or obese; type 2 diabetes mellitus; high levels of *homocysteine*; high levels of *C-reactive protein* (a marker of inflammation); depression. Some researchers include negative emotions and chronic pessimism, as well.

Remember: The recommendation for your daily intake of *saturated fats* (including *trans fats*, which should be as close to zero as possible) is less than 10% of your total calories (about 20 grams per day) and consume no more than 300mg per day of cholesterol.

However: If you have an increased risk for cardiovascular disease, you may need to restrict *saturated* (including *trans fats*) to 7% or 15 grams daily and consume no more than 200mg per day of cholesterol.

If you want to calculate your own or a family member's five-year risk for heart disease, please take the online test at www.med-decisions.com.

Note: A newly recognized risk factor for cardiovascular disease is depression. People with depression have a 70% higher risk of having first heart attack than non-depressed people. Depression also increases by 3.5 times your chance of dying in the first few months after having suffered a heart attack. If you or a family member suffers from depression, make sure your physician takes you seriously. And more especially if you are post-menopausal. Depression is not just another "normal" symptom in postmenopausal women.

If your goal is to prevent or treat cardiovascular disease in yourself or a family member, it is a good idea to begin first with homeopathy, then add the appropriate vitamins and minerals, and then consider nutritional supplements targeted to heart health. Your constitutional homeopathic remedy is the right place to start.

Before you buy a supplement, look for the *USP mark* on the label for quality assurance. If you want to buy a non-USP labeled supplement, please check first with ConsumerLab.com. They performed product reviews of many heart healthy supplements. You can read the results at www. ConsumerLab.com or in their book, ConsumerLab. com's *Guide to Buying Vitamins and Supplements, What's Really in the Bottle?*

When using heart healthy nutritional supplements for self-care you must pay strict attention to the **Guidelines for Consulting Your Health Care Provider** at the end of this chapter. You may want to refer to the last section **Putting It All Together** for ideas on how to integrate the essential natural alternatives, homeopathy, herbal remedies, and nutritional supplements.

Alcoholic beverages

Doctors find themselves in something of a quandary when they recommend that their patients drink alcoholic beverages to better their cardiovascular health. They worry that they may be encouraging alcohol abusers to drink. But, medical evidence points to the fact that a certain dosage level of daily alcohol intake can be associated with a lower incidence of heart attacks and strokes.

The trick in using alcohol for heart health is to understand that doctors recommend a *reasonable amount* of daily alcohol intake for some people. What is a reasonable amount? A "light" amount of alcohol is one standard-sized alcoholic drink per day for men and one every other day for women. A "moderate" amount means no more than 2 standard-sized drinks per day for men and one for women. What is a standard-sized drink of alcohol? For wine it is a five ounce glass of 12% alcohol; for beer a 12 ounce can or bottle of 4.5% alcohol; for distilled ("hard") liquor it is a 1.5 ounce glass of 80 proof or 40% alcohol. You may not increase your alcohol intake beyond "moderate" if you want to reap its health benefits.

Since women and men process alcohol differently and since women usually weigh less than men, the recommended amount of alcohol for heart health differs by gender. Men should limit themselves to 2 drinks per day; women to one.

How does alcohol contribute to heart health? Alcohol's anti-inflammatory properties probably act on the lining of blood vessels (endothelial tissue) helping to keep them atherosclerosis-free. Alcohol's anti-inflammatory effect probably comes into play to explain how it decreases the *C-reactive protein*, a *risk factor* for heart disease.

In addition, alcohol raises the HDL ("good") cholesterol and lowers the LDL ("bad") cholesterol levels in your blood. Alcohol also improves your blood sugar control by decreasing insulin resistance. And if that isn't enough, alcohol acts to decrease platelet stickiness thereby helping to keep your blood flowing. And all this is not even mentioning alcohol's effect on lowering psychological stress.

Although the same heart healthy protective effects have been found with all types of wine, beer, vodka, gin, bourbon, and scotch, it is my recommendation to drink one glass of red wine every day.

Drinking red wine delivers not only the protective effects of alcohol in general, but also the antioxidant phytochemical *resveratrol*. This may help to explain why wine drinkers tend to have less dementia than non-wine drinkers.

Of course my recommendation does not apply to persons who are in danger of alcohol abuse or who have liver damage from any cause. Nondrinkers are not encouraged to begin drinking for health reasons unless they have diabetes or heart disease or 2 or more *risk factors* for heart disease.

Women who have (or had) breast cancer themselves or who have a family history of breast cancer probably should not use alcohol for heart health because of the slight increase in risk for breast cancer associated with even "light" alcohol use.

> **Remember:** Many prescription drugs have the potential to interact with alcohol. If you or your family member is taking any prescription medication, it is necessary to talk with your physician before beginning a program of using alcohol for heart health.

Amino acids

Your body requires 20 *amino acids* to build more than 50,000 different proteins. Your liver manufactures 11 of them, called non-essential *amino acids*. The 9 others, essential *amino acids* are obtained from plant and animal foods in your diet. It is highly unlikely that you have an *amino acid* deficiency, especially if you eat a healthy diet.

Deficiency or not, *amino acid* supplements are being used to prevent and treat congestive heart failure (*taurine*), prevent and treat hypertension (*arginine*), augment the immune system (*glutamine*), decrease anxiety and calm nervous people (*theanine*), prevent recurrent herpes simplex infections (*lysine*), increase muscle mass (*glutamine*), increase libido (*arginine*), and to treat insomnia and depression (*5HTP*).

> **Note:** *Glutamine*'s beneficial effect on the immune system makes it a leading choice for supplementation in persons who have suffered serious burns. *Glutamine* is the most abundant amino acid in all your body's proteins.

Glutamine helps to maintain and increase muscle mass.

Note: *Arginine* has been shown to increase levels of *nitric oxide*, a chemical that keeps your arteries supple so that blood keeps flowing, thus reducing blood pressure. *Arginine* increases the blood flow through the coronary arteries of the heart. *Arginine* supplements help people with cardiovascular disease to exercise more. *Arginine*, as a topical preparation, has been used in diabetics to improve blood flow to their toes and feet. The dose is 2-3 grams daily.

Note: *Arginine* is required for the synthesis of growth hormone in your body so that some people take *arginine* supplements in an effort (albeit misguided) to stave off the aging process. And some sports-minded people take *arginine* supplements to stimulate muscle production. However, *arginine's* effect on sports performance may be due to its connection to creatine synthesis. When used to treat erectile dysfunction, the dose is 2-3 grams daily.

Note: *Theanine* (in the form of *L-theanine*), an *amino acid* derived from the leaves of the tea plant, *Camellia sinensis*, may be used for stress relief. The dosage is 100-400mg daily. But *theanine* has additional actions far beyond calming anxieties. Conventional chemotherapeutic drugs become more effective tumor killers when *theanine* is given too.

Note: The *amino acid tryptophan* is important in brain chemistry because once in the body, it is converted to *5-hydroxytryptophan (5-HTP)*, which is then used to manufacture *serotonin*, the neurotransmitter that affects eating, mood, and depression. The dose is usually 400mg daily.

Note: *Carnosine* is comprised of the *amino acids alanine* and *histadine*. *Carnosine* is present in highest concen-

tration in the brain. It is an antioxidant, protective against damage caused by free radicals. The dose is 500-1000mg daily.

However, some researchers claim that using one or another *amino acid* in large amounts (as in supplements) may create an unbalance and confound protein synthesis in your body. Since the long-term effects of taking *amino acid* supplements are not known, my recommendation is to get your *amino acids* by healthy proteins in food alone and to foreswear *amino acid* supplements.

Note: An exception to relying on healthy foods alone would be taking the amino acid *lysine* as a nutritional supplement. *Lysine* can help to prevent recurrent cold sores that are caused by the herpes virus. Take 500-1000mg of *lysine* daily. There are no significant side effects with long-term use.

Note: *Liquid Aminos* by Bragg is a tasty way to put extra *amino acids* into your daily nutritional program. *Liquid Aminos* is a low sodium (110mg in one-half teaspoon) substitute for soy sauce or tamari. Sprinkle a few drops onto salads, vegetables, stir-frys, tofu and tempeh or add to soups, sauces, rice and beans. It contains these 16 essential and non-essential *amino acids*: *alanine, arginine, aspartic acid, glutamic acid, glycine, histadine, isoleucine, lysine, leucine, methionine, phenylalanine, proline, serine, threonine, tyrosine* and *valine* in naturally occurring amounts. You can contact Bragg at 1-800-446-1990 or www.bragg.com.

Note: HeartBar is a popular soy-based nutritional bar containing *arginine*. Despite the implications of its name, I recommend that you get your *arginine* from a heart healthy diet, especially nuts, poultry, low-fat dairy, and fish.

L-carnitine

L-carnitine is produced inside your liver and kidneys from the *amino acids lysine* and *methionine*. It is considered a "conditionally essential nutrient" because your need may outstrip the supply you are able to naturally synthesize. Under those conditions, you will utilize *L-carnitine* found abundantly in animal and dairy products as well as in some plants like avocados and wheat germ.

L-carnitine is mostly found inside muscles, especially the heart muscle. *L-carnitine* is necessary for optimal functioning of mitochondria, the factories inside our cells that convert glucose and fatty acids into energy in the form of *adenosine triphosphate* (*ATP*). It works in the heart muscle to bring long-chain fatty acids inside cells into the mitochondria where they are oxidized to provide energy.

L-carnitine is sometimes used to augment weight loss since it helps to mobilize fats to be used as an energy source. *L-carnitine* may decrease fatigue and post-exertional fatigue. For this reason, it may be useful as a treatment for chronic fatigue syndrome. *L-carnitine* may increase athletic performance and endurance by preventing the accumulation of lactic acid in muscles. In persons with diabetic neuropathy *L-carnitine* not only decreases pain but also promotes nerve fiber myelination. *L-carnitine*, naturally highly concentrated in the epididymis, may have an effect on male fertility by increasing sperm count, morphology, and motility. It may also have an effect on sperm DNA integrity.

Taking supplements of *L-carnitine* (or the related compound *acetyl-L-carnitine*) may improve the strength of your heart muscle, decrease anginal episodes, and may help to normalize your heartbeat.

> **Note:** Some medical researchers believe that *L-carnitine* may act to prevent structural damage of mitochondria in the heart.

> **Note:** *Carnitine* is the term for a family of compounds that include *L-carnitine* and *acetyl-L-carnitine*. However, once absorbed into the body, *acetyl-L-carnitine* rapidly loses its acetyl group and becomes *L-carnitine*, the biologically active chemical. *Acetyl-L-carnitine* has

been shown to slow the decline in cognitive function in patients with Alzheimer's disease.

> **Note:** The combination of *L-carnitine* 500mg twice daily along with *alpha-lipoic acid* 200mg twice daily is considered by some nutritional experts to be a natural anti-aging remedy. You may buy these 2 supplements separately or together as *Weil Juvenon*. Take one capsule of *Weil Juvenon* twice daily with meals. Each capsule contains 500mg of *acetyl-L-carnitine* and 200mg of *alpha-lipoic acid*.

For persons with congestive heart failure, the dose of *L-carnitine* is 500-2,000mg/day. However, some medical studies showing positive results used 4 grams per day. Side effects are infrequent, and usually limited to the gastrointestinal system with abdominal cramps, diarrhea, nausea and vomiting. In persons suffering from heart disease, *L-carnitine* is often used together with *Coenzyme Q10* and *alpha-lipoic acid*.

> **Note:** The level of *C-reactive protein* (*CRP*) in your blood is being used as a marker for the level of inflammation going on in various organs inside your body. A higher than normal level of *CRP* (normal is less than 3.00mg/L) indicates a higher than normal risk for certain diseases, especially heart disease, stroke, and Alzheimer's disease. Since *L-carnitine* supplements tend to lower *CRP*, this may be the means by which it lowers the risk for heart disease.

Coenzyme Q10

The fat-soluble antioxidant *Coenzyme Q10* (also called *CoQ10* and *ubiquinone*) is found in every cell in your body. It is manufactured inside your body, but the amount declines with increasing age, one reason why *Coenzyme Q10* supplements are sometimes useful.

Coenzyme Q10 is involved in energy production within mitochondria. All enzymes (except one) involved in mitochondrial energy production require *Coenzyme Q10* as the coenzyme. The amount of *Coenzyme Q10* is especially high in heart muscle cells. It has a direct stimulatory action on heart muscle, helping the heart to contract more strongly and efficiently. This is the reason *Coenzyme Q10* supplements are useful in treating congestive heart failure.

Coenzyme Q10 also stabilizes the heart's electrical conduction system which is why *Coenzyme Q10* supplements may be useful in treating arrhythmias. In addition, *Coenzyme Q10* has been shown to increase HDL cholesterol and to lower fasting blood glucose. *Coenzyme Q10* supplements are sometimes used to treat persons with type 2 diabetes mellitus, making them more sensitive to the actions of insulin.

Coenzyme Q10 supplements are also used to treat males with infertility. *Coenzyme Q10* supplements are being used to treat persons who have the very rare diseases of mitochondrial dysfunction. These are "newer" diseases that we are just now "discovering." *Coenzyme Q10* may help to heal periodontal disease.

One proven and particularly important use of *Coenzyme Q10* supplements is to protect the heart from oxidative damage of chemotherapy during and after treatment for cancer.

> **Note:** *Coenzyme Q10* supplements are never used during treatment with the chemotherapeutic agent *adriamycin*; however, it can be safely used afterwards.

Foods containing *Coenzyme Q10* include: meats, nuts, spinach, broccoli, and fish. The dose of *Coenzyme Q10* supplements is 50-150mg/day although 200-300mg/day is sometimes used for more severe heart disease, especially congestive heart failure.

The *Coenzyme Q10* dose to treat Parkinson's disease is 2mg per kilogram of body weight daily. *Coenzyme Q10* supplements have been shown to be more effective when given early in the disease. Using *Coenzyme Q10* to treat Parkinson's disease must be supervised by a physician.

Side effects of *Coenzyme Q10* supplements are mild. Most of the side effects are concerned with the gastrointestinal system, such as abdominal pain, nausea, and vomiting. Even though *Coenzyme Q10*

supplements are considered safe for use during pregnancy and lactation, I recommend that you refrain from self-care with *Coenzyme Q10* supplements during those lifecycles. If you are pregnant or breastfeeding please consult your physician or homeopath before taking *Coenzyme Q10* supplements.

Coenzyme Q10 supplements may interact with the anticoagulant *warfarin* (*Coumadin*). If you or your family member is currently taking any blood thinner prescription medication, please consult with your physician before starting *Coenzyme Q10* supplements.

"Statins" act to lower blood cholesterol by interfering with the enzyme ordinarily required in its manufacture inside the body. Unfortunately, "statins" also interfere with the production of *Coenzyme Q10* inside cells. One of the side effects of "statin" drugs is the depletion of *Coenzyme Q10* levels inside your cells. Persons taking "statin" prescription drugs should consider taking *Coenzyme Q10* supplements.

Enzymes

The function of *enzymes* is to speed up biochemical processes. *Enzymes* control every chemical reaction in your body. They are essential for life. Our bodies utilize more than 3,000 different *enzymes*, each one manufactured according to instructions from your DNA, and each one doing a specific job.

Some *enzymes* come from the pancreas, such as *amylase* (breaks down starch), *lipase* (breaks down fats) and *protease* (breaks down proteins). Other *enzymes* are important in digesting proteins, such as *trypsin* and *chymotrypsin*. *Bromelain* (derived from the pineapple) and *papain* (from the papaya fruit) are *enzymes* that are useful as anti-inflammatory agents.

Oral *enzyme* therapy has been used extensively in Europe, less so here in America, to modulate the effects of inflammation, primarily by regulating anti-inflammatory *cytokines*. Some medical researchers believe that the basis for most cardiovascular disease is inflammation. The *risk factor* for heart disease, *C-reactive protein* is one of the markers of inflammation in the heart. Some alternative medicine providers have been using "systemic oral *enzyme* supplements" as anti-inflammatory agents for many different diseases, including heart disease, arthritis, and cancer. The mechanism by which systemic *enzymes* act may be to break down immune proteins in the blood into harmless chemicals that no longer stimulate the immune response.

One of the most commonly prescribed and widely available systemic pancreatic enzyme supplements is *Wobenzym N* at a dosage of 2 tablets 3 times daily or 3 tablets twice daily.

> **Note:** Systemic pancreatic *enzyme* supplements are not for use by persons with hemophilia, persons taking anticoagulant therapy, or after heart surgery when there is an increased risk of bleeding.

> **Note:** You must take your systemic pancreatic *enzyme* supplements at least 30 minutes before a meal. If you take them with your meal, they will act simply as digestive enzymes, rather than as anti-inflammatory agents.

Fiber

Fiber is the part of plants (vegetables, fruits, nuts, seeds, legumes and whole grains) that give them structure and shape. Once we eat fiber it is not absorbed into our blood stream because our digestive enzymes cannot break it down. Rather, *fiber* remains inside our intestines, forming the bulk of our stool.

Fiber comes in two types, soluble and insoluble. Both types have health benefits, albeit different ones. Insoluble *fiber*, or roughage, is composed of cellulose, hemicellulose, and lignin, those chemical compounds that give plant cell walls their structure. The function of insoluble *fiber* is to move waste material along inside your intestines. Insoluble *fiber* is essential for regular, bulky bowel movements. Too little insoluble *fiber* in your diet can end up causing constipation, hemorrhoids, and diverticulosis. A deficiency of *fiber* is also associated with irritable bowel syndrome. Insoluble fiber is found in nuts, wheat bran, fruits and vegetables.

Soluble *fiber*, on the other hand, dissolves in water, thickening the water and becoming sticky. Soluble *fiber* binds to fats (including cholesterol) in

your intestines, pushing them along towards elimination rather than absorption. This is the reason why increasing soluble *fiber* in your diet has been shown to lower total cholesterol and LDL cholesterol. Soluble *fiber* is found in guar gum, *pectin*, oat bran, rice bran, barley, fruits, and legumes as well as in the herb *Psyllium*. The soluble *fiber* found in oat bran and barley is called *beta glucan*.

> **Note:** *Glucomannan* or *Konjac* (from *Amorphophallus konjac*) is another soluble fiber source, most often used as a weight loss supplement. Please read about it in **Chapter 26: Nutritional Supplements for Healthy Weight Control**.

Many plant foods contain both soluble and insoluble *fiber*, such as legumes (including all types of beans, peanuts and green peas), dried fruits, whole grains and fresh vegetables. Flaxseed not only contains both types of *fiber*, but is also rich in *omega-3 fatty acids* and antioxidants called *lignans*, a type of phytoestrogen. Flaxseeds are available as the whole seed (providing fiber for intestinal health, a natural mild laxative), seeds ground into meal, or as sprouted flaxseeds. Flaxseed oil is also available, but it does not contain *lignans*. Flaxseed oil is a rich source of *omega-3 fatty acids*. Adding whole or ground flaxseeds to your daily diet is a good way to get many health benefits.

> **Note:** *Lignans* in flaxseeds may help to prevent breast cancer in those who have never had it. But, if you or your family member is being treated for breast cancer (or any other hormone-dependent cancer like prostate), you should avoid the *lignans* in flaxseeds. It is a good idea to follow the same recommendation if you are pregnant or lactating or if you are trying to become pregnant. The whole grain rye fiber also contains lignans.

Persons with high blood lipids (hypercholesterolemia) as well as persons interested in preventing cardiovascular disease, promoting weight loss and weight control and controlling diabetes, should consider eating a high *fiber* diet combined with low saturated fats from animal sources. Soluble *fiber* products such as *RiSolubles* made by NutraCea contain rice bran derivatives which have been proven to stabilize blood glucose levels and reduce the need for diabetes medications.

> **Note:** Increasing dietary fiber was of no benefit in preventing colon cancer in a study done by the Harvard School of Public Health. Since this is such a surprising finding, contrary to many other studies, it will have to be duplicated in other studies before the truth in the association between fiber intake and colon cancer is known.

If you or your family member wants to take a soluble *fiber* supplement for bowel regularity, a good choice is *Psyllium*. A popular choice of *Psyllium* is *Metamucil*, made by Procter and Gamble. *Metamucil* comes in capsules, powder, granules, and wafers. Another insoluble fiber product called *RiceMucil* by NutraCea promotes colon health.

But, if you wish to take a soluble *fiber* supplement for cardiovascular health, a good choice is *oat bran*, taking as much as 6 grams per day. Several different individual soluble *fiber* remedies are available such as *guar gum* (in a dissolvable supplement called *Benefiber*), *apple pectin* and *grapefruit pectin*.

A popular combination soluble *fiber* choice is *ProFibe*, made from *guar gum* and *citrus pectin*. The dose of *ProFibe* is one level tablespoon scoop in 10 ounces of water (or any liquid) three times a day. You will get 6 grams of soluble *fiber* per serving. Some people complain of increased gas (flatulence) which can be overcome by beginning slowly and increasing to the recommended amount after one week.

Fiber Force-6 is a popular product by The Vitamin Shoppe. It contains: *oat bran, apple pectin, prune, lactobacillus, rice bran, citrus fiber, Psyllium* and *soy fiber* along with several vegetable extracts. The dose is 3-6 capsules daily, with 8 ounces of water, taken at mealtimes.

Another combination *fiber* product is *Multiple Fiber Formula* by Solgar. It contains: *oat bran, apple pectin, grapefruit pectin, flaxseed meal* and *Psyllium seed husks*. The dose is 2-6 capsules daily, with 8 ounces of water, distributed throughout the day.

The National Cholesterol Education Program recommends that adults eat 20-30 gm/day of total *fiber*. The dose of soluble *fiber* is 10-15 gm/day.

> **Remember:** *Fiber* itself does not add any calories to your nutritional program because it is not absorbed. Persons on weight loss and weight control diets should consider taking a *fiber* supplement because of the beneficial effects on blood sugar and lipids along with the increase in feelings of fullness (satiety).

> **Remember:** When choosing carbohydrates for your family, choose whole grains. Whole grains contain *fiber* and this makes them have a lower *glycemic index* compared to refined grains. The *fiber* slows down the absorption of the carbohydrate portion of the whole grain. This means that your blood glucose level will rise more slowly. This means that smaller amounts of insulin will be needed to keep your blood glucose level steady. Your pancreas will thank you. And so will your health insurance company.

> **Note:** The *glycemic index* is a ranking of foods, from zero, the lowest and healthiest to 100, the highest and least healthy, on the basis of how high they increase your blood sugar and how much insulin is secreted from your pancreas in order to get that blood sugar back into the normal range. A score of high on the *glycemic index* is 70 or more; medium is 56-69; low is 55 or less.

Following a diet based on the *glycemic index* can help people lose weight. For people with type 2 diabetes mellitus a *glycemic index*-based diet can help to stabilize blood sugar levels and decrease the need for diabetes prescription medications. A listing of common carbohydrate-containing foods and their *glycemic indexes* can be found in *The South Beach Diet* and *Eat, Drink, and Be Healthy*. Or you can go to www.glycemicindex.com and www.southbeachdiet.com.

To help you know where different foods fall on the *glycemic index* scale here are two rules-of-thumb: 1) whole foods are lower while refined foods are higher; and 2) foods high in *fiber* are lower on the scale because they convert their carbohydrates into slow-release carbohydrates. For example, the *glycemic index* of white rice is 72 (high) while that of the whole grain brown rice is 54 (low).

Guggulipid

Guggulipid (also spelled *gugulipid*) is derived from the myrrh tree, *Commiphora mukul*, an herb used in Ayurvedic medicine. *Guggulipid* has been used to lower LDL ("bad") cholesterol while at the same time raising HDL ("good") cholesterol. A recent study by medical researchers at the University of Pennsylvania found that *guggulipid* surprisingly had the opposite effect on blood lipids, resulting in a non-healthy change.

However, this same study showed that *guggulipid* decreased *C-reactive protein*, a *risk factor* (please see above) for cardiovascular disease (and for inflammation, in general) by almost 30%. This is a healthy change.

For persons who want to decrease their *C-reactive protein* by taking a *guggulipid* supplement, the dose is 500mg tablets of *guggulipid*, one tablet three times a day, but going up to as much as 3,000-6,000mg total per day.

For persons who want to lower cholesterol, there are more effective products than *guggulipid*, such as *fiber, policosanol* and *red yeast rice*. Persons who suffer from liver disease, thyroid disease, or inflammatory bowel disease should not take *guggulipid*.

Horse chestnut

The herbal remedy *Horse chestnut* seed extract (*Aesculus hippocastanum*) is sometimes used to treat chronic venous insufficiency and varicose veins. *Horse chestnut* seed extract acts to strengthen capillaries and veins. It was found to be as effective as compression stockings in one medical research study.

The dose is 500-600mg twice daily of *horse chestnut* seed extract standardized to 16-20% of *escin* (or *aescin*), the active ingredient. Side effects are minor, mostly headache, stomach upset and nausea.

Although short-term use of *horse chestnut* seed extract is generally safe, the safety of long-term use has not been established.

Phytosterols

Phytosterols are a group of compounds from plants that contain *sterols* and *stanols* that interfere with the absorption of cholesterol from the intestines. *Phytosterols* can lower LDL ("bad") cholesterol by about 10%, but they do not effect HDL ("good") cholesterol or triglycerides. Newer spreads, such as *Benecol, Take Control, OmegaPlus* and *Smart Balance* contain *phytosterols* (nevertheless they are still called margarine). If your own or a family member's total cholesterol is elevated, it is a good idea to use one of these products as a spread on bread or potatoes rather than either margarine or butter. Buy the "Lite" variety to reduce calories. *Phytosterols* are also present in *Heart Wise* a new orange juice by *Minute Maid*. If you prefer to take your plant *sterols* and *stanols* in capsule form, Nature Made makes *Cholest-Off*, containing 900mg in two caplets, to be taken twice daily, for 1-8 grams/day, optimally, 30 minutes before eating. *Phytosterols* may be taken with "statin" drugs. The *National Cholesterol Education Program* (*NCEP*) recommends 2000mg of *phytosterols* daily to lower LDL cholesterol.

Phytosterols are also useful to enhance your immune system. This feature makes them powerful allies in the quest to prevent cancer and other immune system diseases. Nuts and seeds contain phytosterols in relatively large amounts, as do peanuts, the legume that shares many characteristics with nuts. However, you must always balance the healthy choice of nuts, seeds, and peanuts with their caloric density. Remembering portion size will help to keep you in balance.

Note: A specific *phytosterol, beta-sitosterol*, lowers cholesterol. *Beta-sitosterol* is found naturally in high concentration in avocados, nuts, and amaranth (a whole grain). *Beta-sitosterol* also has been found to decrease urinary symptoms stemming from prostate enlargement as well as interfering with the growth of prostate cancer cells. It is likely that it will soon be added to herbal formulations that include: *Saw palmetto, Pygeum* and *Stinging nettle*. *Beta-sitosterol* as a nutritional supplement is available as part of a complex of *phytosterols*. Follow the dosage directions on the bottle.

Policosanol

Policosanol is a compound that is extracted from the outer waxy layers of the sugar cane plant and widely used as a lipid lowering medicine in Cuba. It is becoming more popular in the U.S. *Policosanol* has been found in large, double-blind medical research studies to have the ability to lower total cholesterol, LDL cholesterol, and triglycerides, while raising HDL cholesterol. Some studies comparing *policosanol* to "statin" drugs proved that *policosanol* was as effective as the "statin" drug in changing blood lipids. In addition, patients taking *policosanol* had decreased blood pressure, decreased angina episodes, and less electrocardiogram changes during stress testing than controls. *Policosanol* also helps with vascular insufficiency called intermittent claudication (hardening of the arteries of the legs).

The mechanism of action of policosanol is *probably* the slowing down of the manufacture of cholesterol by the liver. In addition, *policosanol* has a significant anticoagulant effect, similar to *aspirin*'s antiplatelet effect, which is beneficial to your cardiovascular health.

The dose of *policosanol* is 10-20mg/day in 2 divided doses. There are no significant side effects associated with *policosanol* supplement use. The minor side effect of weight loss may actually be beneficial to some people who are trying to lower their blood cholesterols.

Even though no toxic effects were found in pregnant rabbits and rats or their offspring, the safety of *policosanol* use during pregnancy and lactation is not established, especially considering its antiplatelet action. If you use *aspirin* to protect against heart attack, you should use caution when combining with *policosanol*.

> **Remember:** Anticoagulant effects of herbal and nutritional supplements are additive. *Ginkgo biloba, garlic, policosanol*, Vitamin E, and *aspirin* all have similar anticoagulant-antiplatelet

effects. If you or your family member is using some of these supplements in combination, you should be under the supervision of a physician.

Note: Only *policosanol* made from sugar cane has been evaluated in large, double-blind medical research studies. We need to develop the same information on *policosanol* made from beeswax, yams, and brown rice bran. Although *policosanol* made from those plants and *octacosanol* (the active ingredient) alone are being used extensively in the U.S., they may not produce the same lipid-lowering results with the same safety record. *Policosanol* from sugar cane is found in Biotic Research Corporation's product, *PCOH-Plus*.

Red yeast rice

Red yeast rice is a strain of yeast called *Monascus purpureus*, grown on rice and causing a red color. Then the rice together with the yeast are pulverized into a powder. *Red yeast rice* is a remedy in Traditional Chinese Medicine.

Red yeast rice has the ability to lower total and LDL cholesterol but it does not raise HDL cholesterol. It is chemically the same as the "statin" drug *lovastatin* (*Mevacor*) and similar to other "statin" drugs. Therefore, you should not eat grapefruits or drink grapefruit juice if you take *red yeast rice* supplements. *Red yeast rice* should not be used together with "statin" drugs.

Red yeast rice, in contradistinction to "statin" drugs, also contains antioxidants (*isoflavones*) and plant *sterols*, compounds that promote heart health. *Red yeast rice* comes in 600mg capsules. The dose is 2 capsules twice daily. Side effects of *red yeast rice* are mild, including dizziness, heartburn, and abdominal gas. *Red yeast rice* should not be used by people who are allergic to rice or yeast. *Red yeast rice* should not be used during pregnancy or lactation. Do not take *red yeast rice* if you are taking a "statin" prescription medication. Do not mix grapefruits or grapefruit juice with *red yeast rice*.

Guidelines for Consulting Your Health Care Provider

You should consult your health care provider if:
- the patient doesn't look right or act right (trust your instincts!)
- the patient is getting worse instead of better over the course of the illness
- the patient is having trouble breathing or complaining of chest pains or there is mental confusion or lethargy or irritability
- the patient develops allergic symptoms (hives, itchy or watery eyes, runny nose, scratchy throat, asthma, shortness of breath) after taking a nutritional supplement
- after beginning a nutritional supplement the patient experiences *new onset* of any serious symptoms such as:

  paralysis, weakness, tingling, inability to focus or concentrate, blurred or double vision or blindness, slurred speech, severe headaches, seizures, irritability, dizziness, disorientation, memory loss, anxiety, depression, insomnia, blackouts, fainting, or the person complains of not feeling like himself

- the patient is taking *ANY* prescription medication
- the patient is pregnant or breastfeeding
- the patient has any serious, chronic disease which may have complications and become life-threatening, such as:

  autism, cancer, HIV and AIDS, arthritis, multiple sclerosis, coronary artery disease, heart attack (myocardial infarction), blood dyscrasia, cancer (of any type), congestive heart failure, diabetes mellitus, obesity, thyroid disorders, high blood pressure (hypertension), stroke, seizures, acute and chronic kidney (renal) failure, schizophrenia, bipolar disorder, borderline personality disorder, eating disorders, fibromyalgia, chronic fatigue syndrome, Crohn's disease, ulcerative colitis, celiac disease, mental deficiency disorders, chromosomal disorders, infertility, frequent miscarriages, polyneuropathy, cystic fibrosis   [Adapted from *The Merck Manual* at www.merck.com]

Note: Do not discontinue taking any pharmaceutical medication prescribed by your health care provider unless you or your family member is under the supervision of a physician.

Note: Do not take any heart healthy nutritional supplement without first consulting your health care provider if you or your family member is taking a prescription medication for one of the cardiovascular diseases or is pregnant or breastfeeding.

In addition, it is a good idea to check with your health care provider if your family member is either very young or very old because heart healthy nutritional supplements given injudiciously may overwhelm the body's defenses in those age groups.

Remember: Many prescription drugs have the potential to interact with alcohol. If you or your family member is taking any prescription medication, it is necessary to talk with your physician before beginning a program of using alcohol for heart health.

Remember: Anticoagulant effects of herbal and nutritional supplements are additive. *Ginkgo biloba, garlic, policosanol*, Vitamin E, and *aspirin* all have similar anticoagulant-antiplatelet effects. If you or your family member is using some of these supplements in combination, you should be under the supervision of a physician.

Note: Grapefruits and grapefruit juice (and also tangelos, Seville oranges, and limes) contain chemicals (furanocoumarins) that interfere with the metabolism of certain commonly prescribed pharmaceuticals. The result is to potentiate their actions in the body which may result in toxic side effects. Do not eat grapefruits or drink grapefruit juice if you are taking any of the following drugs: *astemizole* (*Hismanal*, an antihistamine); cholesterol-lowering drugs such as *Zocar* and *Lipitor* ("statins"); estrogens, caffeine, *saquinavir* (*Invirase*, for HIV infection); immunosuppressants *cyclosporine* (*Sandimmune*) and *tacrolimus* (*Prograf*); *alprazolam* (*Xanax*) and *triazolam* (*Halcion*); calcium channel blockers *felodipine* (*Plendil*), *nifedipine* (*Adalat, Procardia*), *nimodipine* (*Nimotop*) and *verapamil* (*Calan, Isoptin, Verlan*); *cisapride* (*Propusid*); and *cilostazol* (*Pletal*). If you are taking *red yeast rice* it is a good idea to forego grapefruits and grapefruit juice as well because the active ingredient is a "statin."

Recommendation: *CholestSure* by DaVinci Laboratories contains (in 3 tablets) *Red Yeast Rice* (600mg), *Policosanols* from sugar cane (20mg), *Phytosterols Complex* from soy (500mg), *Coenzyme Q10* (20mg), *Guggul lipids* (200mg), along with *chromium, artichoke leaf extract* and *Eicosapentaenoic Acid* (*EPA*) (180mg).

Putting It All Together

If you are considering using a *heart healthy* nutritional supplement, it is a good idea to familiarize yourself with **Chapter 2: Introduction to Nutritional Supplements**. It makes good sense to understand the role of vitamin or mineral nutritional supplements from **Chapter 23: Vitamins and Minerals**, especially Vitamins B6, B12, and folate as low levels of these vitamins increase *homocysteine*, a chemical that increases the risk for heart disease. Vitamin E is also important in protection from cardiovascular disease.

You will likely want to become familiar with *antioxidant* nutritional supplements from **Chapter 24: Antioxidant Phytochemicals: Natural Anti-Aging Remedies** (for *alpha-lipoic acid, grape seed extract, flavonoids, anthocyanins* and *proanthocyanidins*). You will also want to know about fish oil (*omega-3 fatty acids*) and heart healthy spreads (please see **Chapter 31: Oils and Fats**).

Whenever you have decided to go ahead with a *heart healthy* nutritional supplement, it is a good idea to consider giving the sick person's homeopathic constitutional remedy as well (please refer to **Chapter 9: Homeopathic Remedies for Constitutional Problems in Infants, Children, and Adolescents** or to **Chapter 18: Homeopathic Constitutional Remedies** if you are dealing with an adult; or **Chapter 13: Homeopathy for Elderly Persons** if you are dealing with an elderly person).

Please take a look at **Chapter 20: Herbs You Need to Know** and familiarize yourself with the herbal remedies *Hawthorn, Green tea, Garlic* and *Psyllium*.

Chronic inflammation underlies cardiovascular disease. So it is a good idea to consider nutritional remedies that regulate inflammation. You may want to consider medicinal *mushrooms* (please refer to **Chapter 27: Nutritional Supplements to Prevent Cancer and Augment Your Immune System**). In addition, investigate *prebiotics* and *probiotics* to enhance the immune system (please refer to **Chapter 30: Prebiotics and Probiotics**).

Chapter 26

Nutritional Supplements for Healthy Weight Control

Healthy Weight Loss and Weight Control in General

Ailment/Disorder/Symptom	Nutritional Supplement
Blood sugar and insulin resistance control	*Banaba leaf*
Body fat mass	*Conjugated linoleic acid (CLA)*
Enhance libido and blood sugar control	*Fenugreek*
Obesity, heart and skin diseases	*Forskolin*
Fat storage prevention	*Garcinia cambogia*
Blood sugar control	*Glucomannan*
Lean muscle mass	*L-Glutamine*
Blood sugar control	*Gymnema sylvestre*
Cravings for sweets	*Low carb bars*
Carbohydrate absorption	*Phaseolus vulgaris*
Lean muscle mass	*Pyruvate*
Muscle performance	*Rhodiola*
Blood sugar control	*Vanadium*
Appetite suppressant, increasing feelings of fullness	*Yerba mate*

Guidelines for Consulting Your Health Care Provider
Putting It All Together

Healthy Weight Loss and Weight Control in General

A rational approach to weight loss and weight control is to conquer the elements of healthy diet and exercise before beginning nutritional supplements. Some of the readily available information on diet (better called daily nutritional program) is confusing and some of it may actually be harmful in the long run.

A good place to start is to gather some of the tools necessary to be able to guide yourself and your family through healthy changes in eating. *Fat Land—How Americans Became the Fattest People in the World* by Greg Critser, published by Houghton Mifflin in 2003, provides background material and motivation for changing your family's eating choices.

> **Note:** Greg Critser wrote another book in 2005, called *Generation Rx How Prescription Drugs Are Altering American Lives, Minds, and Bodies*. This one is about how the American public has allowed itself to become chemically "improved," indeed drugged, by "Big Pharma."

If you are interested in a book on proper nutrition for our times, I strongly recommend *Eat, Drink, and Be Healthy*, authored by Walter C. Willett, published by Simon and Schuster in 2001. *Eat, Drink, and Be Healthy* will give you all the nutrition basics you need to make informed healthy choices for yourself and your family. It will introduce you to the *glycemic index*. Understanding the *glycemic index* and putting its concepts to work for you and your family is one of the most important things you could do for health. Dr. Willett presents his own *Food Guide Pyramid* based on current nutritional thinking.

> **Note:** The USDA's *Dietary Guidelines for Americans* is revised every five years to reflect advances in nutritional science. The *Guidelines* in turn are the basis for the *Food Guide Pyramid* which is just a tool to concretize the *Guidelines*. The new 2005 version, nicknamed

MyPyramid, encourages daily physical activity (for 30-90 minutes every day) and makes it clear that weight loss results from fewer calories taken in while more calories are expended. The number of daily servings of fruits and vegetables have increased from five to nine. Whole grains are encouraged (for the first time!) over refined grains. Three portions of dairy is specified daily. Several issues are not dealt with in a definitive manner: limiting *trans fats* to 1% of total calories and setting limits on added sugar. You may read the *Guidelines* free online at www.healthierus.gov/dietaryguidelines. Or call 1-866-512-1899 to purchase the complete 80-page report (costs $12). Please visit www.mypyramid.gov and for kids at www.mypyramid.gov/kids and for Spanish at www.mypyramid.gov/sp-index.html.

> **Note:** If you think that the USDA's *MyPyramid* is not helpful, then you may want to take a look at the *Healing Foods Pyramid* at www.med.umich.edu/umim/clinical/pyramid. The base of this pyramid is water, which is the basis of life itself. The entire pyramid is made up of foods that promote health. The apex of the pyramid is called "personal space," giving you someplace to insert the foods that are healthy and healing for you. Each level of the pyramid is color-coded to indicate daily (blue), weekly (yellow), and optional (red). Unfortunately, this pyramid does not include physical exercise, which should be at the base, along side water.

Another basic book is the *American Dietetic Association Complete Food and Nutrition Guide*, 2nd edition, by R. I. Duff, published by John Wiley & Sons in 2002. This easily read book is written in a friendly manner. The book has well-written chapters about everything you might want to know about nutrition from infancy on up. The book's main deficiencies are: 1) it endorses, indeed extols, the USDA *Food Guide Pyramid* instead of Dr. Walter Willett's more up-to-date pyramid which takes into account healthy fats and whole grains; and 2) it glosses over the problems with sugar, our sugar-centered culture, and our pervasive sugar-based foods.

Note: *The South Beach Diet* by Dr. Arthur Agatston, published by Rodale in 2003 has helped some people lose weight and keep it off. *The South Beach Diet* is a low-carbohydrate, high-protein diet, heart-healthier than the *Atkin's Diet*. *The South Beach Diet* teaches you about healthy carbohydrate choices based on the *glycemic index*.

Note: *The South Beach Diet* has its critics who point out that it contains elements that have not been proven in a scientific manner as well as inconsistencies. However, low-carb diets may be a healthy way to lose weight in the short-term. It is not yet known if a low-carb lifestyle for the long-term will turn out to be healthy and help you not to regain the weight. Some medical researchers stress that there is little evidence to support low-carb diets. They tend to believe that "a calorie is a calorie," meaning that the only healthy way to lose weight is to reduce caloric intake and increase energy output by physical exercise.

Note: Some researchers believe that the added protein in low carb diets works to suppress appetite so the dieter consumes fewer total calories. The bottom line is the total number of calories consumed versus the total number of calories expended in physical activity.

Remember: Diets that exclude any one food group for the long-term are called fad diets. Fad dieting is not a healthy way to lose weight. Fad diets may be associated with quick weight loss and just as quick weight regain, usually to

an even higher set point (sometimes called yo-yo dieting). Unhealthy dieting is one of the main reasons why Americans have been getting steadily fatter and fatter over the last 4 decades.

The healthy way to lose weight is to decrease the amount of calories you eat every day by decreasing *portion size* (and making healthy food choices) while you increase the amount of physical exercise. Portion control and physical exercise are lifestyle changes that will help you to remain healthy throughout your entire lifetime. One of the best nutritional programs to help you readjust your food intake to proper *portion sizes* is *Weight Watchers*. You may contact *Weight Watchers* at www.Weight Watchers.com for online meetings and to find out about meetings in your community. To help you calculate how long it would take you to lose a certain amount of weight, please visit www.caloriesper-hour.com.

Note: Learn about the whole food family of whole grains for powerhouse nutrition at www.wholegrainscouncil. org. Eating whole grains give you vegetable protein, complex carbohydrates, minerals, vitamins, antioxidants, and fiber. Whole grains include: amaranth (actually a seed), barley, buckwheat (or groats) (which contains no wheat or gluten), bulgur (made from wheat kernels), millet, oats, quinoa, brown rice, wild rice, teff, rye, spelt, kamut and wheat berries. Quinoa was the food staple of the Incas. It is actually a seed so it delivers an all-over nutritional punch with high levels of amino acids, magnesium, potassium, vitamin E, B vitamins, copper and zinc. Barley comes pearled (processed for faster cooking) or hulled (contains more fiber). For more information visit www.wholegrainscouncil. org.

Note: General Mills converted all its breakfast cereals into whole grain. But, don't be lulled into believing that their *Brown Sugar and Oat Total* or *Honey Nut*

Cheerios are health foods! At this level of added sugar, it's like eating candy for breakfast. Try delicious and nutritional breakfast choices from unprocessed foods, like low-fat-no-sugar-added yogurt with fresh fruit, or microwaved oats with soy milk and fresh fruit.

Note: White whole wheat called *Ultragrain*, manufactured by ConAgra, is a newcomer in the grocery isles. It is added to whole wheat flour to make the product look and taste more like it contains white flour. But remember that *Ultragrain* flour is more processed than 100% whole wheat flour. *Glycemic index* results for *Ultragrain* are not yet available.

Refined or processed carbohydrates such as products made from white flour (pasta, white breads, baked goods, etc.) have no place in the short or long haul in any healthy diet. Unprocessed carbohydrates are healthy. These include whole grains, legumes, and most fruits. They are healthy because they are low on the *glycemic index*.

Note: The *glycemic index* is a ranking of foods, from zero, the lowest and healthiest to 100, the highest and least healthy, on the basis of how quickly they increase your blood sugar and how much insulin is secreted from your pancreas in order to get that blood sugar back into the normal range. A score of high on the *glycemic index* is 70 or more; medium is 56-69; low is 55 or less.

Following a diet based on the *glycemic index* may help people lose weight. For people with type 2 diabetes mellitus a *glycemic index*-based diet may help to stabilize blood sugar levels and decrease the need for diabetes prescription medications. A listing of common carbohydrate-containing foods and their *glycemic indexes* can be found in *The South Beach Diet* and *Eat, Drink, and Be Healthy*. Or you can go to www.

glycemicindex.com and www.south-beachdiet.com.

To help you know where different foods fall on the *glycemic index* scale here are two rules-of-thumb: 1) whole (unprocessed) foods are lower while refined foods are higher; and 2) foods high in *fiber* are lower on the scale because they convert their carbohydrates into slow-release carbohydrates. For example, the *glycemic index* of white rice is 72 (high) while that of the whole grain brown rice is 54 (low).

Note: All legumes (beans) are low-*glycemic index* foods. Tomatoes have a *glycemic index* of 15 which is one of the lowest of all foods.

Note: High-*glycemic index* diets are associated not only with insulin resistance and type 2 diabetes mellitus but also with the *metabolic syndrome*. The *metabolic syndrome* consists of a constellation of abnormalities in the blood which predispose to heart disease, diabetes, and other chronic diseases. These blood abnormalities are: high triglycerides, low HDL cholesterol, high LDL cholesterol, high fasting blood sugar, and high insulin (leading to the underlying abnormality, insulin resistance). Obesity and hypertension are two conditions commonly found together with the *metabolic syndrome*.

Note: People who have hypertension (high blood pressure) or prehypertension should examine the DASH diet at www.dashdiet.org.

Note: Another way to choose foods for yourself and your family is by their *energy density* (calories per gram). Foods with a higher *energy density* tend to hamper weight loss. Conversely, foods with a lower *energy density* tend to facilitate weight loss. Low *energy density* foods are also called big foods because they are increased in bulk from water and fiber. This figures into greater satisfaction and satiety. You can figure the *energy density* of foods by dividing the total calories by the number of grams. Low *energy density* foods contain up to 1.5 calories per gram. Medium *energy density* foods contain 1.5-4 calories per gram. Everything above 4 are high *energy density* foods.

Insulin from your pancreas quickly metabolizes simple carbohydrates (or "carbs") into sugar which your body uses for energy. The problem with simple carbohydrates comes when insulin converts the leftover sugar just as quickly into fat. And, that's not the end of the sad story. When the quick energy boost from those simple carbohydrates wears off, you start to feel hungry sooner, and this can cause you to grab high *energy density* snacks to satisfy your hunger. You can see how this is apt to cause weight gain. On the other hand, complex carbohydrates are converted into sugar more slowly and we do not feel hungry for a longer period of time. Besides that, complex carbohydrates offer more nutrition than just the carbohydrate portion. We get some fiber, vitamins, minerals, protein, and antioxidants at the same time.

Remember: Nutritional supplements and fast foods do not mix. When you decide to take nutritional supplements for yourself or for family members, it is also a commitment to stay away from fast foods. Fast foods are notoriously high in unhealthy fats, sugars, refined carbohydrates, and total calories, while being low in fiber, healthy fats, and whole, unprocessed foods. Fast foods are not only fast in the sense of easy and convenient but also in how they raise your blood sugar.

If you want to read about how fast foods have changed the way Americans eat (while at the same time changing their waistlines), please read *Fast Food Nation* by Eric Schlosser, published by Houghton Mifflin in 2002.

Note: You may want to learn more about the international movement called *Slow Food* which tries to put quality back into food by using unprocessed, usually organic ingredients. Take a look at www.slowfood.com.

Note: Another reason to stay away from fast foods is that processed meats, like hamburger, hotdogs, and sausage (as opposed to whole, boneless cuts of beef), are manufactured by "automatic meat recovery," forcibly tearing the flesh away from the bone. This results in some inadvertent nervous tissue being intermixed with the muscle. In cattle infected with bovine spongioform encephalopathy (BSE), this practice may increase the risk of transmitting the infection to humans who unwittingly eat those processed meats. And, never eat brains!

Note: If you are concerned about BSE and want to protect against the development of the human form of it (variant Creutzfeldt-Jakob disease) in the future (as much as possible), you may want to consider eating kosher meats. Kosher meats differ from non-kosher in several slaughtering practices. Kosher meats come from young animals only and BSE tends to occur in the older population of animals. "Downer" animals are not considered kosher so they are rejected and do not get into the kosher food supply. Most cattle are killed by injecting pressurized air into the animal's brain, thereby raising the possibility of brain tissue ending up in other organs. Kosher animals are killed by a super-sharp knife cutting the carotid arteries in the neck. And every kosher animal's organs are examined for signs of illness. The animal is rejected as not kosher if such signs are found. These differences may make kosher meat safer than non-kosher, although this is still theoretical.

Once you and your family are no longer eating fast foods, you are ready to make the switch from processed to unprocessed foods. This means that you forego prepared foods like TV dinners, most convenience foods, and perhaps even prepared baby foods. This means that you are cooking "from scratch" so you consciously decide what ingredients to add to your food. This means that you are gaining ground towards healthy nutrition for yourself and your family. (To help you find foods that fulfil your nutritional criteria, go to the USDA's National Agricultural Library Nutrition Database at www.nal.usda.gov.)

> **Note:** Processed foods in the frozen foods isle in your supermarket come in a large variety and they may tempt you with the reflex feel-good words on the package. Just because the package says "wholesome," or "whole grains" or even "natural" or "organic" doesn't mean you're making a healthy choice. The only way to overcome the misuse of language is to read both the Ingredients and the Nutrition Facts labels. Make sure you're not choosing anything that contains partially hydrogenated vegetable oils. Make sure the calorie value is for the entire serving that you're likely to eat. Make sure the saturated fat content is low. Check on the sodium (salt) content. Try to choose fiber-containing foods.

At this stage, you are probably avoiding many foods made with flour because once a grain (even a whole grain) is processed into flour, some of its nutritional value is lost. At the same time, you are finding yourself experimenting with whole grains that you have just "discovered," like amaranth, quinoa, and buckwheat. This is a wonderful nutritional "stage" because you (and likely your whole family) are in harmony with a healthy pancreas. With a healthy pancreas helping your metabolism along, you will find weight loss and weight control to be less gruesome, and sometimes, if you pay attention to portion control and physical exercise, even occurring naturally.

> **Note:** People who have celiac disease (gluten enteropathy), an autoimmune disorder, must eat a gluten-free diet which eliminates wheat, rye and barley (and possibly oats as well). However, they may eat other whole grains, like amaranth, quinoa and buckwheat. They may also eat products made from corn, rice, soy, potato and arrowroot flour.

A prerequisite for healthy weight control and just as important as your nutritional plan is your daily exercise program. My personal experience treating obese patients over many years leads me to the inescapable conclusion that the best way, and indeed it may be the only safe and sure way, to increase one's metabolic rate is to increase one's daily physical activity. The power to speed up your metabolism is in your hands (and feet).

> **Remember:** Metabolic rate means the amount of calories expended for survival functions, like sleep, heart rate, breathing, digesting, cell growth and repair per 24 hours. If you increase the amount of calories you burn for these functions every day, you may lose more weight. A tiny gland in your brain called the hypothalamus is your metabolic rate setter. It is sensitive to the amount of physical activity you do every day. It is also sensitive to the amount of sleep you get at night (don't count daytime naps). You should sleep 7-8 hours every night. This helps to regulate hormones that affect appetite and eating.

> **Note:** People who tend towards restlesness with fidgeting, rocking, tapping, or other rythmic movements (as part of their natural temperament) burn more calories every day.

Your physical fitness program should include flexibility, stability (balance or equilibrium), aerobic (or endurance), and strength training (or weight training) exercises. Walking is one of the best physical fitness exercises. Find something that interests you so you stick with it long-term. And try to be physically active as a family unit. This conveys a sense of joy in the outdoors while at the same time teaches healthy physical activity.

Stability and strength training exercises are very important for older men and women not only for physical fitness reasons, but also because these tend to protect against falls. If you or your family member is an older person with a sedentary lifestyle, it is a good idea to first schedule a visit with your health care provider and a stress test before beginning a new exercise regime.

You may prefer to include mind/body exercises such as any of the several forms of *yoga, tai chi,* or another of the martial arts, with your daily physical fitness routine. These exercises combine an element of meditation with physical activity. They have been proven to relieve stress, release tension, and enhance emotional stability, while they promote cardiovascular fitness.

The *Pilates* system focuses on improving your "core strength" by exercising the muscles of the abdomen, pelvis, and back. *Pilates* will help you to improve flexibility, stability, and endurance.

It is worthwhile to remember that healthy nutritional and physical exercise programs are not the only factors in successful long-term weight control. Healthy eating habits play a significant role too. When eating habits are unhealthy, it is termed disordered eating. Disordered eating includes a whole range of behaviors that have become all too common in our society.

Disordered eating habits include:

eating double portions, bingeing on large quantities of food, skipping meals, snacking much of the day ("grazing"), not eating proper portions of vegetables and fruits, standing up while eating, eating quickly, secret eating in your bedroom, "mindless" eating in front of the television set, vomiting after meals, and many more that you could probably name.

Our society today fosters disordered eating habits because we are pressured into eating vast quantities of calorically dense foods making us fatter and fatter, while at the same time, we are exhorted to fit the ideal, waif-like body type. These two situations simply cannot exist together in harmony. This "schizophrenic" situation may have devastating consequences, perhaps especially for females but they are becoming more and more common among males as well. Disordered eating habits are a prerequisite for eating disorders and obesity.

From my vantage point, anorexia nervosa is the mirror image of obesity. Our obsessive food culture fosters both. Some persons with certain family and personality traits develop one while some others develop the other. Both eating disorders and obesity are a manifestation of our out-of-control eating culture.

There is a complex interrelationship between the eating disorders and overweight/obesity. Overweight and obesity is often the starting point for anorexia nervosa and bulimia nervosa because both these eating disorders usually begin with dieting. Overweight and obesity often co-exist with another of the eating disorders, binge eating disorder (which is essentially bulimia nervosa without the purging part). Again dieting is often a part of the picture because failed diets usually end up with the dieter weighing ever higher and higher. Indeed, the national obsession with dieting is one of the reasons why we are getting fatter and fatter.

I strongly urge you and every member of your family not to diet. Diets don't work. They tend to make dieters fatter and fatter. Rather, make healthy eating changes and make them forever. Let healthy nutrition and physical activity programs become a matter of lifestyle for you and your family. (If you or someone in your family has an eating disorder, you can find reliable information from the National Eating Disorder Association at www.nationaleatingdisorders.org.) The best way to start reducing calories is to eliminate, as much as possible, added sugars and saturated fats.

Although sugar (as well as all its reincarnations, seriously health-damaging high fructose corn syrup being the latest) is partly to blame for many significant health problems such as diabetes and obesity, non-caloric substitutes for sugar may not be the answer we have been waiting for. Despite being used for more than a quarter century, sugar substitutes have not been proven to help with weight loss. This is probably because people tend to make up for the non-caloric sugar substitute in total calories consumed. We just tend to eat more freely when a sugar substitute is on board. This is the same behavior we engage in when eating low-fat and fat-free foods.

> **Note:** The Sugar lobby, disparagingly called Big Sugar, has been engaged in a downhill fight to delude the American public that sugar does not cause disease (other than dental cavities to which they do admit).
>
> As the obesity epidemic gears up, sugar is finally taking its rightful place as one of the contributing demons in our unhealthy food culture.

However, there are times when using a sugar substitute makes good sense, such as sweetening coffee and tea. Some of the commonly used sugar substitutes include:

saccharine (*Sweet 'N' Low*), aspartame (*Equal, NutraSweet*), sugar alcohols (*xylitol, sorbitol, maltitol* and other "ols"), stevia leaf (*Stevita, Sweet Leaf*), acesulfame potassium (*Sweet One, Sunett*) and sucralose (*Splenda*).

Saccharine is not metabolized so it does not contain any calories. Evidence that saccharine caused bladder tumors in mice prevented its use until 2000 when the evidence was reevaluated and it was deemed safe for use in humans. However, there still may be an increased risk for bladder cancer in humans upon heavy consumption.

Aspartame should not be used by persons with phenylketonuria (PKU). Some people report headaches and gastrointestinal upset with aspartame. Animal research with aspartame has resulted in lymphoma, leukemia and brain tumors but the results are questionable so that further research is indicated. Medical research studies on humans have shown no such link so far. The internet is rife with anecdotal reports of aspartame causing such serious ailments as lupus and multiple sclerosis. The way things stand at this time, especially for children, it's probably prudent to stay away from aspartame and chose a safer substitute, like sucralose, instead.

Sugar alcohols have about half the calories of sugar. They may cause bloating, gas, and diarrhea.

Do no use if you have irritable bowel syndrome or inflammatory bowel disease. Stevia leaf comes from a plant found in Brazil and Paraguay. Stevia is an herbal sweetener because it is made from the South American plant *Stevia rebaudiana*. The FDA does not allow Stevia to be used in foods or drinks because of its uncertain safety record. But it is sold as a supplement. However, it has been used for centuries by South American natives. It is not recommended for use during pregnancy and lactation. Acesulfame potassium is not absorbed by the body and hence has no calories. It has not been tested adequately to prove or disprove claims that it causes cancer.

Sucralose tastes like sugar and is made from sugar but is not absorbed from the intestinal tract. Maltodextrin is added for bulk. Since the sweetness of sucralose remains after being heated, it can be used for baking. It has a good safety record. Sucralose (*Splenda*) is the sugar substitute I recommend. *Splenda* has been added to more than 3,000 sugarless or reduced sugar food and drink products.

> **Note:** *Splenda* is not a natural product. Although it starts with sucrose (table sugar), the end product (sucralose) is created artificially. The Center for Science in the Public Interest (CSPI) along with many other watch-dog organizations concluded that *Splenda* is safe to use.

> **Note:** Honey consists mostly of fructose, glucose, and water, but it also has small amounts of vitamins, minerals, amino acids, and a variety of antioxidants. The darker the color of the honey, the higher the antioxidant activity. But don't forget that honey has 64 calories in every tablespoon, even more than table sugar (sucrose) with 48. Honey, even though slightly more healthful than sugar, has no place in a weight-loss program.

> **Remember:** Under one-year-olds may not ingest honey because of the risk that it may contain spores of *Clostridium botulinum*, the causative agent of botulism.

When using nutritional supplements for healthy

weight loss for self-care you must pay strict attention to the **Guidelines for Consulting Your Health Care Provider** at the end of this chapter. You may want to refer to the last section **Putting It All Together** for ideas on how to integrate the essential natural alternatives, homeopathy, herbal remedies, and nutritional supplements.

Banaba leaf

Banaba leaf is an herbal remedy from the plant *Lagerstroemia speciosa*. *Banaba leaf* contains *corosolic acid* which controls blood sugar (hypoglycemic agent) in a way that is similar to the action of insulin, thereby helping persons with type 2 diabetes mellitus to decrease, or in some cases discontinue, oral prescription agents. It may reduce insulin resistance. *Banaba leaf* is also used to control sugar and carbohydrate cravings and to promote weight loss by aiding in reducing hunger and appetite.

The dose of *Banaba leaf* is between 250-1000mg per day, taken in divided doses with meals. You should decrease your daily dose if symptoms of low blood sugar (hypoglycemia) occur such as dizziness and headache. *Banaba leaf* is not to be used during pregnancy and lactation.

> **Note:** *Banaba leaf* is available from Paradise Herbs at www.paradiseherbs.com. The dose is one capsule 3 times daily.

Conjugated linoleic acid (CLA)

Conjugated linoleic acid is a polyunsaturated fatty acid, occurring naturally in meat, dairy products, and eggs. It is manufactured as the nutritional supplement from *safflower oil*. The function of *conjugated linoleic acid* is to increase the amount of sugar that is burned for fuel rather than being sent to your fat tissue to be stored. *CLA* decreases the action of lipoprotein lipase, the enzyme that takes triglycerides from the blood and stores them in fat cells. This may lead to a decrease in body fat mass especially around the midriff.

> **Note:** Abdominal fat is more metabolically active than subcutaneous fat

deposits. For that reason, abdominal fat deposits in obese people are particularly associated with an increased risk for metabolic consequences like heart disease and type 2 diabetes mellitus.

CLA makes your body's cells more receptive to the action of insulin, thereby decreasing insulin resistance, the underlying metabolic defect in the metabolic syndrome.

In addition to its ability to improve body composition (replacing fat with muscle), *conjugated linoleic acid* may also possess anti-cancer properties because of its immunomodulating activity.

Conjugated linoleic acid is available in softgels. The dose is 1000mg, 1-3 times daily. Although it is considered safe and side effects are minimal, there are not enough data to recommend *conjugated linoleic acid* supplements during pregnancy and lactation.

Fenugreek

Fenugreek is the herb *Trigonella foenum-gracecum* a member of the *Leguminosae* botanical family. The ripe seeds are used to make the remedy. The seeds contain a high proportion of *fiber* which gives *Fenugreek* its laxative properties. However, *Fenugreek* also has the ability to reduce blood sugar, probably because the seeds contain a compound (4-*hydroxyisoleucine*) that increases insulin release from the pancreas.

In addition to decreasing insulin resistance, *Fenugreek* is used to improve libido in both men and women.

Fenugreek should not be used during pregnancy. If you or your family member is a diabetic taking blood sugar lowering medications (hypoglycemic agents), you should steer clear of *Fenugreek* because it may potentiate your medications.

Fenugreek is available as a tea, which together with *Green tea* can become your steady beverage, providing you with metabolic enhancers all day long.

Fenugreek is also available as a nutritional supplement for healthy weight loss in 610mg capsules. The dose is 1 or 2 capsules a day. Side effects include abdominal gas with flatulence and diarrhea.

Forskolin

Forskolin is derived from the plant *Coleus forskohli*, a member of the mint family. *Forskolin* is used extensively in Ayurvedic medicine to treat heart and skin diseases such as congestive heart failure, hypertension, angina, eczema, and psoriasis. *Forskolin* increases the activity of an enzyme called adenylate cyclase which in turn increases the amount of cyclic adenosine monophosphate (cAMP) present inside every cell and linked to energy production. In turn, cAMP performs many functions in your body helping you to ward off skin and heart diseases as well as obesity. *Forskolin* may increase metabolic rate, helping you to burn more calories during your daily activities.

Forskolin also relaxes smooth muscles including bronchial muscles, which makes it useful as a treatment for asthma. This action on smooth muscles makes *Forskolin* useful to treat high blood pressure (hypertension).

Forskolin has been shown to possess antidepressant actions, which may make it useful in the treatment of depression in the future. *Forskolin* also possesses hormone-modulating effects. This means that persons with mild hypothyroidism may be able to increase their own production of thyroid hormone without the use of synthetic hormone.

Forskolin has been used to treat obesity, especially in people with lower than normal amounts of cAMP. *Forskolin* has been shown to help in achieving a normal body composition by decreasing the amount of body fat.

Forskolin extract is available in 50 and 100mg capsules. The dose is one capsule twice daily. It is safe and effective for use in the recommended dosage. But, *Forskolin* should not be used in pregnant and lactating women because the effects on the fetus and newborn are unknown.

Garcinia cambogia

Garcinia cambogia is a tropical plant, common name *brindall berry*. The rind of its fruit is used to make the nutritional supplement. The active component of *Garcinia cambogia*a is *hydroxycitric acid* (*HCA*). It has been shown to interfere with fat metabolism and preventing fat storage but without causing a decrease in lean muscle mass. This means that while taking *Garcinia cambogia* your body may burn more calories. However, bear in mind that some studies have not shown positive results on weight loss. This may be true because *Garcinia cambogia* may help only certain people with weight loss. Some people report that *Garcinia cambogia* suppresses appetite.

Garcinia cambogia is available together with *chromium picolinate* in a preparation called *Citrimax*. *Citrimax* contains 1 gram of *Garcinia cambogia*, equivalent to 500mg of *hydroxycitric acid*, with 150 microgram of *chromium picolinate*. Take one tablet 2-3 times daily (never more than 3 times), about one hour before meals.

Garcinia cambogia should not be used in pregnant and lactating women because the effect on the fetus and newborn are unknown.

Glucomannan

Glucomannan (also called *konjac mannan*) is a water-soluble *fiber* made from the root of the plant *Amorphophallus konjac*, common name *elephant yam*. *Glucomannan* not only functions as a laxative, being a healthy way to treat constipation, but also improves glucose control and blood lipids (lowers cholesterol) in persons with type 2 diabetes mellitus. *Glucomannan* also has weight loss activity, possibly due to its bulk effect in the intestines (i.e., it has the ability to absorb many times its weight in water), giving a feeling of fullness (satiety) thereby helping to prevent overeating.

Glucomannan is available in 665mg capsules. The dose is 3 capsules one hour before every meal (2-4 grams per day) along with a full glass of water. Higher dosages are recommended for attaining glucose control in type 2 diabetes mellitus. *Glucomannan* is commonly accepted as safe although long-term studies have not been done.

L-glutamine

L-glutamine is the most common non-essential amino acid in the body, present abundantly in muscle tissue. *L-glutamine* taken as a supplement may help to increase lean muscle mass. More muscle tissue may increase the number of calories your body uses while exercising. This leads to an increase in your metabolic rate which may be beneficial for weight loss.

L-glutamine is available in 500mg and 1000mg capsules. The dose is 1-2 capsules daily. *L-glutamine* is also available in megadoses to be taken just before and just after vigorous workouts as a part of sports nutrition when it acts as an energy source instead of glucose. *L-glutamine* in megadoses comes either as a powder containing 4,500mg per heaping teaspoonful, or as 2000mg capsules where the dose is 2 capsules before and 2 after the workout. *L-glutamine* supplements may improve performance in sports and workouts. Another way to ingest more *glutamine* is to take 20-30 grams of *whey* protein twice daily.

> **Remember:** *L-glutamine* supplements to help with weight loss are useless unless you are engaging in a fairly intensive program of daily physical exercise.

Gymnema sylvestre

Gymnema is an herbal remedy used in Ayurvedic medicine for decreasing blood glucose levels. Persons with type 2 diabetes mellitus may be able to discontinue their oral prescription medications when taking *Gymnema*. Some medical researchers believe that *Gymnema* may help to regenerate the insulin-secreting cells in the pancreas which makes *Gymnema* suitable for persons with type 1 diabetes mellitus as well as type 2. *Gymnema* is known to prevent sugar and carbohydrate cravings, helping dieters keep on track.

Gymnema sylvestre is available in 250mg capsules. The dose is one capsule once or twice daily.

Low carb bars

Low carb bars are usually high protein as well. You will find a bewildering array of *low carb bars* (shakes and powders too) on the market. A popular brand is the *Keto Bar*, available in 7 flavors. They include *glutamine*, *taurine* and *whey peptides* which may be effective against cravings for sweets. In addition,

each *Keto Bar* contains 250mg of *conjugated linoleic acid*. *Low carb bars*s may help people who have insulin resistance and diabetes to normalize their blood sugar.

> **Remember:** Total calories are what count at the end of the day. If you are using *low carb bars* to help you lose weight you need to subtract those calories from the daily total you have set for yourself. The calories in *low carb bars* usually run between 150-300 per bar.

> **Note:** "Net carbs" or "effective carbs" mean only those carbohydrates are counted on the nutrition label that have an impact on blood sugar. So, the grams of glycerine, sugar substitutes (like sucralose and aspartame), alcohols (like sorbitol and xylitol) and fiber are not counted under "carbohydrates" on the nutrition label.

Phaseolus vulgaris

When the kidney bean (*Phaseolus vulgaris*) is made into a protein concentrate, it inactivates one of the enzymes that digest the starch in carbohydrates inside your intestines. This property promotes weight loss because less starch is absorbed into your bloodstream. Less starch means less calories. A brand of kidney bean protein concentrate is called *Phase2 Starch Neutralizer*.

Pyruvate

Pyruvate (*pyruvic acid*) is synthesized inside every cell during energy metabolism as well as being widely distributed in fruits and vegetables. When *pyruvate* is taken as a supplement (often combined with *dihydroxyacetone phosphate* [*DHAP*] to increase the burning of fat) it may help to increase lean muscle mass. More muscle tissue would increase the number of calories your body uses when exercising. This leads to an increase in your metabolic rate which may be beneficial for weight loss.

Pyruvate is available as 500mg and 750mg capsules. The dose is 4-6 capsules daily. Do not use *pyruvate* during pregnancy or lactation.

Rhodiola

Rhodiola rosea, common name *golden root* or *rose root* or *Arctic root* is a member of the botanical family *Crassulaceae*. It is an herbal remedy made from a plant native to China and Siberia. *Rhodiola rosea* is classified as an adaptogen, meaning it may help the body cope with the biochemical effects of stress by boosting energy. It may function by increasing energy synthesis inside mitochondria. More energy manufactured by your body means more ingested calories utilized rather than stored as fat.

>**Note:** Other herbal adaptogens include: *Panax ginseng, Panax quinquefolius, Siberian Ginseng (Eleutherococcus senticosus)* and *Ashwagandha (Withania somnifera*, used in Ayurvedic medicine).

For that reason *Rhodiola* has been used to augment performance capacity (endurance) during sports and to combat depression and fatigue. *Rhodiola* may be helpful in treating fibromyalgia and chronic fatigue syndrome. It may be of benefit in persons with mild depression because of its mood elevating properties. It has also been used to augment libido and sexual functioning.

Rhodiola's active ingredient *rosavin* (or *rhosavin*) may possess weight loss properties. It probably works inside the body by influencing chemicals in the brain called neurotransmitters. It is considered safe at recommended doses of 100-500mg /day of a product standardized to 3% *rosavin* and at least 1% *salidrosides*. This is the same ratio found in nature. Take *Rhodiola* on an empty stomach. At higher dosage levels, irritability and insomnia may occur. The paucity of medical information about *Rhodiola* means that it should not be taken during pregnancy or lactation. Do not use *Rhodiola* together with other adaptogens such as *Ginseng*.

>**Note:** Please do not confuse *Rhodiola rosea* with the herb *Rhodiola crenulata* which is added to some herbal formulas promising longevity. *Prolongeveity Formula* by ProVita includes *Ficus bengalensis (Banyan tree), Angelica keiskei (Ashitaba)* and *Rhodiola crenulata*.

Vanadium

Vanadium is an ultra-trace mineral found in our bodies. *Vanadium*, given as the organic compound *Vanadyl sulfate* helps people with type 2 diabetes mellitus to control their blood glucose levels. That means that less insulin will be necessary to keep blood glucose in the normal range. With less insulin comes less storage of fat, so *Vanadyl sulfate* may decrease body weight by decreasing body fat.

The organic compound *Vanadyl sulfate* is given instead of the inorganic mineral *Vanadium* because it is safer. *Vanadyl sulfate* is not associated with gastrointestinal side effects or liver and kidney toxicity, effects that are sometimes seen with ingesting the mineral *Vanadium*. Due to lack of research information, *Vanadyl sulfate* supplements should not be used by pregnant and lactating women. *Vanadyl sulfate* is available as 2mg and 10mg tablets. The dose is one tablet daily.

Yerba mate

The leaves of the *Yerba mate*, the *Ilex paraguariensis* plant from South America, are made into a weight loss supplement. *Yerba mate* is said to increase energy, decrease fatigue, decrease appetite, and increase feelings of fullness (satiety). It possesses stimulant activity similar to *caffeine*.

Yerba mate is available as 450mg capsules. The dose is 2 capsules 1-2 times daily. *Yerba mate* is also available as a tea made by the Wisdom of the Ancients herbal tea company. *Yerba mate* is not for use during pregnancy and lactation.

>**Caution:** Do not take *Yerba mate* together with *caffeine* or *Bitter orange* because the safety record of such a combination is questionable at best.

Guidelines for Consulting Your Health Care Provider

You should consult your health care provider if:
- the patient doesn't look right or act right (trust your instincts!)
- the patient is getting worse instead of better over the course of the illness
- the patient is having trouble breathing or complaining of chest pains or there is mental confusion or lethargy or irritability
- the patient develops allergic symptoms (hives, itchy or watery eyes, runny nose, scratchy throat, asthma, shortness of breath) after taking a nutritional supplement
- after beginning a nutritional supplement the patient experiences *new onset* of any serious symptoms such as:

    paralysis, weakness, tingling, inability to focus or concentrate, blurred or double vision or blindness, slurred speech, severe headaches, seizures, irritability, dizziness, disorientation, memory loss, anxiety, depression, insomnia, blackouts, fainting, or the person complains of not feeling like himself
- the patient is taking *ANY* prescription medication
- the patient is pregnant or breastfeeding
- the patient has any serious, chronic disease which may have complications and become life-threatening, such as:

    autism, cancer, HIV and AIDS, arthritis, multiple sclerosis, coronary artery disease, heart attack (myocardial infarction), blood dyscrasia, cancer (of any type), congestive heart failure, diabetes mellitus, obesity, thyroid disorders, high blood pressure (hypertension), stroke, seizures, acute and chronic kidney (renal) failure, schizophrenia, bipolar disorder, borderline personality disorder, eating disorders, fibromyalgia, chronic fatigue syndrome, Crohn's disease, ulcerative colitis, celiac disease, mental deficiency disorders, chromosomal disorders, infertility, frequent miscarriages, polyneuropathy, cystic fibrosis [Adapted from *The Merck Manual* at www.merck.com]

Note: Do not discontinue taking any pharmaceutical medication that has been prescribed by your health care provider unless you or your family member is under the supervision of a physician.

Note: Do not take any nutritional supplement for healthy weight control without first consulting your health care provider if you or your family member is taking a prescription medication, has diabetes mellitus, or is pregnant or breastfeeding. Weight loss supplements are never given to young children under the age of 14 because of the lack of information on long-term sequelae in that age group.

In addition, it is a good idea to check with your health care provider if your family member is either an adolescent or older than 65 because nutritional supplements for healthy weight control given injudiciously may overwhelm the body's defenses in those age groups.

Remember: *Ephedra sinica*, also called *Ma Huang* had once been a prominent component in some weight loss remedies, but because of the number of deaths attributed to it from disturbances in heart rhythm, the FDA ordered it removed from all products sold in the U.S. early in 2004. Avoid weight loss preparations that contain *Ephedra*. It has no place in healthy weight loss.

One more herbal product to avoid: The prudent person will also avoid all weight loss products made with *Bitter orange* from the flowers of the plant *Citrus aurantium* because the active compound, *synephrine*, is similar to

Ephedra. The safety record on *Bitter orange* is just not known. *Bitter orange* is on *Consumer Reports'* list of supplements that may cause cancer, kidney or liver damage, or even death.

Do not confuse *Bitter orange* with *Bitter melon* from the plant *Momordica charantia*. *Bitter melon* may actually have some benefits in lowering blood glucose levels and increasing the efficiency of the liver, but medical information is scanty.

Please be vigilant: When it comes to herbal remedies touted for weight loss without any scientific proof of safety. Edita Kaye's *Skinny Pill for Kids* is just such a product. It contains the herbs *Uva ursi*, *Juniper berry* and *Buchu leaf*, all of which act as diuretics, eliminating water from the body. Besides the point that children and teenagers should not be led to believe that taking a pill can make them "skinny," this remedy has the potential to be dangerous.

Environmental Nutrition Newsletter: The January 2006 issue listed nutritional supplements that may help with weight loss by increasing metabolic rate.
  Bitter orange (Citrus aurantium)— uncertain safety
  Caffeine—stimulant on many organs of the body
  Cayenne (Capsaicin frutescens)— decreases body fat
  Green tea (Camellia sinensis)—antioxidant EGCG (at least 90mg/day)
  Ephedrine or *Ma Huang (Ephedra sinica)*—stimulant, banned in U.S. for causing 17 deaths
  Forskolin (Coleus forskohli)—involved in energy production
  Guarana—stimulant containing caffeine
  White willow bark extract or salicin (Salix alba)—anti-inflammatory

agent similar to *acetylsalicylic acid (aspirin)*
  Yerba mate (Ilex paraguariensis)—stimulant similar to *caffeine*
  Yohimbine (Pausinystalia yohimbe)—stimulant that decreases appetite with uncertain safety record, can be dangerous

Remember: Before starting nutritional supplements for weight loss or weight control, it is essential that you first master the elements of healthy eating and healthy exercise.

Note: The brown sea algae *Bladderwrack (Fucus vesiculosus)* contain *iodine* which impacts the thyroid gland. *Iodine* may help to increase the metabolic rate, making you expend more calories without being hungry.

Note: Adolescents tend to use herbal weight loss supplements at particularly high rates. Studies have shown that not only do they tend to not understand what they're taking but they do not generally reveal it to their parents.

Note: Three servings a day of cow's milk dairy products, specifically fat-free milk and yogurt, is being touted as a weight loss strategy. But, the medical evidence (only 3 small studies) is flimsy at best. There's no compelling reason to eat 3 dairy portions a day for weight loss reasons. However, from a calcium intake point of view, it may be healthy to eat 3 dairy portions a day, but make sure you aren't increasing your total daily calories.

Note: A reliable and reader-friendly source of evidence-based nutrition information is *Arbor Clinical Nutrition Updates* available by subscription at www.nutritionupdates.org.

Note: A reliable internet source coming from the National Institutes of Health for information on obesity is the Weight-Control Information Network (WIN) at www.win.niddk.nih.gov.

Note: Please take a look at www.patientINFORM.org. This is a free online service for patients and families to access "the most up-to-date, reliable, and important research available" about diseases like cancer, diabetes, and other serious, chronic diseases. This website is a collaborative effort by the *American Cancer Association*, the *American Heart Association* and the *American Diabetes Association* along with some of our most trusted medical schools and medical journals.

Remember: The emphasis is emphatically not on alternative medicine! But you can learn a lot.

Note: A good book about healthy nutrition for baby and toddler is *Super Baby Food*, 2nd edition, by Ruth Yaron, published by F. J. Roberts in 1998. It contains sound advice on everything from breastfeeding to preparing homemade whole foods for baby, with menus, recipes, and tables of nutrient values in foods.

Another excellent book about nutrition for infants is *What Should I Feed My Baby?* by Suzannah Olivier, published in the United Kingdom by Orion Publishing Group in 1998. Order by email at orders@lbsltd.co.uk or on the web at http://pubeasy/books/lbsltd.co.uk. This is the book that my own grandchildren's nutrition is based upon.

Remember: Once your baby starts eating finger foods at the family table, the lessons he/she learns about eating habits and food choices will last a lifetime. Make sure your family's kitchen teaches your baby healthy nutrition and eating habits from the very beginning.

Look for: A weight loss product with promise for the future is *Ginseng berry* extract. This is the same herb *Ginseng* from which the root is used for energy enhancement. *Ginseng berry* extract possesses the ability to correct the metabolic abnormalities in diabetes and to promote weight loss by decreasing appetite.

Look for: Using the kitchen condiment *cinnamon* has been shown in a medical research study to decrease blood sugar, triglycerides, and LDL cholesterol. The amounts used in that study are 1 gram (equal to about one quarter teaspoon) to 6 grams, every day, in capsule form. *Cinnamon* helps insulin to be more efficiently used in the body. If you or your family member suffers from type 2 diabetes mellitus or any other insulin resistance syndrome, it may be a good idea to begin using *cinnamon* more liberally in your kitchen. Or you may want to consider taking *cinnamon* as a nutritional supplement. *Cinnamon* (125mg in each capsule) is available together with *coffee berry* (extract from *Coffea arabica*, 100mg in each capsule) in *Cinnulin PF* from Life Extension at 1-800-544-4440 or www.lifeextension.com. Take 1 capsule before each meal.

Look for: The *Hoodia* "cactus" (*Hoodia gordonii*) from the African Kalahari Desert possesses anti-appetite effects. It is available as a tea and several different pills. It may also possess sexual stimulant properties. It may exert its action on the appetite center of the brain. Side effects and interactions have not yet been determined. For more information, please see www.hoodia.com. The downside is that preliminary findings suggest a weight loss of about one pound per week, in line with what you would expect with a nutritious but low calorie diet and exercise program.

Look for: The herbal remedy *Mulberry leaf* (*Morus nigra*) is being tested as an agent to decrease insulin resistance by improving insulin sensitivity. It may be helpful in persons with type 2 diabetes mellitus.

Look for: The herbal remedy *Korean pine* (*Pinus koraiensis*) contains *pinolenic acid*, a natural appetite suppressant.

Look for: A combination of herbal remedies *Magnolia officinalis* and *Phellodendron amurense* (from Next Pharmaceuticals, Inc., Irvine, California), has been shown to be effective in preventing weight gain among a small number of premenopausal women who tend to overeat during stressful situations. The herbal combination has an effect on *cortisol* secretion during stress which may be the way it is able to keep body weight in check. The results of this encouraging study was published in *Alternative Therapies in Health and Medicine*, January-February 2006.

Think about: Try putting *mindfulness* into your daily life. If you suffer from life-long overeating (or compulsive overeating or binge eating disorder), then please consider learning about *mindfulness*. There is nothing as powerful as practicing *mindfulness*, a type of meditation, at mealtimes to help you really "see" what, how much, and why you are eating. *Mindfulness* pulls you into the present moment. *Mindfulness* allows you to comprehend the now, the present, leaving out the past and future. When you practice *mindfulness*, you won't be hurrying through your meal, thinking about seconds (or thirds!).

A good way to learn more about *mindfulness* is by reading *Mindful Recovery, A Spiritual Path to Healing from Addiction* by Thomas and Beverly Bien, published by John Wiley & Sons in 2002. Some health care providers (including myself) believe that overeating (or compulsive overeating or binge eating disorder) can be considered as a form of addiction even though it is not, strictly speaking. *Mindful Recovery* teaches you how to employ *mindfulness* in your daily life whether or not you believe you have an addiction to food.

Note: If you or your family member has compulsive overeating or binge eating disorder, you may want to investigate *Food Addicts Anonymous* (called *FAA*), a "12-step" program that has the highest cure rate for BED. You may learn about *FAA* at www.foodaddictsanonymous. org. You may learn more about the food program of *FAA* from reading *Food Addiction: The Body Knows* by Kay Sheppard. You may order this book at the *FAA* website.

Note: If you are overweight and having a difficult time losing weight, you may benefit from calculating your resting metabolic rate (RMR). Ask your fitness center trainer to measure your RMR. It's as simple as breathing into a machine. Once you know your RMR, you will be able to calculate the number of calories you should eat every day to lose weight.

Note: There is no medical evidence that *vinegar* (*acetic acid*, made from any source, apple, wine, potato, other) aids in weight loss or lowers cholesterol. However, if you use *vinegar* on salads along with small amounts of *olive oil* instead of commercially prepared salad dressings, you may consume fewer calories.

Note: *Serotonin* is the brain neurotransmitter involved in complex chemical reactions that regulate feeding and eating as well as mood. (Have you noticed how your mood affects your appetite?) The amino acid *tryptophan* is converted into *serotonin* in your body. If you want to try to stabilize mood to help regulate appetite, it's a good idea to consume *tryptophan*-rich foods. Turkey is highest in *tryptophan* but duck, chicken fish, whole grains, nuts, seeds, eggs, cheese, tofu, fruits and vegetables also have good concentrations. The supplement *5-HTP (5-hydroxytryptophan)* is an *amino acid* that is converted in your body to *serotonin*. The dose is 100mg three times a day. Do not take if you are taking antidepressants or migraine medicines called *triptans*.

Note: Performance-enhancing supplements are sometimes used to increase muscle mass, strength, and endurance. Anabolic steroids (also called androgenic steroids) and prohormones such as androstenedione have not only been banned by all major sports organizations but they are controlled substances so using them is illegal. This is because using them is associated with serious side effects such as testicular atrophy and irreversible breast enlargement in males, and masculinization of females.

Note: The supplement *dehydroepiandrosterone (DHEA)* is exempt to being classified as a controlled substance despite its being a steroid hormone. It is banned by the Olympics and many other sports organizations. *DHEA's* exemption is based on its reputed anti-aging and weight redistribution actions. In a very small study, *DHEA* decreased abdominal fat in elderly men and women. Abdominal fat wreaks metabolic havoc with insulin and makes people prone to diabetes. But, until more is known about *DHEA* and its long-term effects on both men and women, it is still prudent to refrain. (For more information

on *DHEA*, please see **Chapter 24: Antioxidant Phytochemicals: Natural Anti-Aging Remedies.**)

Note: Certain herbal remedies called hormone boosters, such as *Tribulus terrestris* and *Eurycoma longifolia* are touted to increase muscle mass, strength, and endurance. But, these herbs have not been studied for either efficacy or safety in humans. Toxic effects were observed in some animal studies. I strongly recommend that you stay away from these herbal remedies.

Note: The supplement *Creatine* is available for use to decrease muscle fatigue during training. But it has not been shown to increase muscle mass, strength, or endurance. *Creatine* is associated with weight gain from water retention.

Note: Don't fall for the premise behind *CortiSlim* and the cheaper knock-offs, *CortiTone, CortiSol* and others. There is no medical evidence that reducing one's level of *cortisone* (the stress hormone) has any effect on weight or weight loss. There's no evidence that persons with lower *cortisone* levels weigh less than those with higher levels. And similarly, there is no evidence that these products reduce one's level of *cortisone*. So why would you buy it? Maybe because it's hyped on television?

Putting It All Together

If you are considering using a nutritional supplement for healthy weight control, it is a good idea to familiarize yourself with **Chapter 22: Introduction to Nutritional Supplements**. It makes good sense to understand the role of vitamin and mineral nutritional supplements (especially the mineral *chromium picolinate*) from **Chapter 23: Vitamins and Minerals**; *antioxidant* nutritional supplements from **Chapter**

24: Antioxidant Phytochemicals: Natural Anti-Aging Remedies and *omega-3 fatty acids* from **Chapter 31: Oils and Fats**. In addition, you will likely benefit from learning about *L-Carnitine* and *Fiber* in **Chapter 25: Heart Healthy Nutritional Supplements**.

Whenever you have decided to go ahead with a nutritional supplement for healthy weight control, it is a good idea to consider giving the sick person's homeopathic constitutional remedy as well (please refer to **Chapter 9: Homeopathic Remedies for Constitutional Problems in Infants, Children, and Adolescents** or to **Chapter 18: Homeopathic Constitutional Remedies** if you are dealing with an adult; or **Chapter 13: Homeopathy for Elderly Person**s if you are dealing with an elderly person).

Specifically, please take a look at **Chapter 15: Homeopathy for Eating Disorders and Weight Control**. Homeopathic remedies may be used in conjunction with herbal medicines and nutritional supplements.

Please investigate **Chapter 20: Herbs You Need to Know** and familiarize yourself with the herbal remedies *Green tea* and *Psyllium*. You will need to incorporate *probiotics* (please refer to **Chapter 30: Prebiotics and Probiotics**) into your daily supplements to optimize the functioning of your gastrointestinal system and provide support for your immune system while you restrict calories. It is very important to understand healthy oils and fats, found in **Chapter 31: Oils and Fats** in order to make good choices for yourself and your family.

Chapter 27

Nutritional Supplements to Prevent Cancer and Augment Your Immune System

Cancer and the Immune System in General

Ailment/Disorder/Symptom	Nutritional Supplement
Immune system function	*Colostrum*
Immune system and inflammation	*Enzymes*
Quality of life during chemotherapy	*Essiac tea*
Anti-cancer activity	*Mistletoe*
Cancer metastases	*Modified citrus pectin*
Immune system function	*Mushrooms*
Immune system function	*Phytosterols*
Anti-inflammatory and anti-cancer activity	*Propolis*
Immune system function	*Whey*

Guidelines for Consulting Your Health Care Provider
Putting It All Together

Cancer and the Immune System in General

You might think that the prevention of cancer and the treatment of cancer are two completely opposite situations. But, as strange as it might seem, prevention and treatment come together in many areas. I call the point where prevention and treatment come together the *Fabulous Four*.

What are the *Fabulous Four*?

FIRST and foremost, the same healthy nutritional program is the cornerstone for prevention and treatment (as well as for relapse prevention for people who have had cancer and want to prevent metastases).

Optimal nutrition is the key to mitigating genetic predisposition towards cancer. Your nutritional state also affects hormones and growth factors which either promote or inhibit tumor cell division. And if you have/had cancer, your nutritional state has over-arching influence on whether or not metastases will occur.

A healthy nutritional program is the single most important step you can take to enhance the functioning of your immune system. If your cellular milieu contains toxic products of metabolism due to poor nutritional choices, you may be in a state of immune system suppression. If this state is allowed to continue for a prolonged period of time, low-level inflammation, unchecked by your immune system malfunction, may allow cancerous cells to develop and flourish. The anti-inflammation and anti-cancer nutritional programs are one and the same.

> **Note:** The healthy dietary plan for the prevention and treatment of cancer to consider is, according to Dr. Andrew Weil, the anti-inflammatory diet, which is based on the Mediterranean diet. The anti-inflammatory diet depends heavily on whole foods that grow from the earth like whole grains, fresh fruits and vegetables, with *olive oil* as your fat source. In addition, you will need to consume foods high in *omega-3 fatty acids*, like walnuts and flaxseeds. Animal protein is at a minimum except for cold water

fatty fish, again supplying *omega-3 fatty acids*. You may add *ginger* and *turmeric* to your food for their anti-inflammatory effects as well as antioxidant vitamins and minerals. You must limit or eliminate your intake of processed foods and sugar.

The *American Institute for Cancer Research* (*AICR*) has reported evidence that one's childhood diet directly influences one's adult cancer risk. I look forward to the *AICR*'s recommendations on optimal childhood nutrition designed to prevent cancer. It is likely that maintenance of normal weight (for age and gender) will be a prominent feature.

> **Note:** *AICR* has published a cookbook, *The New American Plate Cookbook*, available through their website www.aicr.org that helps you to learn how to cook and eat in a cancer-preventive way.

> **Note:** Although a recently published study by the *Women's Health Initiative* (*WHI*) following almost 49,000 women reported that a low fat diet (20-30% versus almost 40%) did not prevent cancer, it is possible that the study did not follow the women long enough to show a statistically significant difference. It is noteworthy that a subgroup of women in the study who ate the lowest fat diet (20%) did develop fewer breast cancers. These results tell us that there are multiple factors that influence the development of cancer in an individual so that changing just one factor in one's diet may not be sufficient for prevention.

SECOND, healthy lifestyle practices are the same for prevention and treatment (as well as for relapse prevention for people who have had cancer and want to prevent metastases). When considering the treatment or prevention of cancer, it is imperative that you and your family members heed the **good health practices**:

—no smoking, moderate alcohol, nutritionally healthy diet, adequate daily physical exercise, adequate sleep, time for daily relaxation techniques, seeking humor and love in everyday life, engaging in activities for intellectual stimulation, doing things for other people, and participating in preventive health testing.

THIRD, the same nutritional supplements are useful for both prevention and treatment in many cases. A good example is antioxidant phytochemicals, found in good foods and supplements and uniquely useful to prevent and treat cancer and enhance your immune system. Another example is antioxidant vitamins and minerals. Some herbal remedies are also useful for both prevention and treatment of cancer and enhancing the function of the immune system. *Prebiotics* and *probiotics* have been proven to augment your immune system and may decrease the risk of some cancers.

FOURTH, homeopathic remedies offer both prevention and treatment for cancer in the form of one's constitutional remedy.

But, there are major differences too, in the prevention and treatment of cancer. Cancer is such a life-threatening condition that it does not make sense to consider self-care for its treatment even though it makes perfect sense to consider self-care for its prevention. If you or a family member has cancer, it is essential that you obtain oncology health care services from a M.D. or D.O. specialist in the cancer you are trying to treat or the recurrences you are trying to prevent. It is irresponsible to "go it alone" when the diagnosis is cancer. The patient with cancer needs an exact diagnosis, then the proper surgery, chemotherapy and/or radiation therapy, and then the proper follow-up care designed to prevent recurrences and metastases. Within all of this, there will be a place for homeopathy, herbal medicines, and nutritional supplements, but you will need to consult with your health care provider.

What causes cancer?
Why do people get cancer?
Since cancer is the second leading cause of death among adult Americans, it is prudent to endeavor to understand its causation. One and a half million people are diagnosed with a new case of cancer every year (excluding the more than one million skin cancers).

Cancer is a complex of different diseases and consequently, there is no single cause that explains all cancer. The best way to think about the causes of cancer is along the lines of the *multifactorial* basis of causation. This means that there are many different factors that come together in one person to cause cancer, or considering the opposite side of the coin, to prevent cancer from developing.

Those *multifactorial* reasons fall into 3 categories: genetic, environmental and psychological. These 3 different categories of factors interact with each other inside the same body over a prolonged period of time. Cancer may result when genetic, environmental, and psychological factors converge at a particularly crucial time.

GENETIC or familial causes of cancer refer to specific genes that are passed down through the generations that tend to trigger cancerous growths. There are certain genes that tend to inhibit cancerous growths too. The list of cancers with known genes that trigger them is getting longer every year. Perhaps the most famous is BRCA1 and BRCA2 found in familial breast cancer.

ENVIRONMENTAL factors not only include exposures to toxins but also to lifestyle factors. Environmental factors include exposure to such cellular poisons as:

cigarette smoke and other tobacco products; x-rays, ultraviolet radiation, high-calorie and high-fat diets, obesity, low physical activity, consumption of salt-cured and charcoal-broiled foods, consumption of alcohol, and inflammatory processes such as infection with *Helicobactor pylori* bacteria inside the stomach or *Human Papilloma Virus* inside the cervix, or chronic periodontal gum disease, as well as numerous other toxic factors.

Note: So far there is no solid medical evidence that exposure to pesticides, herbicides, fungicides, pollutants, solvents, dyes, food additives, genetically modified foods, hormones in beef and poultry, proximity to power lines, cell phones, artificial sweeteners, and breast implants provides an increased risk for cancer. However, it is prudent to try to limit your exposure to these more controversial environmental factors until good evidence for their safety (or their carcinogenic toxicity) becomes available.

Note: When meats are cooked over an open flame at high temperatures (charbroiled) they produce *heterocyclic amines* which are proven carcinogenic chemicals.

PSYCHOLOGICAL factors refer to those aspects of your personality, behavior, thoughts, and feelings that enhance or compromise the functioning of your immune system. The term for the interplay between your psychological and immunological systems is psychoneuroimmunology. Much is being learned about the way in which stress hormones influence the immune system.

Psychological factors include:
temperament especially in one's handling of anger responses, optimism and positivity vs negative thinking, one's ability to cope with chronic stress and anxiety, one's ability to relax and meditate, resiliency in the face of great emotional trauma such as divorce, death of a spouse, or a financial crisis, hopelessness, degree of social isolation, and history of bodily trauma and assault.

Note: Although current wisdom acknowledges the effects of emotions on the onset and outcome of cancer, some medical researchers have found no increase in cancer incidence in people with depression or after death of a spouse. And some studies show no relationship between one's attitude and survival. However, these results are considered preliminary since they need to be replicated in studies of large numbers of people. A meta-analysis (pooled analysis of the results of many studies) of 58 studies showed that persons with cancer have a lower suicide rate than persons without cancer. People with cancer who scored higher on happiness measures tended to live longer than those who scored lower. The Mayo clinic study (published in 2000) showed that pessimists were more likely to die prematurely than optimists.

Remember: Our emotional outlook may have a lot to do with the chronic physical diseases we will develop in later life. Negative emotions probably begin to influence our health starting in adolescence. The success of cognitive-behavioral therapy in changing behaviors (such as in substance abuse and eating disorder therapy) taught us that our thought patterns can be changed and this will allow our behaviors to change. If you want to enhance positive thinking and positive emotions, please investigate the different methods available. Stress reduction strategies may be helpful. You may want to start with www.authentichappiness.org.

After reading these lists of causative factors, I hope you have come to the conclusion that *cancer is largely a preventable disease.* This is the same conclusion reached by the *American Cancer Society* and the *American Institute for Cancer Research* (*AICR*). In fact, 80% of all cancers would be prevented if people would eat at least 9 servings of vegetables and fruits each day (called a "plant-based diet"), avoid all tobacco products, consume only small amounts of animal products, perform regular physical exercise, and maintain a healthy body weight.

Note: Dr. Andrew Weil will email you his *Daily Tips* at www.DrWeil.com. He stresses diet and nutrition in the prevention of breast cancer. He has 7 important dietary practices that may help you to prevent breast cancer: keep your daily fat content below 25% of total calories; avoid animal fats and hydrogenated vegetable oils; use healthy fats especially monounsaturated oils like *olive oil* and eat oily fish rich in *omega-3 fatty acids*; avoid alcohol; decrease animal protein (beef, poultry, eggs, and dairy) and buy organic for the small amounts that you do eat; increase the amounts of fruits and vegetables in your daily diet for their naturally occurring, protective antioxidants.

Throughout this book I have extolled the virtues of the **essential natural alternatives**, namely homeopathy, herbal medicine, and nutritional supplements. I told you that in most cases, you would not need any other kind of alternative and complementary medicine. However, when you need to put out the fires of *cancer treatment's side effects*, now may be the time to consider several other modalities for relief.

> **Note:** The *side effects* of the treatment of cancer first need to be met with the *Fabulous Four*, namely a nutritional diet, healthy lifestyle practices, nutritional supplements and homeopathy. When you have all that in place, it may be necessary to consider other modalities of treatment.

What about other alternative modalities to treat cancer?
If the *Fabulous Four* and *ginger* do not provide relief for the nausea that often accompanies chemotherapy and radiation therapy, then please consider acupuncture. Acupuncture may be helpful to relieve some of the pain as well. Guided imagery and meditation techniques may be useful to treat depression, anxiety, and pain. Cancer support groups may be helpful for some people to relieve depression and anxiety. However, contrary to conventional wisdom, the results of medical research do not show better survival in cancer patients who attend support groups. *Slippery elm* lozenges or chewable tablets of *deglycyrrhizinated licorice* (*DGL*) are helpful to treat mouth sores.

When considering nutritional supplements for self-care to prevent cancer and augment your immune system you must pay strict attention to the **Guidelines for Consulting Your Health Care Provider** at the end of this chapter. You may want to refer to the last section **Putting It All Together** for ideas on how to integrate the essential natural alternatives, homeopathy, herbal remedies, and nutritional supplements.

Colostrum

Colostrum is the very first milk that is secreted in the breast after birth. Breastfeeding mothers have learned that offering the breast shortly after birth will give the newborn *colostrum*, that special, nutrient-rich, pre-milk, containing natural antibodies and glycoproteins. This pre-milk fluid will help baby to protect itself from the onslaught of antigens as it faces its new world. The *colostrum* from cows (*bovine colostrum*) and goats is used in humans to enhance immunity.

Colostrum contains a special group of chemicals called *cytokines* which in turn include *interleukins*. *Interleukins* help in regulating the immune response to foreign matter. They are particularly concerned with preventing the development of cancer and if it has already developed, with the fight to stop it from flourishing. In addition, *colostrum* contains a high titer of *immunoglobulins*. *Immunoglobulins* are proteins in your blood which help to repel viruses and bacteria from overwhelming your immune system.

Colostrum is also known to contain several growth factors, such as *insulin-like growth factor-1* and *-2* (*IGF-1* and *IGF-2*). Since growth factors are important in reparative functions, the anti-aging or rejuvenation medicine proponents tend to use *colostrum*.

Colostrum has no known side effects. The dose is 2-10 grams/day in capsule form. *Colostrum* from bovine source is lactose-free. *Colostrum* from goat source is also available.

> **Note:** *Transfer factor* is a molecule composed of immune messenger chemicals (*peptides* and *amino acids*), isolated from bovine *colostrum*. *Transfer factor* enhances the immune system much the way *colostrum* does. However, it is more expensive.

Enzymes

Systemic oral *enzymes* that degrade proteins are called *proteolytic enzymes*. Each *enzyme* targets a specific protein and digests it. Systemic pancreatic *proteolytic enzymes* are used as nutritional supplements to modulate the immune response to inflammation. Chronic inflammation is considered to be one of the underlying causes of cancer, heart disease, and arthritis.

Upon swallowing an oral *enzyme* nutritional supplement, it is absorbed intact into your bloodstream. It is there that the *enzyme* supplement acts to trigger *cytokines*, the immune system's cascade of chemicals that work towards optimal immune system function. Systemic oral *enzymes* act to maintain a balance between *cytokines* that dampen inflammation (anti-inflammatory, called downregulation) and those that are pro-inflammatory (called upregulatation).

The Gonzalez-Isaacs Program for the control and cure of pancreatic cancer consists in large part of systemic oral *enzymes* which are taken in large doses as nutritional supplements. The Gonzalez-Isaacs Program includes other nutritional supplements (vitamins, minerals, and antioxidants) as well as a completely organic, vegetarian diet. The Gonzalez-Isaacs Program currently receives grant money from the National Cancer Institute to perform a clinical trial of its alternative treatments. The unconventional use of alternatives by Dr. Gonzalez is based on a book published in 1911 by John Beard called *The Enzyme Treatment of Cancer*.

> **Note:** Pancreatic cancer is a particularly brutal form of cancer. The average length of survival is about 5 months. Pancreatic cancer patients treated with conventional methods of surgery and chemotherapy have 25% one-year and 10% two-year survival rates.

One of the most commonly prescribed and widely available systemic oral *enzyme* supplements is *Wobenzym N* at a dosage of 2 tablets 3 times daily or 3 tablets twice daily. Another way to obtain enzymes on a daily basis is to consider taking *Ultra Source of Life* by Nature's Plus, 3 tablets daily. *Ultra Source of Life* is a complete multivitamin-multimineral supplement (except you would need to take additional calcium) laced with whole foods, herbs, complete amino acids, essential fatty acids, *modified citrus pectin*, and *enzymes*.

> **Note:** Systemic oral *enzyme* supplements are not for use by persons with hemophilia, persons taking anticoagulant therapy, or after heart surgery when there is an increased risk of bleeding.

Essiac tea

Essiac tea is an herbal remedy composed of *Burdock root* (*Arctium lappa*), *Indian rhubarb root* (*Rheum palmatum*), *Sheep sorrel* (*Rumex acetosella*), and *Slippery elm* (*Ulmus fulva* and *Ulmus rubra*).

> **Note:** A related product, *Flor Essence Tea* contains the same herbs as above with the addition of *Watercress* (*Nastrurtium officinale*), *Blessed thistle* (*Cnicus benedictus*), *Red clover* (*Trifolium pratense*) and *Kelp* (*Laminaria digitata*).

Medical research data on *Essiac tea*'s effectiveness are scanty. Quality of life may improve while using *Essiac tea* during conventional cancer therapy. There are some reports that tumor size may be decreased. It is sometimes used to treat acquired immunodeficiency syndrome (AIDS). It is available in health food stores and online.

Mistletoe

Mistletoe extract (*Viscum album*, European *Mistletoe*, not the decorative plant *American Mistletoe*) is commonly used in Central Europe as therapy for a wide range of cancers. *Mistletoe* extract is marketed under several brand names, the best known being *Iscador*. *Mistletoe* is a semiparasitic plant that grows on several different trees like apple, oak, pine and others. The chemical composition of the extract varies depending on the host tree. Chemical compounds in the *viscotoxin* and *lectin* groups are probably responsible for its in-vitro cancer killing effects. *Mistletoe* is available in both forms, either as the homeopathic remedy or herbal extract. *Mistletoe* is usually administered by subcutaneous injection. However, the injectable form is not available in the U.S.A. because it is not a *FDA*-approved drug.

Mistletoe 's safety and efficacy has been an open

question. A review of 23 controlled clinical trials using *Mistletoe* was published in 2003. No major side effects were reported. Twelve studies had positive results, 7 showed a positive trend, 3 showed no effect, and 1 showed a negative trend. However, all the studies had methodological flaws that preclude a firm determination of the effectiveness of *Mistletoe* for the treatment of cancer at this time. The best I can say is that *Mistletoe* has potential as anti-cancer therapy.

> **Note:** Currently, the anticancer property of *Mistletoe* is the subject of a well-designed clinical trial under the auspices of *The National Center for Complementary and Alternative Medicine* (*NCCAM*). In this study, *Mistletoe* is combined with *gemcitabine*, a chemotherapy drug. People with advanced, recurrent, or metastasized pancreatic, colorectal, non-small cell lung, and breast cancer are being recruited. If you want more information about participation in this clinical trial, you may call 1-800-411-1222 and visit http://nccam.nih.gov/health/ eurmistletoe/.

Modified citrus pectin

Pectin, a form of soluble *fiber* present in plants, helps them to maintain their shape and structure. Chemically, *pectin* is a water-soluble *polysaccharide* (complex carbohydrate). *Modified citrus pectin* comes from the pulp and peel of citrus fruits.

There is some experimental data in animals (not yet in humans) that suggests that *modified citrus pectin* prevents secondary cancers (metastases) from developing. Metastases, in contradistinction to the original cancer, are most often the feared killers of people with cancer. *Modified citrus pectin* binds to specialized proteins located on cell surfaces called *galectins*. *Galectins* are involved with creating new blood vessels, an essential part of cancer growth. *Modified citrus pectin*'s ability to prevent metastases is based on its interference with *galectins*.

Modified citrus pectin is non-toxic in large amounts and not associated with any serious side effects. The dose for cancer prevention is 3-5 grams/day in 3 divided doses, for cancer treatment 15-25 grams/day. *PectaSol* is a popular product, manufactured by EcoNugenics.

> **Note:** The book *Modified Citrus Pectin, A Super Nutraceutical* by Fuchs, published by Basic Health in 2003 is a good choice if you want to learn more.

Mushrooms

Medicinal *mushrooms* contain chemicals that augment immunity called *beta glucans* which are *polysaccharides* (complex carbohydrates). *Beta glucans* are one of a group of important precursor-nutrients because they activate the components of the immune system. *Beta glucans* increase the numbers of *natural killer cells* which are the body's main defense against cancer cells. They also augment the immune response by causing *cytokines* to be produced by the immune system. *Cytokines* are messenger chemicals that are mobilized to fight off invading predators.

There are many medicinal *mushrooms* containing *beta glucan* that are available in liquid extract to be taken as supplements. Some of them are eaten as foods as well.

The *Cordyceps mushroom* comes from the fungus *Cordyceps sinensis*, common name *Caterpillar fungus*. It is used to increase energy in people with chronic illnesses and to enhance athletic performance. The *Cordyceps mushroom* is used in Traditional Chinese Medicine to lower total cholesterol. The *Cordyceps mushroom* acts to increase production of *superoxide dismutase*, an antioxidant enzyme that prevents cholesterol from layering onto the walls of arteries. Some health care providers use *Cordyceps* to improve heart and lung function especially in asthma and tuberculosis.

The *Enoki mushroom* (also called *Enokitake*) from the fungus *Flammulina velutipes* contains *flammulin* which demonstrates anti-cancer activity. The *Enoki mushroom* also shows activity in lowering blood pressure and cholesterol. This *mushroom* is good to eat.

The *Lion's mane mushroom* from the fungus *Hericium erinaceus* contains *erinacines* which cause nerve cells to grow. The *Lion's mane mushroom* is recommended as adjunctive treatment for amyotrophic lateral sclerosis (Lou Gehrig's disease) and multiple sclerosis. It may be possible to use extracts of this *mushroom* in patients with Alzheimer's disease to improve cognitive function. This *mushroom* may one day be used to help regenerate nerve tissue after spinal cord injury. This *mushroom* is good to eat.

The *Maitake mushroom* comes from the fungus *Grifola frondosa*, common name in Japan *dancing mushroom*. A chemical in the *Maitake mushroom* called *Maitake D-Fraction* possesses anti-cancer activity (proven for breast, colon, and prostate cancers) and augments immune function. It shows a regenerative effect on tissues which have been subjected to chemotherapy and radiation. The *Maitake mushroom* may also have a beneficial effect on blood sugar. It lowers triglycerides and LDL cholesterol while promoting a lower blood pressure. For those reasons, the *Maitake mushroom* is useful for persons with cardiovascular disease. This *mushroom* is used to increase energy, vitality, stamina, athletic performance, and mental functioning. The *Maitake mushroom* is good to eat.

The *Reishi mushroom* comes from the fungus *Ganoderma lucidum*. It augments the function of the immune system and shows anti-cancer activity. It shows a regenerative effect on tissues which have been subjected to chemotherapy and radiation. Since it possesses anti-inflammatory activity, it is sometimes recommended to treat arthritis and heart disease. The *Reishi mushroom* has been used in China for over 2,000 years to promote longevity. You may find *Reishi mushrooms* in liquid extracts, capsule form, and as an ingredient in teas.

The *Royal sun agaricus mushroom* comes from the fungus *Agaricus brasiliensis* (called the *Brazilian blazei* so as not to be confused with *Agaricus blazei* which is actually a separate species). It possesses anti-cancer properties and augments the immune system. It reduces cholesterol and modulates blood sugar. This *mushroom* contains chemicals that decrease the activity of *aromatase*, an enzyme that enhances the growth of cancers.

The *Shiitake mushroom* comes from the fungus *Lentinula edodes*. It is the most studied medicinal *mushroom*. This remarkable *mushroom* possesses the chemical *eritadenine* which lowers LDL cholesterol and triglycerides. It is useful to treat cardiovascular disease. It also possesses the chemical *lentianan* which activates the immune system (increases T-cell and natural killer cell production) as well as demonstrating anti-cancer activity. It is useful in treating immune system diseases such as HIV/AIDS. The *Shiitake mushroom* is good to eat.

The *Zhu ling mushroom* comes from the fungus *Polyporus umbellatus*. This *mushroom* is being used to increase immune response in patients with lung cancer. It is useful to help patients regenerate tissues after chemotherapy and radiation. In addition this mushroom contains potent antibiotics and is sometimes used to treat urinary tract infections.

Dr. Andrew Weil is a proponent of medicinal *mushrooms* to prevent and treat cancer and augment immunity in ailments like cancer, arthritis, HIV/AIDS, and heart disease. He recommends *Fungi Perfecti* at 1-800-780-9126 or www.fungi.com as a reliable source for *medicinal mushroom* supplements. He recommends taking a combination product (*Stamets 7 Mushroom Blend* or *MycoSoft Gold* from *Fungi Perfecti*) which may be more effective than taking any one single *mushroom*. *Stamets 7 Mushroom Blend* is a blend of 7 *mushroom* species while *MycoSoft Gold* contains 13. These products come in liquid drop form. The dosage is 15-30 drops twice daily. You may call *Fungi Perfecti* and order a copy of the book *MycoMedicinals* by Stamets, published by MycoMedia in 2002. Another reliable source for hot water extracts of *mushrooms* is *Mushroom Science* at www.mushroomscience.com.

Note: Dr. Weil's *Self-Healing Newsletter* provided some of the information on *medicinal mushrooms*. You can order his newsletter at www.drweilselfhealing.com.

Note: Our most commonly eaten *mushrooms*, *Button mushrooms* do not contain *beta glucans*.

Note: Information on whether *mushrooms* extracts taken as nutritional supplements are safe during pregnancy and lactation is scanty. I recommend that you stay with *mushrooms* as food during pregnancy and lactation.

Phytosterols

Phytosterols are plant *sterols* and *sterolins* (such as *beta-sitosterol* and *beta-sitosterolin*). *Phytosterols* show anti-inflammatory as well as cholesterol-lowering activity. *Phytosterols* are immune system regulators.

Moducare, manufactured by Essential Phyto-sterolins, Inc., contains *sterols* (20mg) and *sterolins* (0.2mg) in a 100:1 ratio. The dose is one capsule three times daily before meals. *Moducare* is useful to restore normal functioning of the immune system as a result of cancer, HIV/AIDS, autoimmune diseases, arthritis, heart disease, fibromyalgia, and chronic fatigue syndrome, as well as many other chronic diseases.

> **Note:** Medical research on patients with chronic fatigue syndrome showed that patients taking homeopathic treatment for CFS had significantly greater improvement that those taking placebo.

Propolis

Propolis is a complex chemical compound derived from bees. Since *propolis* possesses antibacterial, antifungal, and antiviral activity, it is used by bees as a "cement" to seal and repair their hives. By stimulating the immune system, *propolis* also has anti-inflammatory and anti-cancer properties.

Propolis comes in a wide variety of different forms from lozenges (to enhance the immune system) to creams (to enhance wound healing, treat acne and Athlete's foot) to toothpaste and mouth rinse. The most prudent approach would be to follow the directions on the label for dosage recommendations.

Propolis has not been shown to be safe if used by pregnant or lactating women. People who are allergic to bees should not take *propolis*.

> **Note:** Other products derived from bees are *bee pollen* and *Royal Jelly*. *Bee pollen* is rich in minerals and vitamins so it may be useful for elderly persons who have trouble digesting multivitamin-multimineral supplements. *Royal Jelly* is the food fed to the queen of the hive, enabling her to live for years rather than just weeks. It may be helpful to improve energy. However, serious allergic reactions have been reported so people with allergy to bees should not take any bee-derived supplement (except honey).

Whey

Whey is the high quality protein fraction that results from the manufacture of cheese from milk. Cow's milk contains 2 proteins, casein (80%) and *whey* (20%). *Whey* contains no lactose or fat. *Whey* contains a very high concentration of *glutamine*, the amino acid found in the highest amount in your body.

Whey protein contains other chemical compounds, besides healthy *glutamine*, like immunoglobulins, that augment the functioning of your immune system. *Whey* protein may be used to boost immune function during the debilitation phase after chemotherapy or radiation treatment for cancer. *Whey* protein may act to decrease the amount of the antioxidant *glutathione* inside cancer cells, making them more susceptible to destruction by chemotherapy and radiation. At the same time, *whey* increases the amount of *glutathione* in normal cells.

Whey protein supplements are often used as performance-enhancing supplements. They tend to increase strength, lean muscle mass, and overall weight. Persons prone to kidney problems should not take *whey* or any protein supplement because they may suffer from a serious condition called protein overload.

Whey protein supplements come in different flavors to mix with water. The dose is 20-30 grams twice daily.

> **Remember:** Most people need between 50 and 65 grams of protein daily. Males need more than females. Older people need more than younger. Protein synthesis is occurring all the time inside your body, directed by your nuclear DNA that sends chemical messages to your RNA, located in the cytoplasm of every cell. People on higher protein diets tend to consume fewer total calories which is helpful in weight loss.

Guidelines for Consulting Your Health Care Provider

Note: Never self-prescribe homeopathy, herbal remedies, or nutritional supplements for a person with cancer without the expert guidance of a health care provider. Always disclose your homeopathic remedies, herbal medicines, and nutritional supplements to your health care provider.

You should consult your health care provider if:
• the patient doesn't look right or act right (trust your instincts!)
• the patient is getting worse instead of better over the course of the illness
• the patient is having trouble breathing or complaining of chest pains or there is mental confusion or lethargy or irritability
• the patient develops allergic symptoms (hives, itchy or watery eyes, runny nose, scratchy throat, asthma, shortness of breath) after taking a nutritional supplement
• after beginning a nutritional supplement the patient experiences *new onset* of any serious symptoms such as:

   paralysis, weakness, tingling, inability to focus or concentrate, blurred or double vision or blindness, slurred speech, severe headaches, seizures, irritability, dizziness, disorientation, memory loss, anxiety, depression, insomnia, blackouts, fainting, or the person complains of not feeling like himself
• the patient is taking *ANY* prescription medication
• the patient is pregnant or breastfeeding
• the patient has any serious, chronic disease which may have complications and become life-threatening, such as:

   autism, cancer, HIV and AIDS, arthritis, multiple sclerosis, coronary artery disease, heart attack (myocardial infarction), blood dyscrasia, cancer (of any type), congestive heart failure, diabetes mellitus, obesity, thyroid disorders, high blood pressure (hypertension), stroke, seizures, acute and chronic kidney (renal) failure, schizophrenia, bipolar disorder, borderline personality disorder, eating disorders, fibromyalgia, chronic fatigue syndrome, Crohn's disease, ulcerative colitis, celiac disease, mental deficiency disorders, chromosomal disorders, infertility, frequent miscarriages, polyneuropathy, cystic fibrosis [Adapted from *The Merck Manual* at www.merck.com]

Note: Do not discontinue taking any pharmaceutical medication prescribed by your health care provider unless you or your family member is under the supervision of a physician.

Note: Self-care for persons who already had/have cancer is not a sound practice in any case. Do not take any nutritional supplement to prevent or treat cancer or augment your immune system without first consulting your health care provider especially if you or your family member is taking a prescription medication to treat cancer or its complications or is pregnant or breastfeeding.

In addition, it is a good idea to check with your health care provider if your family member is either very young or very old because nutritional supplements given injudiciously may overwhelm the body's defenses in those age groups.

Note: If you or your family member requires diagnostic testing or treatment for cancer, I recommend that you investigate the cancer treatment centers that incorporate integrative medicine units. A good example is the *Zakim Center for Integrated Therapies at the Dana Farber Cancer Institute* in Boston. Oncologists who do not practice in a setting with an integrative medicine unit are less likely to help you with your quest for healthy adjunctive therapies such as homeopathy, herbal medicines, and nutritional supplements. If your philosophy of health embraces the tenets of self-care, you will never need a partner more than for the treatment of cancer.

Note: If you want a virtual second opinion, a good place to start is *Partners Online Specialty Consultations* at https://econsults.partners.org. This gives you the benefits of the major Boston hospitals (including *Dana Farber Cancer Institute, Brigham and Women's Hospital* and *Massachusetts General Hospital*). You will need a referral from your primary health care provider and the complete report is sent to that doctor.

Note: The most important thing to understand about using *homeopathy, herbal remedies, and nutritional supplements* for the treatment of cancer is that these must **not** be given during chemotherapy or radiation therapy. This is because the effects of *homeopathy, herbal remedies, and nutritional supplements* may actually go against the action of chemotherapy or radiation therapy. For this reason *homeopathy, herbal remedies, and nutritional supplements* are taken after the chemotherapy or radiation therapy sessions are finished, or during the respite between sessions.

However: More and more evidence is accumulating to contradict this conventional wisdom. Read about the controversial issues in articles from the Simone Protective Cancer Institute published in *Alternative Therapies in Health and Medicine*, January/February 2007 and March/April 2007.

Note: Do not use any nutritional supplements to augment the immune system if you or your family member is taking a drug for immunosuppression (usually prescribed to treat autoimmune diseases or to prevent organ transplant rejection).

Note: Contrary to its past categorization as an anti-nutrient, *phytic acid* (also called *inositol hexaphosphate* or *IP6*) may also possess anti-cancer properties, in large part due to its antioxidant content. Although *phytic acid* does bind to minerals decreasing their absorption from the intestines, it's probably insignificant among persons eating a nutritious diet. However, nutritional supplements of *phytic acid* and *inositol* are not recommended at this time. The best food sources are whole grains, beans, and nuts.

Note: *Oleander* extract (*Nerium oleander*, a member of the *Apocynaceae* botanical family) contains a cytotoxic agent *oleandrin*. *Oleander* extract has been used to treat prostate cancer. It is available as *Xenavex* by ShimodaAtlantic. It should be used only under a doctor's supervision because of its potential toxicity and drug interactions.

Note: *Shark cartilage* may have anti-cancer properties, although it is important to recognize that no study has ever proven any benefit of using it in the treatment of cancer. *Shark cartilage* probably acts by interfering with creation of new blood vessels (angiogenesis). *Shark cartilage* powder is expensive and the taste is so bad that it is mixed with juice and flavorings. Since so little is known about its advantages and disadvantages, I do not recommend using it unless you are on a research protocol. Certainly, pregnant women should not take *shark cartilage* because of the possibility of interference with creation of new blood vessels in the fetus. The same is probably true with people who have heart disease.

Note: If you are unsure about a nutritional program to treat and/or prevent cancer, you may obtain further information from the *American Institute* *for Cancer Research* 1-202-328-7744 or www.aicr.org. They are the leading nonprofit organization doing research (and translating it into consumer-friendly terms) into nutritional ways to treat and prevent cancer. The *AICR* publishes a free, worthwhile newsletter *AICR Science Now,* that has always been helpful to me. You may order toll-free at 1-800-843-8114. You may also find that the reader-friendly *How to Prevent and Treat Cancer with Natural Medicine* by Murray, Birdsall, Pizzorno and Reilly, published by Riverhead Books in 2002 to have all the nutritional information you need. It's a good investment.

Note: For reliable information on cancer research as well as online answers to your general questions about cancer, try *The Cancer Information Service* (*CIS*) of the National Cancer Institute at http://cis.nci.nih.gov.

The *American Cancer Society* is a good place to go for a survivor's network at www.cancer.org or 1-800-ACS-2345. But I do not recommend everything that the *American Cancer Society* publishes. I do not recommend their overly conservative and often out-of-date advice on homeopathy, herbal remedies, and nutritional supplements for the prevention and treatment of cancer.

Beware: of the *American Cancer Society's Guide to Complementary and Alternative Cancer Methods.* It is ultra-conservative and ultra-negative. The book's 2-page review on homeopathy is filled with misinformation and untruths.

Note: You may want to investigate the *National Cancer Institute* (*NCI*), part of the *National Institutes of Health* (*NIH*). The *NCI* funds cancer research using complementary and alternative medicines (CAM) and provides information about CAM to practitioners and the public at www.cancer.gov/cam.

Note: You or your family member may want to investigate participating in a cancer treatment clinical trial. A good place to start is the NCCAM Clinical Trials website at http://nccam.nih.gov/clinicaltrials/.

Beware: *PC-SPES,* a product containing 7 herbs and *Reishi mushrooms,* made by BotanicLab, had been designed to treat prostate cancer in men. But it was found to contain many impurities including DES (*diethylstilbesterol,* a synthetic estrogen). It was ultimately taken off the market in 2002.

Note: For recommendations about cancer detection tests and procedures, please contact the *National Foundation for Cancer Research* 1-800-321-CURE and the *American Cancer Society* at www.cancer.org or 1-800-ACS-2345.

Note: For reliable information on herbal remedies and nutritional supplements for persons with cancer, visit the *Memorial Sloan-Kettering Cancer* Center online at www.mskcc.org.

Note: Reliable online information on cancer and alternative medicine can be found at *The National Foundation for Alternative Medicine* at www.nfam.org (1-202-463-4900) and the *Annie Appleseed Project* at www.annieappleseedproject.org.

Note: You may learn about reliable alternative remedies for the treatment of cancer at www.ralphmoss.com and www.cancerdecisions.com. He has written many books, like *Herbs Against Cancer, Antioxidants Against Cancer, Questioning Chemotherapy, Alternative Medicine Online, Cancer Industry* and *Cancer Therapy: The Independent Consumer's Guide.* You may sign up for his free newsletter.

Note: *Avemar* is fermented wheat germ extract which may turn out to have some value in the treatment of cancer in humans. It probably works by its high concentration of *benzoquinones* helping to increase the body's natural killer cells.

Note: *Acai* (*Euterpe oleracea*) is a fruit from the Brazilian amazon region whose juice has become a popular treatment for cancer. *Acai* berries are rich in antioxidants (anthocyanins), but other fruits are richer. According to *Moss Reports* at www.cancerdecisions.com/020506_page.html no clinical research data exist that justifies using *Acai* juice as an anti-cancer treatment.

Note: Dr. Andrew Weil's skin care products, *Origins*, include several mushroom species in their formulations. *Plantidote Mega Mushroom Face Serum* includes *Hypsizygus ulmarius, Cordyceps* and *Reishi mushrooms* along with the herbal remedies *Ginger, Turmeric* and *Holy Basil*, and the antioxidant *resveratrol*, and *Argan nut oil*. *Plantidote Mega Mushroom Supplement* includes *Hypsizygus ulmarius, Cordyceps* and *Lion's mane mushrooms*, with *Ginger, Turmeric, Holy Basil* and *Flaxseed oil*. Use the face serum topically and the supplement by mouth (one dropperful daily) together.

Putting It All Together

In addition to the nutritional supplements to prevent cancer and augment your immune system in this chapter, there are others that may be found in different chapters in this book.

If you are considering using a nutritional supplement to prevent cancer and augment your immune system, it is a good idea to familiarize yourself with **Chapter 22: Introduction to Nutritional Supplements**. It makes good sense to understand the role of vitamin and mineral nutritional supplements from **Chapter 23: Vitamins and Minerals**; antioxidant nutritional supplements from **Chapter 24: Antioxidant Phytochemicals: Natural Anti-Aging Remedies** and *omega-3 fatty acids* from **Chapter 31: Oils and Fats**. In addition, you will likely benefit from learning about *Coenzyme Q10, systemic Enzymes* and *Fiber*, and the amino acid *theanine* in **Chapter 25: Heart Healthy Nutritional Supplements**. Please consider taking *prebiotics* and *probiotics* to enhance the digestive and immune systems (please refer to **Chapter 30: Prebiotics and Probiotics**). Please be sure you understand when to discontinue taking antioxidants and nutritional supplements during chemotherapy and radiation treatments.

Whenever you have decided to go ahead with taking nutritional supplements to prevent cancer and augment your immune system, it is a good idea to consider giving the sick person's homeopathic constitutional remedy as well (please refer to **Chapter 9: Homeopathic Remedies for Constitutional Problems in Infants, Children, and Adolescents** or to **Chapter 18: Homeopathic Constitutional Remedies** if you are dealing with an adult; or **Chapter 13: Homeopathy for Elderly Persons** if you are dealing with an elderly person). In addition, you will want to read **Chapter 17: Homeopathy for Persons with Cancer**. Homeopathic remedies may be used in conjunction with herbal medicines and nutritional supplements. Please be sure you understand when to discontinue taking homeopathic remedies during chemotherapy and radiation treatments.

Please investigate **Chapter 20: Herbs You Need to Know** and familiarize yourself with the herbal remedies with anti-cancer properties such as *Astragalus, Cat's Claw, Garlic, Ginseng* and *Green tea*. Then take a look at *soy isoflavones* in **Chapter 21: Herbal Remedies for Women's Health**. Please be sure you understand when to discontinue taking herbal remedies during chemotherapy and radiation treatments.

Chapter 28

Nutritional Supplements for Diseases of Joints, Bones and Muscles

Musculoskeletal Ailments in General

Ailment/Disorder/Symptom	Nutritional Supplement
Anti-inflammatory and analgesic (pain relief) activity	*Cetyl myristoleate (CMO)*
Pain relief and joint function	*Chondroitin*
Pain relief and joint function	*Glucosamine*
Anti-inflammatory and analgesic activity	*Devil's claw*
Anti-inflammatory activity	*Enzymes*
Immune system regulation	*Green foods*
Joints, skin, and hair	*Methylsulfonylmethane (MSM)*
Pain relief and joint function, depression	*S-adenosylmethionine (SAMe)*
Pain relief and joint function	*Stinging nettle*

Guidelines for Consulting Your Health Care Provider
Putting It All Together

Musculoskeletal Ailments in General

The list of diseases of joints, bones, and muscles includes the more common ailments such as arthritis, osteoarthritis, gout, osteoporosis, lower back pain, and fibromyalgia, as well as the less common autoimmune connective tissue diseases such as rheumatoid arthritis, systemic lupus erythematosus, polymyalgia rheumatica, and many others.

Bones connect to each other by way of joints. Joints are composed of cartilage situated on each end of the connecting bones with synovial fluid in between. Joints are designed to absorb the shock to your bones delivered every time you move. When joints undergo the process of inflammation, arthritis results. Forty-three million Americans suffer from arthritis (of which there are over 100 different types). The usual symptoms are stiffness, pain, and swelling with progressive disability in movement. Sometimes there is disfigurement of the joints. The most common form of arthritis is osteoarthritis affecting twenty-one million Americans. The joints commonly involved in osteoarthritis are knees, hips, and spines.

Rheumatoid arthritis, affecting 3-5 million Americans, is an autoimmune disease with an underlying immune system dysfunction. It affects not only joints but also other tissues in the body. The most common joints involved in rheumatoid arthritis are fingers, hands, and feet. Stiffness, pain, and swelling of the joints may be accompanied by more general symptoms like fatigue, weakness, and low-grade fevers.

The majority of the serious musculoskeletal diseases are caused by lifestyle factors superimposed on a genetically susceptible person. The most important things you can do to prevent these diseases in yourself or a family member are stop smoking, follow a healthy, anti-inflammatory dietary program, and exercise at least 30 minutes on most days.

> **Note:** The healthy dietary program to prevent and treat musculoskeletal diseases to consider is, according to Dr. Andrew Weil, the anti-inflammatory diet, which is based on the Mediterranean diet. The anti-inflammatory diet depends heavily on whole foods that grow from the earth like whole grains, fresh fruits and vegetables, with *olive oil* as your fat source. In addition, you will need to consume foods high in *omega-3 fatty acids*, like walnuts and flaxseeds. Animal protein is at a minimum except for cold water fatty fish, again supplying *omega-3 fatty acids*. You may add *ginger* and *turmeric* to your food for their anti-inflammatory effects as well as antioxidant vitamins and minerals. You must limit your intake of processed foods and sugar.

Osteoarthritis is an age-related degenerative arthritis of the weight bearing joints (knees, hips). More than twenty million Americans suffer from this form of arthritis. It is present to some degree in almost one of every two persons older than 65. It is often associated with excess body weight. The best way to prevent this type of arthritis is to engage in healthy nutrition and exercise for the long-term.

When taking nutritional supplements for self-care to treat diseases of joints, bones, and muscles you must pay strict attention to the **Guidelines for Consulting Your Health Care Provider** at the end of this chapter. You may want to refer to the last section **Putting It All Together** for ideas on how to integrate the essential natural alternatives, homeopathy, herbal remedies, and nutritional supplements.

Cetyl myristoleate (CMO)

Cetyl myristoleate (CMO) is a synthetic product manufactured from myristoleic acid. Then it is chemically changed into *cetyl myristoleate*. *Cetyl myristoleate* possesses anti-inflammatory and analgesic properties. The results of double-blind placebo-controlled studies of *cetyl myristoleate* in humans showed that the majority of patients derived considerable benefit such as increased mobility and decreased joint pain. Side effects include nausea and diarrhea. A popular brand is *Myristin* made by EHP Products, 550mg capsules containing 110mg of *CMO*. The dosage is 2 capsules 3 times daily.

Chondroitin

Chondroitin is a chemical compound (*mucopolysaccharide*) present in the type of *collagen* (type 2 *collagen*) that holds cartilage together. It is responsible for the elasticity of cartilage and helping to absorb shock. *Chondroitin* helps to relieve pain and improve function in joints damaged by osteoarthritis. *Chondroitin* increases the production of *hyaluronic acid*, a chemical compound present in synovial fluid which acts to reduce friction between the two bones forming the joint.

Chondroitin sulfate is manufactured from the tracheal cartilage of cows and pigs so there is some concern that the product may contain the infective particles (called prions) of "mad cow disease." However, this remains, at this point, a theoretical concern. *Chondroitin sulfate* made from shark cartilage is not recommended because of the likelihood of heavy metal contamination.

The dosage of *chondroitin* is 800-1,200mg daily split into 2 equal doses. It is considered safe for long-term use. There may be gastrointestinal side effects such as diarrhea or constipation. *Chondroitin* as the nutritional supplement may take 2 months or more to see its full effect on joints. The chemical structure of *chondroitin* is similar to *heparin*. Persons taking anti-coagulants like *warfarin* (*Coumadin*) or *heparin* to thin their blood should not take *chondroitin* unless supervised by their physician.

Chondroitin may be taken alone but it is often combined with *glucosamine* (please see below) for presumed increased effectiveness. Medical research studying the effectiveness of the combination is in progress.

> **Note:** Results of a large study done by the National Center for Complementary and Alternative Medicine showed that *glucosamine* with and without *chondroitin sufate* did not decrease knee pain better than placebo in patients with osteoarthritis. But some patients with more severe pain did benefit.

Sometimes both *glucosamine* and *chondroitin* are combined together with *methylsulfonylmethane* (*MSM*) (please see below) in an effort to increase effectiveness.

Insufficient medical data exists on the use of *chondroitin* during pregnancy and lactation so it is not recommended. The same is true for the use of *chondroitin* in children.

Glucosamine

Glucosamine, as the chemical compounds *glucosamine hydrochloride* and *glucosamine sulfate*, are found naturally throughout all the tissues of the body. *Glucosamine* is an integral part of cartilage. Chemically, it is the amino acid *glutamine* combined with glucose. It not only relieves pain, but also functions to repair, restore, and rebuild cartilage. *Glucosamine* is used as a nutritional supplement to alleviate the joint deterioration, destruction, and pain of osteoarthritis. Medical studies have shown that *Glucosamine* may perform better than NSAIDs in alleviating pain, improving function, and restoring joints to a healthier state.

There is no toxicity reported with *glucosamine*. However, there is some controversy about the effect of *glucosamine* on blood sugar. Studies done on animals show an increased insulin resistance when *glucosamine* is used over a long period of time. A supplement that increases insulin resistance in animals might increase the risk of type 2 diabetes mellitus. However, it is important to recognize that this remains a theoretical risk in humans because a recent medical study found *glucosamine* had no effect on blood sugar. If you or your family member has type 2 diabetes, and you do choose to take *glucosamine* you will need to monitor your blood sugars closely.

> **Note:** *Glucosamine* is not recommended for persons who require insulin to regulate blood sugar.

The dosage is 1,500mg per day (or 2,000mg per day for persons weighing more than 200 pounds) split into 2 equal doses. It is considered safe for long-term use. There may be gastrointestinal side effects such as indigestion, nausea, and vomiting. *Glucosamine* as the nutritional supplement may take 2 months or more to see its full effect on joints. *Glucosamine* may be taken alone but it is usually taken with *chondroitin sulfate* (please see above) because it is believed (although not yet proven; studies are being done) that the combination is more effective than either one alone. Sometimes both *glucosamine* and *chondroitin* are combined together with methylsulfonylmethane (MSM) (please see below) in an effort to increase effectiveness.

Glucosamine supplements are made from chitin in the shells of crustaceans (shellfish) such as crabs, lobsters and shrimp. People who are allergic to shellfish should take glucosamine with caution because they may experience an allergic reaction. People who have experienced life-threatening (anaphylactic) allergic reactions to shellfish should not take glucosamine.

Insufficient medical data exists on the use of glucosamine during pregnancy and lactation so it is not recommended. The same is true for the use of glucosamine in children.

> **Note:** Topical glucosamine is not effective because glucosamine is not absorbed through the skin.

> **Note:** When ConsumerLab.com performed product reviews of glucosamine and chondroitin supplements they found that one-third failed to contain the labeled amounts of the active ingredients. This means you need to be particularly vigilant. You should not buy a product without reading the results at www.ConsumerLab.com or in their book, ConsumerLab.com's Guide to Buying Vitamins and Supplements, What's Really in the Bottle?

> **Note:** ArthroMax manufactured by Life Extension contains glucosamine sulfate (derived from shellfish), methylsulfonylmethane (MSM) (please see below), nobiletin and tangeretin (from natural citrus and palm fruit extracts), and 5-loxin from Boswellia extract (please see below). Nobiletin and tangeretin inhibit cytokines involved in inflammation while 5-loxin reduces the level of 5-lipooxygenase, an enzyme involved in inflammation. Do not use ArthroMax if you are allergic to shellfish. Do not use tangeretin if you are being treated with tamoxifen to prevent breast cancer relapse. Take 2 capsules of ArthroMax twice daily.

Devil's claw

Devil's claw (Harpagophytum procumbens) is an herbal remedy. The plant is a native of Africa. The medicinal part is the root. Devil's claw is approved by German Commission E on herbal medicines for rheumatism. It possesses anti-inflammatory and analgesic activity. Medical research shows that Devil's claw provides relief of the knee pain of osteoarthritis in about 50% of patients. It is being used today to treat osteoarthritis, rheumatoid arthritis, gout, and back pain. It is also used to stimulate appetite, so this herbal remedy is not a good choice for persons who need to lose weight to be healthy.

Devil's claw should not be used in people with stomach or duodenal ulcers because the herb stimulates the secretion of acidic gastric juice. It should not be given to women during pregnancy or lactation nor to young children because information on safety is not known.

The dosage is 600-1,200mg of a preparation containing 1%-3% harpagosides three times daily. Devil's claw is often used along with NSAIDS to achieve pain relief. Devil's claw supplements enable you to use a lower dose of NSAIDs to obtain a superior level of relief.

Enzymes

Systemic enzyme nutritional supplements are used to modulate the immune system thereby reducing chronic inflammation. Chronic inflammation underlies rheumatoid arthritis and osteoarthritis as well as heart disease and cancer.

Systemic enzyme nutritional supplements are also used to treat fibromyalgia and the ailments commonly associated with it such as irritable bowel syndrome and chronic fatigue syndrome. People with fibromyalgia tend to suffer from disturbed or disordered sleep which is best treated by safe and effective homeopathic remedies.

Systemic enzymes that break down proteins are called proteases. They have the ability to interfere with inflammatory processes by disrupting pathways that are triggered by inflammatory chemicals called cytokines.

One of the most commonly prescribed and widely available systemic pancreatic enzyme supplements is *Wobenzym N* at a dosage of 2 tablets 3 times daily or 3 tablets twice daily.

> **Note:** Systemic pancreatic *enzyme* supplements are not for use by persons with hemophilia, persons taking anticoagulant therapy, or after heart surgery when there is an increased risk of bleeding.

> **Note:** To use systemic *enzymes* as anti-inflamatory agents, you must take them at least 30-60 minutes before eating. Otherwise, they function to aid digesetion.

> **Note:** If you want to explore the use of *enzyme* nutritional supplements for the treatment of arthritis, please read *The Aspirin Alternative—the Natural Way to Overcome Chronic Pain, Reduce Inflammation and Enhance the Healing Response* by Loes and Steinman, published by Freedom Press in 2001.

> **Note:** For more information on Systemic pancreatic *enzymes*, please see **Chapter 27: Nutritional Supplements to Prevent Cancer and Augment Your Immune System**.

Green foods

Green foods refer to nutritional supplements that contain chlorophyll, that remarkably complex chemical that is the energy factory for green plants. Chlorophyll is the photoreceptor for photosynthesis. But as miraculous as chlorophyll is for plants, it plays no metabolic role in humans.

Green foods that come from the sea (such as *Kelp*, other seaweeds, the microalgae *spirulina*, and *chlorella*) are called sea vegetables. They contain certain nutrients that may alleviate degenerative joint diseases. *Spirulina* inhibits viral penetration into cells. *Chlorella* may alleviate symptoms of fibromyalgia. *Chlorella* stimulates T-cell activity and increases interferon levels thus augmenting the immune system.

Green foods that do not come from the sea such as *wheat grass* and *barley grass*, may be used to help peo-

ple ingest the recommended daily servings of leafy green vegetables. *Green foods* both sea-based and non-sea-based possess immunomodulatory activity. This means that the nutrients in *green foods* strike a balance in the body between pro- and anti-inflammatory *cytokines*. *Green foods* may be useful to treat chronic inflammatory ailments such as arthritis, fibromyalgia, and cancer.

There are many different preparations of *green foods* so that specific dosage recommendations cannot be made. It is prudent to follow the directions on the label of the nutritional supplement that you have chosen.

> **Note:** When we realize that our own health and survival are based on chlorophyll, the powerhouse of plants, we recognize our interdependence on the green plants of this planet. We each of us should do as much as we can to preserve the health and well being of green plants.

Methylsulfonylmethane (MSM)

Methylsulfonylmethane (MSM) is an organic form of the mineral element sulfur (also spelled sulphur). It occurs naturally in plants and animals. *MSM* releases bioactive and bioavailable sulfur, which may help to make joints, skin, and hair healthier. Its mechanisms of action possibly include inhibition of pain impulses, decreasing inflammation, and increasing blood flow among others. *MSM* is used to treat osteoarthritis and rheumatoid arthritis as well as to thicken and strengthen hair and nails. However, medical research on effectiveness is scanty and long-term studies of safety are lacking.

Side effects of *MSM* include diarrhea, upset stomach, headache, and rash. *MSM* should not be used by people who are taking anticoagulants such as *warfarin (Coumadin)* or *heparin* unless supervised by their physicians. I recommend that you first check with your physician before starting *MSM* if you are taking *aspirin*, *Ginkgo biloba*, *Garlic*, or high doses of Vitamin E. The dosage 2-8 grams daily, depending on response, in divided doses with meals. You will also find *MSM* in topical form to treat muscle and bone pain. *MSM* is often combined with *chondroitin* and *glucosamine* (please see above) in an effort to increase effectiveness (still unproven).

S-adenosylmethionine (SAMe)

SAMe is a synthetic form of a naturally occurring compound that helps your body to produce dopamine, norepinephrine, and serotonin, chemicals that send messages in your brain (neurotransmitters). SAMe is manufactured from the essential amino acid methionine and the energy storage molecule adenosine triphosphate (ATP). SAMe is present in every cell in your body. It functions as a methyl donor in more than 100 chemical reactions.

SAMe has been proven to be a useful adjunctive treatment for most forms of arthritis as well as for depression. It possesses anti-inflammatory and analgesic properties. In some medical research studies the effect of SAMe on decreasing joint pain and increasing mobility in persons with osteoarthritis was equivalent to NSAIDs (without the side effect of gastrointestinal bleeding). It may take up to 4 weeks for SAMe to have a beneficial effect in treating osteoarthritis. The same is true when treating depression.

SAMe may be particularly useful in people with fibromyalgia because it reduces trigger-point tenderness, decreases joint pain and stiffness, while it reduces the depression (a usual accompaniment).

The dose of SAMe is 400-600mg daily although for severe osteoarthritis 1,600mg daily may be necessary. It is taken in 1-2 divided doses on an empty stomach. It may take 1- 4 weeks for the beneficial effects of SAMe to manifest in treating depression and joint pain. The side effects of SAMe include stomach upset, headaches, insomnia, dizziness, diarrhea, and over-stimulation. The safety of taking SAMe long-term is unknown. The safety of SAMe during pregnancy and lactation is unknown. SAMe is not recommended for use in children. There are no allergic reactions from taking SAMe.

> **Note:** Persons who suffer from bipolar disorder should not take SAMe because it may trigger manic episodes. The safety of SAMe in treating Parkinson's disease is unknown. Persons who are taking an antidepressant prescription medication of the MAO inhibitor type should not take SAMe. I do not recommend taking SAMe along with specific serotonin reuptake inhibitors (SSRIs) because of the theoretical possibility of increasing serotonin levels. High serotonin levels may precipitate the serotonin syndrome (sweating, confusion, twitching and hyperthermia).

> **Note:** SAMe is converted into the amino acid homocysteine in the body. High levels of homocysteine are a risk factor for heart disease, stroke, Alzheimer's disease, and certain cancers. It is not known if your homocysteine level increases as a result of taking SAMe supplements. However, to minimize this possibility, when using SAMe it is recommended to take supplemental amounts of certain B Vitamins such as B6 and B12 and folic acid (folate) which act to metabolize homocysteine.

> **Note:** SAMe is also useful to promote liver health. This may be related to SAMe increasing the amount of the antioxidant glutathione inside your body which helps your liver to function better.

> **Note:** When ConsumerLab.com performed product reviews of SAMe supplements they found that one-half failed to contain the labeled amounts of the active ingredients. A popular brand is SAMe by Nature Made. You can get more information on SAMe by Nature Made by calling their information line 1-800-276-2828 or visiting online at www.naturemade.com.

Stinging nettle

Stinging nettle (Urtica dioica) is an herbal remedy. The medicinal part is the leaves of the plant. Stinging nettle possesses anti-inflammatory properties. It is useful to control the pain and swelling of rheumatoid arthritis. *Stinging nettle* interferes with the actions of histamine, thereby reducing pain and swelling.

Stinging nettle is often used along with NSAIDS to achieve pain relief. *Stinging nettle* supplements enable you to use a lower dose of NSAIDs to obtain a superior level of relief.

Other herbal remedies for arthritis
You may find *Stinging nettle* combined with other herbal remedies that affect joint health.

White willow bark (Salix alba) contains *salicin*, a naturally occurring salicylic acid, the compound in aspirin which has anti-inflammatory and analgesic properties.

Ginger (Zingiber officinale) is an antioxidant herb with anti-inflammatory activity. It may be used for the pain and swelling of osteoarthritis and rheumatoid arthritis. The dose is 500mg 2-4 times daily.

> **Note:** *Zyflamend* is a popular, natural, anti-inflammatory, combination, herbal remedy manufactured by New Chapter that, according to medical research evidence, acts like Cox-2 inhibitors on joints and muscles. *Zyflamend* contains the herbal ingredients *Rosemary, Turmeric, Ginger, Holy Basil, Greet tea, Hu Zhang, Chinese Goldthread, Barberry, Oregano* and *Scutellaria baicalensis*. Since *Zyflamend* comes in several different dosage levels, as well as capsules and liquid, it's best to follow the directions on the bottle. You my order at 1-866-963-9675 or www.new-mark.com. It may take up to two months to see results.

Boswellia gum-resin extract *(Boswellia serrata)*, common name *Indian frankincense*, possesses both anti-inflammatory and analgesic actions, making it useful to treat osteoarthritis and rheumatoid arthritis. Taking *Boswellia* may enable you to decrease the dosage of NSAIDs while achieving the same relief from pain, swelling, and morning stiffness. The dose of *Boswellia* containing a standardized extract of 37.5% *boswellic* acids is 300-400mg three times daily.

The kitchen spice *turmeric (Curcuma longa)*, a potent anti-cancer antioxidant, contains the anti-

inflammatory compound *curcumin*. *Turmeric* and *Boswellia* are sometimes combined to achieve a higher level of effectiveness. It is a healthy step to increase your use of *turmeric* in your cooking. When you take *turmeric* as the nutritional supplement, the dose of *curcumin* is 400mg three times daily.

> **Note:** Do not use *turmeric* along with NSAIDs because both inhibit platelet aggregation. This combination may cause an increased risk of bleeding. But you may continue to season your foods with *turmeric* as the spice.

Ashwagandha root *(Withania somnifera)* is an herbal remedy popular in Ayurvedic medicine. *Ashwagandha* exerts an anti-inflammatory effect. Its use allows some people to decrease their reliance on NSAIDs and steroids. An ayurvedic formula to treat rheumatoid arthritis consists of *ginger, Boswellia, turmeric* and *Ashwagandha*.

Zostrix cream contains *capsaicin*, a chemical found naturally in the hot-pepper plant. It relieves painful joints associated with osteoarthritis. You must apply it 4 times daily. Do no apply to broken or irritated skin and avoid getting any into your eyes.

Guidelines for Consulting Your Health Care Provider

You should consult your health care provider if:
- the patient doesn't look right or act right (trust your instincts!)
- the patient is getting worse instead of better over the course of the illness
- the patient is having trouble breathing or complaining of chest pains or there is mental confusion or lethargy or irritability
- the patient develops allergic symptoms (hives, itchy or watery eyes, runny nose, scratchy throat, asthma, shortness of breath) after taking a nutritional supplement
- after beginning a nutritional supplement the patient experiences *new onset* of any serious symptoms such as:
  > paralysis, weakness, tingling, inability to focus or concentrate, blurred or dou-

ble vision or blindness, slurred speech, severe headaches, seizures, irritability, dizziness, disorientation, memory loss, anxiety, depression, insomnia, blackouts, fainting, or the person complains of not feeling like himself
- the patient is taking *ANY* prescription medication
- the patient is pregnant or breastfeeding
- the patient has any serious, chronic disease which may have complications and become life-threatening, such as:

autism, cancer, HIV and AIDS, arthritis, multiple sclerosis, coronary artery disease, heart attack (myocardial infarction), blood dyscrasia, cancer (of any type), congestive heart failure, diabetes mellitus, obesity, thyroid disorders, high blood pressure (hypertension), stroke, seizures, acute and chronic kidney (renal) failure, schizophrenia, bipolar disorder, borderline personality disorder, eating disorders, fibromyalgia, chronic fatigue syndrome, Crohn's disease, ulcerative colitis, celiac disease, mental deficiency disorders, chromosomal disorders, infertility, frequent miscarriages, polyneuropathy, cystic fibrosis [Adapted from *The Merck Manual* at www.merck.com]

Note: Do not discontinue taking any pharmaceutical medication prescribed by your health care provider unless you or your family member is under the supervision of a physician.

Note: Do not take any nutritional supplements for diseases of joints, bones, and muscles without first consulting your health care provider especially if you or your family member is taking a prescription medication to treat cancer or its complications or is pregnant or breastfeeding.

In addition, it is a good idea to check with your health care provider if your family member is either very young or very old because nutritional supplements given injudiciously may overwhelm the body's defenses in those age groups.

Note: Do not use any nutritional supplements to enhance the immune system if you or your family member is taking a drug for immunosuppression (usually prescribed to treat autoimmune diseases or to prevent organ transplant rejection).

Note: If you or your family member has arthritis in any form, please call the *Arthritis Foundation* at 1-800-283-7800 or visit online at www.arthritis.org. You will find information on alternative therapies here.

Recommended reading: *Maximizing The Arthritis Cure: A Step-By-Step Program to Faster, Stronger Healing During Any Stage of the Cure* by Theodosakis, Adderly and Fox, published by St. Martin's Press in 1998.

Recommended reading: *Conquering Arthritis: What Doctors Don't Tell You Because They Don't Know: 9 Secrets I Learned the Hard Way* by Barbara D. Allan for nutritional advice and a diet that has helped cure some of my patients with arthritis.

Remember: People with gout should beware of eating certain foods high in purines, including certain vegetables like asparagus and spinach, legumes (especially peas), meat (including beef, pork, and poultry), nuts, and seafood. Eating low-fat dairy products and simple carbohydrates (made of white flour) seem to decrease the number of gout flare-ups. Since some of these dietary changes are not healthy, it's a good idea to seek the help of a nutritionist who specializes in treating people with gouty arthritis.

Note: Some people with gout use *Cherry extract*, 1000mg twice daily because the plentiful *anthocyanins* act as natural anti-inflammatory agents.

Note: Some people with arthritis tend to have increased joint pain after eating nightshade family vegetables (which include tomatoes, eggplant, potatoes, and peppers). You may eliminate all the nightshade family vegetables from your diet for a period of 3 weeks or so to see if that alleviates your joint pain.

What about other alternative modalities to treat ailments of joints, bones, and muscles?

Although this book does not go into detail about other alternative methods besides homeopathy, herbal medicine, and nutritional supplements, it is a good idea to keep acupuncture in mind for people with painful arthritis. Other possibly helpful alternative therapies include massage therapy and mind-body techniques for relaxation.

If you want to learn more about other beneficial alternative therapies beyond the essentials (homeopathy, herbal remedies, and nutritional supplements), then read *Own Your Health: Choosing the Best from Alternative and Conventional Medicine* by Weisman and Berman, published by Health Communications, Inc. in 2003. You can use this book to learn about acupuncture, Traditional Chinese Medicine, mind-body therapies such as Shiatsu massage, Alexander Technique, Feldenkries, yoga and meditation.

Putting It All Together

In addition to the nutritional supplements for diseases of joints, bones, and muscles in this chapter, there are others that may be found in different chapters in this book.

If you are considering using a nutritional supplement for diseases of joints, bones, and muscles, it is a good idea to familiarize yourself with **Chapter 22: Introduction to Nutritional Supplements**. It makes good sense to understand the role of vitamin and mineral nutritional supplements from **Chapter 23: Vitamins and Minerals** (especially Vitamins C and D, calcium and magnesium as well as trace minerals); *antioxidant* nutritional supplements from **Chapter 24: Antioxidant Phytochemicals: Natural Anti-Aging Remedies** (because they possess anti-inflammatory properties, and especially *curcumin* in the spice *turmeric*), and *omega-3 fatty acids* from **Chapter 31: Oils and Fats**. In addition, you will likely benefit from learning about the anti-inflammatory effects of *systemic enzymes* in **Chapter 25: Heart Healthy Nutritional Supplements**. Please consider taking *prebiotics* and *probiotics* to enhance the digestive and immune systems (please refer to **Chapter 30: Prebiotics and Probiotics**). You will want to learn about augmenting the immune system with *medicinal mushrooms* (please see **Chapter 27: Nutritional Supplements to Prevent Cancer and Augment Your Immune System**).

Whenever you have decided to go ahead with to the nutritional supplements for diseases of joints, bones, and muscles, it is a good idea to consider giving the sick person's homeopathic constitutional remedy as well (please refer to **Chapter 9: Homeopathic Remedies for Constitutional Problems in Infants, Children, and Adolescents** or to **Chapter 18: Homeopathic Constitutional Remedies** if you are dealing with an adult; or **Chapter 13: Homeopathy for Elderly Persons** if you are dealing with an elderly person).

In addition, you will want to read **Chapter 14: Homeopathy for Problems in Joints, Bones, and Muscles**. Homeopathic remedies should be considered first line defense to treat musculoskeletal system injuries (please refer to **Chapter 3: Homeopathic Remedies for Traumatic Injuries**). Homeopathic remedies may be used in conjunction with herbal medicines and nutritional supplements. And they may be used together with non-steroidal anti-inflammatory drugs (NSAIDs) and COX-2 inhibitors.

Please investigate **Chapter 20: Herbs You Need to Know** and familiarize yourself with the herbal remedies with anti-inflammatory properties such as *Astragalus, Cat's claw, Garlic, Ginseng* and *Green tea*.

Remember: Anxiety and depression tend to make pain worse. If you or your family member suffers from anxiety or depression, it is a good idea to take control of those symptoms as you treat the musculoskeletal pain and stiffness. (For more information on treating anxiety and depression with homeopathic remedies, please refer to **Chapter 8: Homeopathic Remedies for Emotional Problems** and **Chapter 18: Homeopathic Constitutional Remedies**. For more information on *St. John's Wort*, please see **Chapter 20: Herbs You Need to Know.**)

Chapter 29

Nutritional Supplements for Neurologic Disorders

Neurologic Disorders in General

Ailment/Disorder/Symptom	Nutritional Supplement
Memory and thinking	*Dimethylaminoethanol (DMAE)*
Epilepsy	*Gamma-aminobutyric acid (GABA)*
Speech and seizures in autistic children	*Dimethylglycine (DMG)*
Depression	*5-Hydroxytryptophan (5-HTP)*
Memory and concentration	*Huperzine*
Memory, thinking, and muscle activity	*Lecithin*
Memory, learning, and thinking	*Phosphatidylserine*
Brain circulation and stroke prevention	*Vinpocetine*

Guidelines for Consulting Your Health Care Provider
Putting It All Together

Neurologic Disorders in General

There are many different forms of neurologic disorders, such as:

> attention deficit/hyperactivity disorder (and other developmental and behavioral problems like autism and related autistic spectrum disorder), amnesia, coma, dementia (Alzheimer's, Huntington's, and Pick's diseases, and others), headaches (migraine, cluster, tension), insomnia, Parkinson's disease (and other movement disorders), multiple sclerosis, muscular dystrophy, peripheral neuropathy, restless legs syndrome, seizures (also called epilepsy or convulsions), stroke (ischemic and hemorrhagic), and malformations, injuries, infections, and tumors of the brain and spinal cord.
> [Adapted from *The Merck Manual* at www.merck.com]

From this list you can appreciate that neurologic disorders range from the uncomfortable and rarely serious (insomnia, headache, and restless legs syndrome) to the very serious and life-threatening (stroke and dementia). Some brain ailments are considered under emotional disorders, such as anxiety, depression, and eating disorders.

Attention deficit/hyperactivity disorder (ADHD) (consisting of various degrees of inattention, impulsivity, and hyperactivity) is currently being diagnosed in 4-12% of school-aged children! Pharmaceutical medications used to treat this condition come with associated side effects so there are some parents who seek alternatives. Taking the pathway of the *essential natural alternatives*, homeopathy, herbal medicines, and nutritional supplements, offers the best options available, especially for long-term treatment.

Another reason why some parents seek a non-pharmaceutical pathway is the fear that the particular medicines employed to treat ADHD are begun so early in human brain development that they may have long-lasting effects. This fear has some teeth in it. There is the disconcerting fact that when Ritalin is administered to juvenile rats, there is evidence of permanent alterations in their brain chemistry.

These juvenile rats tend to grow up to be prone not only to depression but also to be over-sensitive to stimulation.

It is important to remember that ADHD is a chronic, incurable condition. It can last a lifetime, affecting not only children but also adults. Some women of childbearing age who have ADHD do not want to take prescription medications during pregnancy and lactation. Again, the *essential natural alternatives* may offer a safer option.

The controversy surrounding autism and autistic spectrum disorder (ASD) focuses on whether or not vaccines (immunizations) given during childhood, particularly the MMR (mumps-measles-rubella) are the cause for the increasing incidence and prevalence of this devastating disorder. However, multiple medical research studies involving millions of children have conclusively shown that childhood immunizations are *not* the cause of this increase. Other environmental factors such as pesticides and heavy metals are now being studied as possible causes of autism. And we are learning more about the genetic determinants for autism as well.

Note: Studies done before 1985 showed the prevalence of autism had been 5 cases per 10,000 children. Studies done after 1996 showed the prevalence to be about 7 times greater at 34 cases per 10,000 children. This is a real difference, more than can be attributed to better awareness and diagnosis.

Note: Ethyl mercury, a toxic form of the heavy metal, is a metabolite of thimerosal (also spelled thiomersal) which had been used as a vaccine preservative, particularly for DPT (diphtheria-whooping cough-tetanus) from the 1930s until 1999 when it was removed from most vaccines in the United States. Medical research studies showed that there was no difference in blood levels of mercury between children who had been given thimerosal containing vaccines and those who had not. Thiomersal was excreted by the body and did not accumulate.

Note: Methyl mercury, even a more toxic form of the heavy metal, is found in fish from polluted waters. Both ethyl and methyl mercury are forms of organic mercury which are toxic to neural tissue, more especially in the fetus and young infant. For recommendations on eating fish in pregnant and lactating women, please see **Chapter 31: Oils and Fats**.

Dementia is the loss of cognitive (thinking) abilities. One increasingly common form of dementia is Alzheimer's disease, a chronic and progressive degeneration of the brain. The current wisdom about preventing Alzheimer's disease in people older than 50 includes such "intellectual exercises" as reading and doing crossword puzzles and other word games, staying socially active, stimulated, and involved, and keeping your creative juices flowing. Prevention of dementia must also include the elements of a healthy lifestyle.

Note: Age-associated memory impairment (AAMI) (affectionately known as "senior moment") is a benign decline in thinking abilities that gets more common the older you get. The most important distinguishing feature from Alzheimer's disease is that AAMI does not interfere with your quality of life. In AAMI, the word or event is temporarily forgotten ("on the tip of your tongue") and is usually recalled later. In Alzheimer's disease it is not recalled later and memory creation and retrieval for recent events and experiences are impaired.

Remember: Our emotional outlook may have a lot to do with the chronic physical diseases we will develop in later life. A 2003 study of elderly people showed that those who reported the most anxiety, depression, and anger were doubly prone to develop Alzheimer's disease than those who reported the least. Negative emotions probably begin to influence our health starting in adolescence. The success of cognitive-behavioral therapy in changing behaviors (such as in substance abuse and eating disorder therapy) taught us that our thought patterns can be changed and this will allow our behaviors to change. If you want to enhance positive thinking and positive emotions, please investigate the different methods available. Stress reduction strategies may be helpful. You may want to start with www.authentichappiness.org.

The most important things you can do to prevent deterioration in cognitive (thinking) abilities and to enhance brain function in conditions like ADHD in yourself or a family member are:

stop smoking, follow a brain healthy, anti-inflammatory dietary plan, drink alcohol in moderation (1 drink per day for women, 2 for men), exercise at least 30 minutes on most days, ensure that you get consistent good quantity and good quality sleep, and reduce stress by practicing yoga, meditation, or prayer.

This brain healthy lifestyle plan forms the backbone for your cardiovascular, joint, and immune systems as well.

A brain healthy, anti-inflammatory dietary program means a vitamin-, mineral-, and antioxidant-rich diet. A recent medical study showed that persons who took at least 400 IU of Vitamin E with more than 500mg of Vitamin C every day had lowered their risks for Alzheimer's disease by almost 80%.

You may want to take a look at the nutritional program of the *American Heart Association* as well as the *American Institute for Cancer Research*. The main differences between them are the number of recommended daily portions of fruits and vegetables, (5 and 10, respectively).

It is a good idea to become familiar with the Mediterranean diet to learn about its emphasis on non-animal protein sources, such as legumes, as well as healthy fats and oils, all important features of a brain healthy diet.

Note: Please consider using the *glycemic index* approach to eating carbohydrates. For more information on the *glycemic index*, please see **Chapter 26: Nutritional Supplements for Healthy Weight Control**.

It is never too late to make these important lifestyle changes. But, it is fruitless and foolish to take brain healthy nutritional supplements without taking these steps first. These particular lifestyle changes will also help to make your nervous system more resistant to the evils of chronic stress.

When taking nutritional supplements for self-care to neurologic disorders you must pay strict attention to the **Guidelines for Consulting Your Health Care Provider** at the end of this chapter. You may want to refer to the last section **Putting It All Together** for ideas on how to integrate the essential natural alternatives, homeopathy, herbal remedies, and nutritional supplements.

Dimethylaminoethanol (DMAE)

Dimethylaminoethanol (also called *Deanol*) is similar in chemical structure to *choline*, one of the B Vitamins. *DMAE* is administered rather than *choline* because it passes the blood-brain barrier more easily than *choline*. *DMAE* is then readily converted to *choline* in the brain and used for chemical reactions. *Choline* is required to make *acetylcholine*, the neurotransmitter involved in memory, thinking, and muscle activity, and *lecithin* (please see below), a component of all cells. *DMAE* is used to improve memory, cognitive (thinking) performance, speed of thinking, and focusing of thoughts (concentration) even though research studies have shown mostly negative results using *DMAE* for these purposes. *DMAE* may improve both learning and behavior in children with ADHD.

The dosage of *DMAE* is 100-200mg daily. Side effects include insomnia, headaches, and constipation. Pregnant and lactating women should not take *DMAE* because safety studies have not been done. *DMAE* metabolic pathway involves *betaine*, a chemical involved in *homocysteine* metabolism. Persons with high *homocysteine* levels should not take *DMAE*.

Gamma-aminobutyric acid (GABA)

GABA is a neurotransmitter that controls inhibitory actions. It has been found to be deficient in some people with seizures (epilepsy). Epilepsy can be viewed as a hyper-excitatory state. The amount of *GABA* in the brain is related to the levels of zinc and Vitamin B6.

The dosage of *GABA* is 500-1000mg daily.

Dimethylglycine (DMG)

Dimethylglycine is a compound found inside your body that possesses two methyl groups, making it a methyl group donor. Methyl group donation is important for many metabolic reactions in your body. *Dimethylglycine* has been used in autistic children to improve speech and seizures, but it does not appear to improve behavior.

The dose of *dimethylglycine* is 60mg to start daily given at breakfast so as not to interfere with sleep, and gradually increasing to 200-500mg daily. To decrease the possibility of hyperactivity as a side effect of *dimethylglycine* administration, it must be given along with folic acid and Vitamin B12.

5-Hydroxytryptophan (5-HTP)

5-Hydroxytryptophan (*5-HTP*) has been used to treat depression. It works by increasing *serotonin* and perhaps other mood enhancing neurotransmitter chemicals in the brain. The body produces *5-HTP* from *tryptophan*, the essential amino acid involved in the production of *serotonin*. Molecules of *5-HTP* are small enough to *penetrate* the blood-brain barrier.

The dosage of 5-HTP is 50mg three times daily with meals. It is possible to see improvement in depression within two weeks, whereas SSRIs can take up to 6 weeks. If there is no or minimal improvement, you may double the initial dose to 100mg three times daily. Do not take *5-HTP* if you are taking a SSRI (like Prozac, Zoloft, Celexa, Paxil, Luvox). *5-HTP* promotes healthy sleep and decreases panic and anxiety.

> **Note:** Food sources of *tryptophan* are chicken, turkey, beef, dairy products,

and fish. *5-HTP* as a supplement usually comes from the seeds of the African plant, *Griffonia simplicifolia*.

Huperzine

Huperzine is a chemical compound found in *Huperzia serrata*, the *Chinese Club Moss*. It is used to improve memory and concentration in elderly persons with Alzheimer's disease and other dementias as well as hyperactivity in persons older than 12 years. The chemical *huperzine A* inhibits the action of the enzyme *acetylcholinesterase*, the enzyme that degrades the neurotransmitter chemical *acetylcholine*. *Huperzine A* acts to increase the amount of *acetylcholine* available to your neurons (nerve cells) thereby increasing memory functions. *Huperzine* crosses the blood-brain barrier.

The dosage of *huperzine* is 10-60 micrograms daily. People with seizures, asthma, and heart arrhythmias should not take *huperzine*. Pregnant and lactating women should not take *huperzine*. Overdosage has not been reported. Some health care providers use *huperzine* along with other *acetylcholinesterase* inhibitors in an effort to enhance the effect.

Lecithin

Lecithin (also called *phosphatidylcholine* and *polyenylphosphatidylcholine*) is found in every cell in your body, playing a myriad of roles in every vital organ. It is a major component of cell membranes. *Lecithin* is a complex *phospholipid* that includes the B Vitamin *choline*, in the form of *phosphatidylcholine* along with two fatty acid molecules. One end of the *lecithin* molecule attracts water and the other end, oil. This characteristic allows *lecithin* to function as a fat emulsifier.

In the brain *lecithin* is transformed into *acetylcholine*, the neurotransmitter chemical involved in memory, thinking, and muscle activity. *Lecithin* forms a part of the myelin sheath of nerve cells (neurons). Your brain weighs in at 30% *lecithin*! *Lecithin* also plays a role in the metabolism of fat and prevents fat from clogging your arteries by dissolving fat deposits. *Lecithin* may also protect your liver from toxins, alcohol and viral hepatitis. There has been some suggestion that *lecithin* may protect against some cancers.

Food sources rich in dietary *lecithin* include soybeans, oats, cruciferous vegetables (cabbage, cauliflower, broccoli), eggs, meat. *Lecithin* as a nutritional supplement should be taken in the form of granules to be sprinkled onto food. *Lecithin* from Lewis Labs is a reliable, high-quality source of *lecithin*, containing 80 calories in 2 tablespoons, the recommended daily dose, although many times this dose poses no safety hazards. Cooking does not change its nutritional value. The dose is 3-9 grams daily in divided doses. Overdosage and drug interactions have not been reported.

Note: *Inositol* functions together with *choline* (a member of Vitamin B complex) and is necessary for the production of *lecithin*. *Inositol* is a component of cell membranes. *Inositol* has been used to treat depression and panic disorders. It is being investigated for its anti-tumor activity as well.

Phosphatidylserine

Phosphatidylserine resembles *lecithin* except that it contains the amino acid *serine* in place of *choline*. *Phosphatidylserine* is converted to *phosphatidylethanolamine* which is then converted to *phosphatidylcholine* (*lecithin*).

Phosphatidylserine plays an integral role in cell membranes, especially in the brain. As we grow older, "mistakes" in cell membrane construction may result in cognitive deficits. *Phosphatidylserine* as a nutritional supplement may enhance memory, learning, and thinking abilities. In addition, *phosphatidylserine* may act as an antioxidant by protecting nerve cells (neurons) from damage by free radicals. It is used primarily to maintain cognitive function in the elderly and to treat patients with Alzheimer's disease.

The dose is 100mg 1-3 times daily, taken with meals. Large doses taken close to bedtime have sometimes caused sleeplessness so do not take *phosphatidylserine* later than dinnertime. Take 200-300mg daily for the first month, decreasing to 100-200mg daily thereafter. Nausea and indigestion are occasional side effects. Long-term safety studies have not been done so it is prudent not to give *phosphatidylserine* to pregnant or lactating women or to children. Overdosage and drug interactions have not been reported.

Vinpocetine

Vinpocetine is derived from the chemical *vincamine*, found in *Vinca minor*, the *periwinkle* plant. It acts to enhance cerebral circulation and by increasing the flow of oxygen to brain cells, it increases brain energy production. *Vinpocetine* is used to treat cerebral circulatory problems, especially stroke. It is useful for the kind of dementia that results from cerebral blood flow deficiencies (called vascular dementia) but studies have not yet shown benefits for patients with Alzheimer's disease. *Vinpocetine* decreases fatality in victims of ischemic stroke. *Vinpocetine* is also used to enhance cognitive function in the elderly. It is useful to treat hearing loss and ringing in the ears (called tinnitus) especially resulting from an injury.

The dosage of *vinpocetine* is 5-10mg daily, although some people recommend 20mg daily. Overdosage has not been reported. *Vinpocetine* has been noted to very slightly change prothrombin time in persons taking *warfarin* (*Coumadin*). There are no other drug interactions. No safety record has been established for pregnant and lactating women so it is best for them to avoid *vinpocetine*. People who have had allergic reactions to other *vinca alkaloids* such as *vinblastine* and *vincristine* (cancer chemotherapy agents) should not take *vinpocetine*.

Guidelines for Consulting Your Health Care Provider

You should consult your health care provider if:
- the patient doesn't look right or act right (trust your instincts!)
- the patient is getting worse instead of better over the course of the illness

- the patient is having trouble breathing or complaining of chest pains or there is mental confusion or lethargy or irritability
- the patient develops allergic symptoms (hives, itchy or watery eyes, runny nose, scratchy throat, asthma, shortness of breath) after taking a nutritional supplement
- after beginning a nutritional supplement the patient experiences *new onset* of any serious symptoms such as:

  paralysis, weakness, tingling, inability to focus or concentrate, blurred or double vision or blindness, slurred speech, severe headaches, seizures, irritability, dizziness, disorientation, memory loss, anxiety, depression, insomnia, blackouts, fainting, or the person complains of not feeling like himself

- the patient is taking *ANY* prescription medication
- the patient is pregnant or breastfeeding
- the patient has any serious, chronic disease which may have complications and become life-threatening, such as:

  autism, cancer, HIV and AIDS, arthritis, multiple sclerosis, coronary artery disease, heart attack (myocardial infarction), blood dyscrasia, cancer (of any type), congestive heart failure, diabetes mellitus, obesity, thyroid disorders, high blood pressure (hypertension), stroke, seizures, acute and chronic kidney (renal) failure, schizophrenia, bipolar disorder, borderline personality disorder, eating disorders, fibromyalgia, chronic fatigue syndrome, Crohn's disease, ulcerative colitis, celiac disease, mental deficiency disorders, chromosomal disorders, infertility, frequent miscarriages, polyneuropathy, cystic fibrosis [Adapted from *The Merck Manual* at www.merck.com]

Note: Do not discontinue taking any pharmaceutical medication prescribed by your health care provider unless you or your family member is under the supervision of a physician.

Note: Do not take any nutritional supplements for diseases of the nervous system without first consulting your health care provider especially if you or your family member is taking a prescription medication to treat cancer or its complications or is pregnant or breastfeeding.

In addition, it is a good idea to check with your health care provider if your family member is either very young or very old because nutritional supplements given injudiciously may overwhelm the body's defenses in those age groups.

Note: If you or your family member has chronic pain consider contacting the American Academy of Pain Management at 1-209-533-9744 or online at www.aapainmanage.org. If you want an integrative approach to pain management you may request an integrative pain management center.

Note: For more information on ADHD, visit online www.kidsmeds.org/adhd. In addition to Western medicine approach to ADHD, you will find some alternative therapy options. Pediatric OnCall at www.pediatriconcall.com is another excellent site for information on ADHD (and all the other pediatric ailments). The information on alternative medicine is rudimentary.

Note: A small subset of children with ADHD may respond to the *Feingold Diet* (not a relative of this author!) which eliminates certain chemicals in food. You can find information on the *Feingold Association* at www.feingold.org.

Note: *Children and Adults with ADD (CHADD)* at www.chad.org or 1-301-306-7070, Ext. 102, is the place to go for support, encouragement, and enlightened information. You are likely to find a chapter near you.

Note: The best parent-centered book available is *The ADD Answer* by Dr. Frank Lawlis, Viking Books in 2004. He encourages a non-pharmaceutical, holistic approach to the management of the ADD/ADHD child. Another book, *Ritalin-Free Kids* by Judyth Reichenberg-Ullman and Robert Ullman focuses on the homeopathic treatment of children with ADD/ADHD.

Note: For persons seeking abstinence from substance abuse and/or alcoholism, as well as freedom from eating disorders, I recommend that you investigate *Desert Canyon's* nutritional program. *Desert Canyon*, located in Sedona, Arizona, is a non-twelve-step program. You may want to read the book *End Your Addiction Now: The Proven Nutritional Supplement Program That Can Set You Free* by Charles Gant and Greg Lewis, published by Warner Books in 2002.

Note: If you or your family member needs help for alcoholism (or suspected alcoholism), you may depend on Alcoholics Anonymous (1-212-870-3400 or www.alcoholics-anonymous.org). Family members may find support at Al-Anon (1-888-425-2666 or www.al-anon.org). Youngsters and adolescents may turn to Alateen at 1-888-425-2666 or www.alateen.org. Recovering drug addicts may depend on Narcotics Anonymous at 1-818-773-9999 or www.na.org.

All these programs utilize the same method, the "12-step" program method, incorporating emotional support from a recovery community to help the addicted person help him or herself. These "12-step" programs have higher success rates than any other type of program for addictive diseases. Often, the addicted person would need to be detoxified first in a hospital or clinic setting and then he would join the appropriate "12-step" program to continue his recovery.

Active membership in the "12-step" program in many cases may need to be life-long to prevent recurrence.

Note: Some people suffering from alcohol addiction have been able to decrease the amount of their drinking by half by taking *Kudzu root*, an herbal remedy. (Yes, the same *Kudzu*, the invasive vine that has destroyed gardens throughout southern America.) Long-term side effects are not known but it is safe in the short-term.

Note: A small subset of children with autism may benefit from a wheat- and milk-free diet called the *gluten-free-casein-free diet*. Some children with autism may actually have an increased intestinal permeability that, in theory, would allow certain absorbed compounds to affect behavior. Your child may need to remain on this diet for 8 months before you would be able to judge whether behavioral benefits occurred or not. I recommend that you do not attempt this diet on your own, but rather work with a nutritionist, because of the opportunity for calcium and protein deficiencies to develop in your child.

You may also be interested in experimenting with a sugar-free and artificial-sugar-free diet (called *sugar avoidance diet*) for your child with autism because of the beneficial behavioral changes noted by both parents and clinicians.

Note: If your child has been diagnosed with autism, please read Amy Lansky's book, *Impossible Cure, The Promise of Homeopathy*, published by R. L. Ranch Press, California in 2003. It is the story of how her son Max was cured from autism by homeopathy. Yes, cured. After reading this book you will have new respect for homeopathy and understand it better too.

But, please skip all the malarkey about vaccinations causing autism. Dr. Andrew Wakefield (and colleagues) published a study supposedly linking autism and MMR (measles-mumps-rubella) vaccine in 1998 in the *Lancet*. Since then any association of autism and vaccines has been soundly disproved not only by our foremost scientific agency the *Institute of Medicine*, but also a gigantic Scandinavian study of approximately 500,000 children. The prestigious British medical journal *Lancet* has since discovered Dr. Wakefield's study to have serious methodological flaws. Worse than that, Dr. Wakefield did not reveal a conflict of interest. While performing the study, he was also financially involved in the legal battle of parents against the MMR vaccine companies. Ten of the original 13 authors of that paper have since retracted their conclusions.

You will also want to use the information and services of Cure Autism Now at www.cureautismnow.org.

Note: You may want to investigate the link between exposure to mercury and autism by reading David Kirby's book, *Evidence of Harm*. Since childhood immunizations no longer contain mercury (except for some brands of influenza vaccine), this link may now be moot. Medical researchers did not find high-quality evidence to support the link between mercury and autism. If you are convinced of the link in your child, please be very careful of having mercury removed because the detoxification process, called chelation, is likely itself to be harmful to health.

Note: You can read about the homeopathic treatment of autism and Asperger's syndrome in *A Drug-Free Approach to Autism and Asperger's Syndrome* by Robert and Judyth Reichenberg-Ullman.

Note: If you or your family member has any neurologic disease, especially autism, it is wise to aim for zero exposure to heavy metals such as mercury, lead, aluminum, and cadmium. Ingestion of seafood contaminated with mercury exposes us to undesirably high levels. Pregnant women must be careful to avoid mercury-contaminated seafood so as not to inadvertently expose the developing fetus.

Note: The culinary herb *sage* may have a place in the prevention of Alzheimer's disease because it inhibits the breakdown of *acetylcholine*, the brain chemical (neurotransmitter) involved in memory and thinking. You may use *sage* as the herb in your cooking or you may take *sage oil* as a supplement.

Note: *Melatonin* is a naturally occurring hormone that is involved in regulating your circadian rhythm. I do not recommend using *melatonin* for sleep disorders/insomnia because, simply, it is a hormone and we don't have enough long-term data to make recommendations. However, *melatonin* can be useful as a short-term remedy to get over jet lag. A dose of just 0.3mg was found to be just as effective as taking 5mg. So take the smallest dose that does the job for you.

Note: The herbal remedy *Butterbur* (*Petasites hybridus*), can be effective in preventing migraine headaches. The herbal preparation by Life Extension includes *Butterbur*, Vitamin B_2 (*Riboflavin*) and *Ginger* (*Zingiber officinale*).

Putting It All Together

In addition to the nutritional supplements for neurologic diseases in this chapter, there are others that may be found in different chapters in this book.

If you are considering using a nutritional supplement for neurologic diseases, it is a good idea to familiarize yourself with **Chapter 22: Introduction to Nutritional Supplements**. It makes good sense to understand the role of vitamin and mineral nutritional supplements (especially the *B vitamins, choline* and *zinc*) from **Chapter 23: Vitamins and Minerals**; *antioxidant* nutritional supplements from **Chapter 24: Antioxidant Phytochemicals: Natural Anti-Aging Remedie**s; and *omega-3 fatty acids* from **Chapter 31: Oils and Fats**. In addition, you will likely benefit from learning about *amino acids, L-carnitin*e and *systemic enzyme*s in **Chapter 25: Heart Healthy Nutritional Supplements**. Please consider taking *prebiotics* and *probiotics* to enhance the digestive and immune systems as they impact the neurologic system (please refer to **Chapter 30: Prebiotics and Probiotics**). People with depression may benefit from *Rhodiola rosea*, a weight loss herbal remedy that has anti-depressant action as well (please see **Chapter 26: Nutritional Supplements for Healthy Weight Control**). *SAMe* is another remedy for depression (please see **Chapter 28: Nutritional Supplements for Diseases of Joints, Bones and Muscles**).

Whenever you have decided to go ahead with using nutritional supplements for diseases of joints, bones, and muscles, it is a good idea to consider giving the sick person's homeopathic constitutional remedy as well (please refer to **Chapter 9: Homeopathic Remedies for Constitutional Problems in Infants, Children, and Adolescents** or to **Chapter 18: Homeopathic Constitutional Remedies** if you are dealing with an adult; or **Chapter 13: Homeopathy for Elderly Persons** if you are dealing with an elderly person).

In addition, you will want to read **Chapter 16: Homeopathy for Neurologic Disorders**. Homeopathic remedies may be used in conjunction with herbal medicines and nutritional supplements as well as prescription pharmaceuticals.

Please investigate **Chapter 20: Herbs You Need to Know** and familiarize yourself with the herbal remedies that affect the neurologic system such as *Ginkgo biloba, St. John's Wort* and *Valerian*.

Chapter 30

Prebiotics and Probiotics

Prebiotics and Probiotics in General

Ailment/Disorder/Symptom	Nutritional Supplement
Immune system function, digestion, diarrhea	*Acidophilus*
Digestion	*Inulin*

Guidelines for Consulting Your Health Care Provider
Putting It All Together

Prebiotics and Probiotics in General

Prebiotics are foods that stimulate the growth and reproduction of your beneficial, intestinal bacteria. *Prebiotics* are certain soluble *fibers* that are not absorbed into the bloodstream because they cannot be digested by human beings. *Prebiotics* make their way to the large intestine where they are used as an energy source for the multiplication of "good" bacteria.

Probiotics are bacterial cultures found in foods, drinks, and nutritional supplements. When *probiotics* are eaten, they reintroduce or promote the health of the "good" bacteria in your intestinal tract (intestinal flora). There are about 100 trillion bacteria living in your gut, lungs, and skin. This is ten times the number of cells in your body! Your body's bacteria are categorized into more than 500 different species.

Yogurt, kefir, and other fermented dairy foods containing live cultures of *Lactobacillus bulgaricus* and *Streptococcus thermophilus* (and some contain *Bifidobacterium* as well) are *probiotics*. Each genus, *Lactobacillus* and *Bifidobacterium*, contain many different species. *Lactobacillus casei* and *Lactobacillus acidophilus* are two of the best-studied *probiotics*.

> **Note:** The fat in yogurt is saturated fat. Yogurt comes in 4 different fat levels. Whole milk yogurt contains 3% fat. Low-fat yogurt contains 0.5-2% fat. Nonfat yogurt contains less than 0.5% fat. Light yogurt refers to nonfat yogurt that contains artificial sweeteners instead of added sugar.

Your digestive health is dependent in large measure, on *probiotics*, the "good" (or "beneficial" or "friendly") bacteria living there. "Good" bacteria suppress the growth of "bad" bacteria, called pathogenic organisms. *Probiotics* have their most pronounced effects on intestinal health. They can decrease the time a child suffers with diarrhea from rotavirus infection, especially when given along with oral rehydration therapy (ORT). In fact, *probiotic* nutritional supplements have been proven to decrease the duration of diarrhea from any cause in all age groups.

Probiotics are able to produce Vitamin B12 and other vitamins as well. *Probiotics* produce *cytokines*, chemicals that fight infection. *Probiotics* stimulate antibody production in the gut. *Probiotics* live on the lining of your intestines and physically keep out infecting organisms as well as certain proteins. *Probiotics* may protect the liver from the chronic inflammation seen with alcohol intoxication and obesity. *Probiotics* tend to prevent recurrent vaginal yeast infections.

An imbalance of "good" and "bad" bacteria in your intestinal tract has been associated with several disease states, ranging from yeast infections to colon cancer. In addition, those beneficial bacteria help to break down milk sugar, lactose, in your gut, so when you develop a bacterial imbalance, you may have difficulty digesting lactose. This can be the reason why lactose intolerance develops, especially after treatment with antibiotics.

> **Remember:** Antibiotics kill indiscriminately. *Probiotic* bacteria disappear along with the pathogenic bacteria that are causing the infection. You can replace *probiotic* bacteria by taking a *probiotic* nutritional supplement before, during, and after the antibiotic. *Probiotics* help to reduce some side effects of antibiotics, like diarrhea and upset stomach. You can help your *probiotic* bacteria to flourish by taking a *prebiotic* nutritional supplement. In addition, it's a good idea to eat cultured foods labeled "Live and Active Cultures."

Prebiotics and *probiotics* have been proven not only to promote healthy digestion but also to enhance the functioning of your immune system. Due to their effect on the immune system, *prebiotics* and *probiotics* are thought to play a role in the prevention of cancer. *Prebiotics* and *probiotics* may also reduce symptoms of irritable bowel disease and help to prevent recurrences of Crohn's disease. They possess antiallergenic and antioxidant activity as well. They are helpful during treatment of food allergies, and they may prevent the onset of food allergies as well as eczema. Supplementation with *probiotics* has been shown to be effective treatment for eczema, allergic atopy in infancy, and allergic asthma.

Note: Together, *prebiotics* and *probiotics* are sometimes called *synbiotics*.

Since chronic inflammation is the likely culprit underlying such seemingly diverse ailments as asthma, eczema, arthritis, heart disease, cancer, diabetes, and Alzheimer's disease, it is prudent to consider a nutritional supplement designed to prevent such inflammation. *Prebiotics* and *probiotics* have been proven to decrease chronic inflammation. They accomplish this feat by helping to eliminate the "leaky gut syndrome." This is a gastrointestinal ailment that occurs as a result of bacterial and fungal overgrowth. It can lead to malnutrition (by blocking nutrients) and toxin exposure (by unblocking the usually impermeable intestinal lining).

When taking *prebiotic* and *probiotic* nutritional supplements for self-care you must pay strict attention to the **Guidelines for Consulting Your Health Care Provider** at the end of this chapter. You may want to refer to the last section **Putting It All Together** for ideas on how to integrate the essential natural alternatives, homeopathy, herbal remedies, and nutritional supplements.

Acidophilus

Acidophilus is the common name for the *probiotic* bacterium *Lactobacillus acidophilus*. People tend to use *acidophilus* as a shorthand way to communicate the whole range of beneficial *probiotic* bacteria found in our intestinal tract.

Acidophilus and *probiotic* nutritional supplements in general, come in an array of capsules, tablets, powders, and drinks. Many products are mixtures of several strains of *Lactobacillus* and *Bifidobacterium*, along with others like *Streptococcus, Lactococcus, Enterococcus* and *Saccharomyces* (a yeast). *Bifidobacterium infantis* has been identified as the strain of *probiotic* bacteria that normalizes bowel function in people with irritable bowel syndrome (IBS).

Lactobacillus rhamnosus is especially effective for treating diarrhea in children. *Lactobacillus reuteri* is the only *Lactobacillus* species to secrete *reuterin*, a chemical that has been proven to prevent colonization in the gastrointestinal tract by "bad" (pathogenic) bacteria. *Probiotica*, manufactured by McNeil

Consumer Healthcare contains *Lactobacillus reuteri*, 100 million colony-forming units (CFU) in every tablet. *Lactinex* contains *Lactobacillus acidophilus* and *Lactobacillus bulgaricus*. It comes as a tablet or as granules in a packet that can be mixed with food or beverage as long as it is not heated or cooled.

There are no harmful effects from taking *acidophilus* or any *probiotic* nutritional supplement. Since there are so many different preparations on the market, you should follow the dosage and storage instructions on the label. Side effects are minor and include constipation and increased intestinal gas. Pregnant and lactating women should use *acidophilus* or any *probiotic* nutritional supplement only under the care of a physician.

A popular brand of *probiotics* is *Primal Defense* manufactured by Garden of Life. It contains "homeostatic soil organisms" (*probiotics*), as well as enzymes, vitamins, minerals, amino acids, antioxidants, and *phytosterols*. The dose is one capsule 3 times daily for adults and 1 capsule daily for children.

> **Note:** To read more about the type of *probiotics* called "homeostatic soil organisms" and their effects on health, please read *Patient Heal Thyself* by Jordan Rubin, published by Freedom Press in 2003.

> **Note:** Dannon manufactures a drink called *DanActive* (called *Actimel* in Europe and Latin America) with 10 times the "good" bacteria than yogurt.
> Dannon also manufactures *Activia* which is a *probiotic* that contains *Bifidus regularis*. It is promoted to treat constipation. The downside is that there are 100 calories in 4 oz., with 17 grams of sugar, most from fructose syrup and sugar.

Inulin

Inulin is a soluble fiber. It is a non-digestible, complex fructose sugar belonging to the chemical group of fructo-oligosaccharides (or *fructans*). *Inulin* is often extracted from the root of the Jerusalem artichoke. Manufacturers of *inulin* or other *prebiotic* nutritional supplement stress that they may actually be more effective than *probiotics* in promoting a healthy digestive tract. However, this has not been proven by medical research studies.

The commonly prescribed brand of *inulin* for use as a *prebiotic* nutritional supplement is *Inuflora*, manufactured by Naturally Vitamins (www.naturallyvitamins.com). The dosage is 1 gram per tablet 1-5 times daily, taken with meals, or 5 grams/teaspoon of the powder (containing 8 calories) sprinkled on food or dissolved in hot or cold drinks. Side effects include those that are known to accompany fiber-containing foods, such as bloating, diarrhea, and increased intestinal gas. *Inulin* may increase the absorption of calcium and magnesium when taken together.

> **Note:** *Nutraflora* is a yogurt with added *inulin* as a *prebiotic* nutritional supplement. Some cookies and breads are being fortified with *inulin*.

> **Note:** The Vitamin Shoppe manufactures the sugar substitute *Stevia* in packets together with *inulin*, 475mg in every one-half packet. *Stevia* leaf comes from a plant found in Paraguay. It has been used as a sweetener for thousands of years and is considered safe.

> **Note:** Fibersure is *inulin* from *Chickory* root giving you 5 grams of fiber (and 25 calories) in every tablespoon of powder.

Guidelines for Consulting Your Health Care Provider

You should consult your health care provider if:
• the patient doesn't look right or act right (trust your instincts!)
• the patient is getting worse instead of better over the course of the illness
• the patient is having trouble breathing or complaining of chest pains or there is mental confusion or lethargy or irritability
• the patient develops allergic symptoms (hives, itchy or watery eyes, runny nose, scratchy throat,

asthma, shortness of breath) after taking a nutritional supplement
• after beginning a nutritional supplement the patient experiences *new onset* of any serious symptoms such as:

> paralysis, weakness, tingling, inability to focus or concentrate, blurred or double vision or blindness, slurred speech, severe headaches, seizures, irritability, dizziness, disorientation, memory loss, anxiety, depression, insomnia, blackouts, fainting, or the person complains of not feeling like himself

• the patient is taking *ANY* prescription medication
• the patient is pregnant or breastfeeding
• the patient has any serious, chronic disease which may have complications and become life-threatening, such as:

> autism, cancer, HIV and AIDS, arthritis, multiple sclerosis, coronary artery disease, heart attack (myocardial infarction), blood dyscrasia, cancer (of any type), congestive heart failure, diabetes mellitus, obesity, thyroid disorders, high blood pressure (hypertension), stroke, seizures, acute and chronic kidney (renal) failure, schizophrenia, bipolar disorder, borderline personality disorder, eating disorders, fibromyalgia, chronic fatigue syndrome, Crohn's disease, ulcerative colitis, celiac disease, leaky gut syndrome, mental deficiency disorders, chromosomal disorders, infertility, frequent miscarriages, polyneuropathy, cystic fibrosis

[Adapted from *The Merck Manual* at www.merck.com]

> **Note:** Do not discontinue taking any pharmaceutical medication prescribed by your health care provider unless you or your family member is under the supervision of a physician.

> **Note:** Do not take any *prebiotic* or *probiotic* nutritional supplements without first consulting your health care provider especially if you or your fami-

ly member is taking a prescription medication to treat cancer or its complications or is pregnant or breastfeeding.

In addition, it is a good idea to check with your health care provider if your family member is either very young or very old because nutritional supplements given injudiciously may overwhelm the body's defenses in those age groups. However, *prebiotics* and *probiotics* have a very consistent safety record. They are usually considered safe even for the very elderly.

Note: when you first begin taking *prebiotic* or *probiotic* nutritional supplements, you might feel bloated and pass more gas than usual. These symptoms are usually temporary, until your intestinal tract adjusts. If the symptoms do not abate, please stop taking that supplement and consult with your physician. Perhaps a different preparation with different bacteria would be easier on your intestinal tract.

Note: For more information please go to www.usprobiotics.org.

Putting It All Together

In addition to the *prebiotic* and *probiotic* nutritional supplements for digestive and immune system health in this chapter, there are others that may be found in different chapters in this book.

If you are considering using a *prebiotic* and *probiotic* nutritional supplements for digestive and immune system health, it is a good idea to familiarize yourself with **Chapter 22: Introduction to Nutritional Supplements**. It makes good sense to understand the role of vitamin or mineral nutritional supplements from **Chapter 23: Vitamins and Minerals**; *antioxidant* nutritional supplements from **Chapter 24: Antioxidant Phytochemicals** and *omega-3 fatty acids* from **Chapter 31: Oils and Fats**. In addition, you will likely benefit from learning about *systemic enzymes* and *fiber* in **Chapter 25: Heart Healthy Nutritional Supplements**.

Please consider taking *prebiotics* and *probiotics* to enhance the digestive and immune systems. You should read about *systemic oral enzymes*, medicinal *mushrooms, modified citrus pectin* and other immune system modulators in **Chapter 27: Nutritional Supplements to Prevent Cancer and Augment Your Immune System**.

Whenever you have decided to go ahead with *prebiotics* and *probiotics* to enhance the digestive and immune systems, it is a good idea to consider giving the sick person's homeopathic constitutional remedy as well (please refer to **Chapter 9: Homeopathic Remedies for Constitutional Problems in Infants, Children, and Adolescents** or to **Chapter 18: Homeopathic Constitutional Remedies** if you are dealing with an adult; or **Chapter 13: Homeopathy for Elderly Persons** if you are dealing with an elderly person).

It is likely that **Chapter 11: Homeopathy for Digestive Tract Ailments** and **Chapter 15: Homeopathy for Eating Disorders and Weight Control** will help you to decide on a relevant homeopathic remedy. Homeopathic remedies may be used in conjunction with herbal medicines and nutritional supplements as well as prescription pharmaceuticals. In those chapters you will read about *peppermint oil* as an herbal remedy for irritable bowel syndrome.

Please investigate **Chapter 20: Herbs You Need to Know** and familiarize yourself with the herbal remedies that affect the neurologic system such as *Milk thistle* and *Psyllium*.

Chapter 31

Oils and Fats

Oils and Fats in General

Ailment/Disorder/Symptom	Nutritional Supplement
Skin, brain, heart, ADD/ADHD, anti-inflammator activity	*Omega-3 fatty acids*
Monounsaturated fat source	*Olive oil*
Monounsaturated fat source	*Canola oil*
LDL ("bad") cholesterol lowering	*Walnut oil*

Guidelines for Consulting Your Health Care Provider
Putting It All Together

Oils and Fats in General

The topic of *fats and oils* can be bewildering. But only until we slip them into categories and then we find the whole matter is simplified. It is a good idea to try to understand the basic rudiments of *fats and oils* because they are so important to healthy nutrition.

> **Remember:** Fats are made up of *fatty acids*. *Fatty acids* are a component of the cell membrane in every cell in your body. They help to transmit chemical messages from outside the cell (the extracellular space) to inside the cell (the intracellular space). They are crucial to the production of many hormones including male and female sex hormones, prostaglandins, leukotrienes, and others. They are involved in modulating inflammatory reactions which are the underlying basis for many chronic ailments like cancer, cardiovascular disease, arthritis, Alzheimer's disease, and many, many others. *Fatty acids* are essential for the health of every organ in your body from your immune system to your brain and heart to your hair and nails.

> **Note:** The fats you eat are broken down into component *fatty acids* in your intestines and absorbed into your bloodstream. *Fatty acids* are used by the body in 3 ways: they are used in vital body processes; they can be burned as an energy source; or they can be stored as fat in *adipose* tissue.

There are 4 basic categories of dietary fats (*saturated, trans, mono-* and *polyunsaturated fatty acids*) depending on the number of carbon atoms in a chain and how many hydrogen atoms are attached to the carbon bonds. *Saturated* and *trans fats* are solid at room temperature while *mono-* and *polyunsaturated fats* are liquid.

> **Note:** *Fats and oils* contain a mixture of *saturated, mono-* and *polyunsaturated fatty acids* but they are grouped into the type they contain the most of.

> **Note:** Some authors have joked that fats can be classified as good (*mono-* and *polyunsaturated*), bad (*saturated*) and awful (*trans*).

> **Remember:** Although *fats and oils* differ markedly in their health benefits, they are created equal with only minor differences in the number of calories they contain: nine per gram. Every tablespoon contains 120 calories and 14 grams of fat.

Saturated fats

FIRST of all, *saturated fats* have hydrogen taking up places in all the carbon bonds, meaning all the carbon atoms are "saturated" with hydrogen. *Saturated fats* are associated with an increased risk for cardiovascular disease and some cancers because they tend to increase LDL cholesterol.

Saturated fats are found in all animal products as well as chocolate and some tropical plant oils such as coconut and palm. Most (but not all) *saturated fats* contribute to your total cholesterol, raising both LDL ("bad" cholesterol) and HDL ("good" cholesterol). The main *saturated fat* in chocolate is *stearic acid* which does not raise or lower total cholesterol. But *palmitic acid*, the main *saturated fat* in dairy foods does increase total cholesterol.

> **Note:** Most dietary guidelines recommend that *saturated fats* make up 10% or less of your total daily calories. All fats, regardless of type, provide 9 calories per gram. So, for a 2,000-calorie diet, you should not consume more than 20 grams of *saturated fats* (including *trans fats*) per day.

Trans fatty acids

SECONDLY, *trans fatty acids* (also called *trans fats*) are produced when *monounsaturated* or *polyunsaturated* vegetable fats are *partially hydrogenated*, and in the process becoming *saturated fats*. The *hydrogenation* process stabilizes and solidifies the fat. This extends the shelf life of the baked goods that contain the *trans fats*. *Trans fats*, listed separately on the nutrition label as of January 1, 2006, are associated with an increased risk for cardiovascular disease because they increase total and LDL ("bad") cholesterol while decreasing HDL ("good") cholesterol (a double whammy).

Note: All molecules (not only fats) exist in space in certain shapes (spatial configurations). These configurations are either *trans* or *cis* or both. When a *trans fat* is created by either high temperatures (frying) or *hydrogenation*, the configuration of the molecule resembles a *saturated fat* more closely.

Remember: Most *trans fats* are created artificially. They fall into the category of processed foods.

Unfortunately: *Trans fats* are allowed to be listed on the label as 0 grams per serving if the serving contains less than 0.5 grams. So to ensure that you get actually zero grams you need to read the ingredients label. Do not buy any products with hydrogenated vegetable oil.

Unfortunately: Although you can steer clear of buying supermarket foods containing *trans fats* by reading labels, no such luck (or protection) in restaurant food since they're not included in the labeling law. Some cities have enacted laws to prohibit *trans fats* in their restaurants.

Dr. Willett in his book *Eat, Drink, and Be Healthy*, calls for zero tolerance for *trans fats*. This means that there is no safe level for *trans fats*. My recommendation (the same as the *National Cholesterol Education Program*) is to avoid *trans fats* as much as possible even if you cannot eliminate it completely. They lurk in many unhealthy stick margarines, solid shortenings (like *Crisco*), deep fried foods (just think about fast food! And donuts!), most baked goods (breads, cakes, cookies, crackers, cupcakes, pastries), salad dressings, dips, and snack foods.

Note: Looks like the food industry is responding to the *trans fats* labeling issue by duping us into believing we'll actually be healthier. The food industry is replacing partially hydrogenated oils with *palm oil* and *palm kernel oil*. This is unfortunate, a missed opportunity to improve the health of the public. *Palm oil* and *palm kernel oil* (both are saturated vegetable oils) act on your arteries much the same as butter and cheese. *Palm kernel oil* has twice the saturated fat level (about 80%) of lard (about 40%)! To add insult to injury, in the process of clearing forests to make way for *palm oil* plants, wildlife habitats are being seriously threatened in Malaysia and Indonesia. Try to steer clear of all tropical oils, including coconut (containing about 85% saturated fat). You can make healthy choices at the supermarket by always reading and comparing nutritional labels.

Note: *Fractionated palm kernel oil* is highly processed. The fractionation process makes the saturated fat content even more concentrated. This is unlikely to be healthy, but there is very little medical evidence so no one really knows what it does in the body! My advice is to stay away from *fractionated palm kernel oil*.

Note: A substitute for hydrogenated vegetable oil may be *Natreon*, manufactured by Dow AgroSciences and derived from *canola oil*. *Natreon* is lowest in saturated fat compared to other vegetable oils and has virtually no *trans fats*. Another is *NuSun*, a sunflower oil that is lower in saturated fat than the naturally occurring sunflower oil, with zero *trans fats*.

Remember: The recommendation for your daily intake of *saturated fats* (including *trans fats*, which should be as close to zero as possible) is less than 10% of your total calories (about 20 grams per day). If you have an increased risk for cardiovascular disease, you may need to restrict *saturated* and *trans fats* to 15 grams daily.

Note: *Trans fats* may interfere with fertility, so women who wish to remain fertile should avoid them completely.

Note: If you are interested in a book on proper nutrition for our times, I strongly recommend *Eat, Drink, and Be Healthy* by Walter C. Willett, published by Simon and Schuster in 2001. *Eat, Drink, and Be Healthy* will give you all the nutrition basics you need to make informed healthy choices for yourself and your family. It will help you to replace unhealthy fats with healthy ones. It will introduce you to the *glycemic index*. Understanding the *glycemic index* and putting its concepts to work for you and your family is one of the most important things you could do for health. Dr. Willett presents his own *Food Guide Pyramid* based on current nutritional thinking.

Monounsaturated fats

THIRD, *monounsaturated fatty acid*s have one carbon bond in the chain unfilled with hydrogen. *Monounsaturated fatty acids* promote cardiovascular health by decreasing LDL ("bad") and increasing HDL ("good") cholesterol. They may also help to prevent cancer. *Monounsaturated fatty acids* are found in olive, canola, safflower, and sunflower oils, nuts (cashews, walnuts, macadamias, and almonds) and avocados. *Oleic acid* is the main *monounsaturated fatty acid* in our diets.

Polyunsaturated fats

FOURTH, *polyunsaturated fatty acids* (often called *PUFAs*) have two or more carbon bonds in the chain unfilled with hydrogen. *Polyunsaturated fatty acids* are further subdivided into *omega-3* and *omega-6 fatty acids* (and other types too).

Polyunsaturated fatty acids, especially *omega-3 fatty acids* have a protective effect on cardiovascular disease (especially sudden death from heart arrhythmias), stroke, cancer (while also decreasing side effects from chemotherapy), arthritis (by anti-inflammatory actions), neurologic ailments (like Alzheimer's disease and ADHD), dermatological ailments (like psoriasis and eczema), and mental illnesses (like behavioral problems, depression, and schizophrenia). *Omega-3 fatty acids* are required for the synthesis of "good" prostaglandins which are important anti-inflammatory chemicals.

There are 3 types of *omega-3 fatty acids*: *eicosapentaenoic acid* (*EPA*), *docosahexaenoic acid* (*DHA*), and *alpha-linolenic acid* (*ALA*). *EPA* and *DHA* are found in oily, cold-water fish while *ALA* is found abundantly in flaxseeds (and flaxseed oil), walnuts (and walnut oil), soy (and soy oil, and tofu), and *canola oil*. *ALA* is converted inside the body to *EPA* and *DHA*, albeit probably only in small amounts; the exact amount is as yet unknown.

Omega-3 fatty acids are important in brain function. *DHA* is a major component of cell membrane *phospholipids*, present abundantly in the gray matter in your brain. Just eating one portion of fish per week may lower your risk for Alzheimer's disease. Some persons with ADHD and autism are found to be deficient in *omega-3 fatty acids*. When children with ADHD as well as autistic children took *omega-3 fatty acid* supplements, they showed improvements in concentration, behavior (especially aggressive behavior), and sleep. *DHA* is a major component of the retina in your eyes.

> **Note:** *The Food and Behavior Research* website www.fabresearch.org is the place to start to learn about the links between nutrition and neurological ailments like ADHD and autistic spectrum disorder, and mental health ailments like depression, anxiety, bipolar disease, and schizophrenia.

Omega-3 fatty acids are protective against sudden death because they tend to stabilize the heart against the development of arrhythmias.

> **Note:** People who have implanted cardioverter defibrillators (ICDs) should not take *omega-3 fatty acid* supplements because, for as yet unknown reasons, they tended to have more episodes of

ventricular tachycardia and fibrillation while taking such supplements. But, it is safe for people with ICDs to continue to eat fish to supply their *omega-3 fatty acids*.

Note: You can read about *omega-3 fatty acids'* effects on cardiovascular disease as well as on other conditions at the website of the *National Center for Complementary and Alternative Medicine*, part of the *National Institutes of Health* at http://nccam.nih.gov/health/bytreatment.htm.

The *American Heart Association* recommendation is to eat at least two portions (3-ounce servings) of oily fish a week. The fish with the most *omega-3 fatty acids* are salmon (farmed and wild), sardines, trout, herring, mackerel, halibut, albacore tuna and oysters. Other fish, like scallops, perch, cod, haddock, catfish, crab, shrimp, clams, and lobster contain smaller amounts of *omega-3 fatty acids*. Canola, walnut, and olive oils should be the main cooking and salad oils in your kitchen.

Environmental pollutants like mercury, polychlorinated biphenyls (PCBs), and dioxins are concentrated in certain predator fish. This contamination can make the recommendation to eat at least two portions of fish a week dangerous! We need to choose the fish in our diet very carefully. The main method to avoid pollutants while eating the recommended amount is to *vary the types* of fish you choose to eat and to refrain from eating predator fish.

In a 2004 study published in the prestigious journal, Science, farmed salmon were shown to contain 8 times the level of PCBs (as well as higher levels of dioxin) than wild. This is because the fish fed to farmed salmon are contaminated with PCBs and other pollutants whereas wild salmon eat a more varied diet of fish as well as algae. Differences in *omega-3 fatty acid* concentration between farmed and wild salmon vary also according to the processed feed the farmed salmon are fed. Canned salmon is wild so it is a healthier choice. Canned tuna contains lower levels of mercury than tuna steaks. Canned white albacore tuna contains about three times the level of mercury than the cheaper light meat tuna (actually the smaller skipjack and yellowfin fish). Canned tuna should be packed in water rather than oil, because fat-soluble *omega-3 fatty acids* tend to migrate from the fish into the oil and are then discarded.

Note: PCBs, organochlorine compounds once used as coolants and lubricants, have been banned for industrial use since 1976. But, they still contaminate the environment from plastics and waste incinerators. The risk to human health has not been fully delineated but there is enough information according to the *Environmental Protection Agency*, to consider that PCBs "probably" cause cancer, although this has not been proven. Women with higher concentrations of PCBs tend to have infants with more neurological problems than women with lower levels. So women who are pregnant or who desire to become pregnant should not eat farmed salmon so as not to expose the fetus to a significant level of PCBs. PCBs accumulate in fat tissue and skin. So, always remove the skin and the visible fat just underneath before eating the fish. Although this method also reduces the amount of *omega-3 fatty acids*, plenty will remain.

If you buy farmed salmon, those with the least PCB contamination come from Chile and the state of Washington, according to the study published in Science. Farmed salmon from Scotland and the Faroe Islands contained the highest levels of contamination. Salmon labeled "Atlantic'" and "Icelandic" are generally farmed.

The authors of the study published in Science recommend eating farmed salmon no more than once a month. But others disagree and recommend that we continue eating farmed (and wild) salmon more often because of the health benefits (especially cardiovascular) of *omega-3 fatty acids*. They point out that the levels of PCBs found in the study were well within the tolerable range according to the *Food and Drug*

Administration (FDA). But, just to make matters even more confusing, the PCB levels were outside the tolerable range according to the *Environmental Protection Agency* (EPA) which has tougher standards than the FDA because it considers only cancer risk. Not only do salmon farmers have to clean up their industry, but the FDA and the EPA need to come to a consensus on standards of pollutants!

Note: Mercury, a heavy metal, emitted from coal-burning power plants, tends to concentrate in the flesh of predator fish like shark, swordfish, king mackerel, fresh albacore tuna, and tilefish (also called golden bass and golden snapper). When mercury is converted into methyl mercury by the action of bacteria it becomes particularly toxic to the developing brain and nervous system of humans (and other animals). Lower concentrations can cause problems with learning, memory, coordination, depression, speech, and vision. Higher concentrations can cause death.

For this reason, my recommendation for women who are pregnant, lactating, or trying to become pregnant is *not to eat any predator fish*. These women should get their *omega-3 fatty acids* from other non-predator fish (no more than 2 portions per week) and from fish oil nutritional supplements taken every day (please see below). Young children under the age of 2 years also should not eat any predator fish. In addition all children under the age of 12 should limit their consumption of other fish to no more than 2-3 portions per week. The secret to safe fish consumption is to eat a *wide variety* of different fish, preferably those low in mercury.

Adults should eat no more than 12 oz of fish a week (2 or 3 servings) and this should come from a *wide variety* of different fish. Non-predator fish with the lowest concentrations of mercury are the smaller ones with shorter life spans, like sardines, perch, cod, black cod (also called sable and butterfish), sole, haddock, flounder, halibut, whitefish, herring, tilapia, pollock (in most fish sticks), mahi-mahi, anchovies, and shellfish. For up-dated fish advisory on pollutant levels, visit the *Environmental Protection Agency* (EPA) at www.epa.gov/ost/fish. For a list of best and worst fish go to www.blueocean.org/seafood and www.seafoodwatch.org.

Note: Two brands of tuna fish containing certified low levels of mercury are *Carvalho Coastal Albacore* and *King of the Sea*.

Remember: Canned salmon and canned bony sardines are good sources of calcium too, if you eat the tiny bones.

Note: If you catch fish yourself for eating and you want to know whether it is in danger of coming from highly mercury-contaminated waters, please check with *The Environmental Protection Agency* (EPA) at www.epa.gov/mercury.

Note: Eating shrimp is heart healthy because it is a rich source of *omega-3 fatty acids*, but on the other hand, it contains more cholesterol per serving than any other shellfish. But overall, shrimp is low in *saturated fat*. *Saturated fat* raises blood cholesterol more than dietary cholesterol does.

Note: The possibility of bacterial contamination causing food-borne poisoning is increased when eating raw or smoked fish.

Note: For information on endangered fish and making ecological choices, please contact *Living Oceans Society* at www.livingoceans.org (1-250-973-6580) or the *Natural Resources Defense Council* at www.nrdc.org (1-212-727-2700).

I recommend the magazine *Environmental Nutrition* as a reliable source of information on how environment and nutrition interconnect at www.environ-mentalnutrition.com.

WildCatch and *Dave's Hook and Line Caught* are brands of canned and fresh salmon which are comprised of wild Alaskan salmon, a non-endangered population.

Omega-6 fatty acids are involved in cell membrane structure, cholesterol manufacture and transport, and the synthesis of anti-inflammatory molecules. The main *omega-6 fatty acid* found in foods is called *linoleic acid (LA)*. It is found in corn (and corn oil), sesame seeds (and sesame oil), soybeans (and soybean oil), sunflower seeds (and sunflower oil) and cottonseed oil.

Consumption of *omega-6 fatty acids* is associated with decreased total cholesterol. *Gamma-linolenic acid (GLA)*, (found in borage, evening primrose, and black currant seed oils), protects against cancer and some psychiatric disorders. *GLA* is used to thicken hair growth on the scalp. It is the precursor chemical for the synthesis of "good" prostaglandins which are anti-inflammatory. *Arachidonic acid (ARA)* is the precursor chemical for the synthesis of certain "bad" prostaglandins which increase platelet stickiness (aggregation). However, *ARA* protects against cancer. Both *GLA* and *ARA* may protect the liver against toxic damage from alcohol.

Note: The ratio of *omega-3* to *omega-6 fatty acids* is important to health. The typical Western diet provides 20-30 times as much *omega-6 fatty acids* than *omega-3 fatty acids*. This imbalance actually interferes with the formation of *EPA* and *DHA* inside the body from *ALA*. This process prevents *omega-3 fatty acids* from being incorporated into cell membranes and from performing their other vital functions. This imbalance makes us prone to chronic ailments like obesity, cardiovascular disease, depression, and schizophrenia. The *World Health Organization (WHO)* recommends a diet providing a ratio of 5:1 to 10:1 *omega-6 fatty acids* to *omega-3 fatty acids*.

Canola oil has a very favorable ratio of 2:1. *Olive oil*, on the other hand, has a ratio of 11:1, but it contains a high proportion of very heart healthy *monounsat-*

urated fatty acids. This is why using a mixture of different healthy oils in your kitchen is important.

Note: Many infant formulas, both cow-milk based and soy-based, have been supplemented with *omega-3 (DHA)* and *omega-6 fatty acids (ARA)* to more closely resemble breast milk. Higher *ARA* blood levels in infants are directly related to better weight gain. But so far, there have been conflicting results as to enhanced cognitive or visual development in infants who have been fed supplemented formulas compared with those who have not. Long-term studies may show that supplementation prevents the development of heart disease.

When using *fats and oils* as nutritional supplements for self-care you must pay strict attention to the **Guidelines for Consulting Your Health Care Provider** at the end of this chapter. You may want to refer to the last section **Putting It All Together** for ideas on how to integrate the essential natural alternatives, homeopathy, herbal remedies, and nutritional supplements.

Omega-3 fatty acids

Omega-6 fatty acid (GLA) and *omega-3 fatty acid* (EPA) taken as nutritional supplements may allow you to decrease or stop the non-steroidal anti-inflammatory drugs (NSAIDs) you may be using. This has been shown to occur in rheumatoid arthritis, asthma, and eczema. The same may be said of decreasing long-term steroid drugs.

EPA and *DHA* taken as nutritional supplements (fish oil capsules) may augment certain chemotherapeutic agents used to treat cancer. They may decrease the risk of sudden death (due to heart arrhythmia) in persons who have had a heart attack (myocardial infarction) as well as in those who have never had heart disease. Fish oil supplements decreased the frequency, duration, and severity of migraine headaches in adolescents. They lower the risk of stroke and certain cancers, notably prostate cancer. There is some medical evidence that children with ADD/ADHD treated with fish oil capsules containing *EPA* and *DHA* show improvement in behavior and cognition.

For people who do not eat seafood, the recommendation for taking *omega-3 fatty acids* as nutritional supplements is to take fish oil pills containing 1000mg (1 gram) of *DHA* combined with *EPA* daily. This is the same dosage recommended by the *American Heart Association* to prevent cardiovascular disease. However, to lower triglycerides, you may need 2,000-4,000mg of combined *EPA* and *DHA* daily. If you take fish oil supplements at this high dosage level, you will need supervision by your physician because of the possibility of an increased risk of bleeding, especially if you are taking *warfarin* (*Coumadin*) or another anticoagulant.

The side effects of fish oil pills include nausea, fishy tasting burps, and diarrhea. Vegetarians are able to choose an algae-derived *DHA* (but not *EPA*) supplement. Refrigeration of the fish oil capsules may prevent the fishy aftertaste in the mouth that can occur. If you find you're experiencing some uncomfortable symptoms with your fish oil pills, sometimes just changing the brand eliminates the problems.

> **Note:** Flaxseeds (whole and ground) contain 1,800mg of *ALA* (an *omega-3 fatty acid*) per teaspoon. But there are restrictions on using flaxseeds because of its *lignan* content. *Lignans* are antioxidant phytochemicals with phytoestrogen activity. They may help to prevent breast cancer in those who have never had it. But, if you or your family member is being treated for breast cancer (or any other hormone-dependent cancer like prostate), you should avoid the *lignans* in flaxseeds. It is a good idea to follow the same recommendation if you are pregnant or lactating or if you are trying to become pregnant. One way to avoid *lignans* while at the same time getting the abundance of *ALA* is to consume *flaxseed oil*. But *flaxseed oil* is not considered tasty for cooking. You may want to add it in teaspoonful amounts directly to foods for its *ALA* content.

> **Note:** Another rich source of *ALA* is *perilla oil* from the seeds of *Perilla frutescens*. *Perilla oil* is available from Life Extension, with 1000mg per softgel providing 550mg of *ALA*. Take 3 softgels twice daily. The richest source of *ALA* is *Chia seed* (*Salvia hispanica*), known to Native North and South American peoples as a high energy food. *Chia seeds* contain a high percentage of *omega-3 fatty acids* as *ALA*. You can find out more about *Chia seed* at www.eatchia.com and www.chiaseedandoil.com.

> **Note:** Since mercury does not dissolve in oil, it is unlikely that your fish oil capsules (as *omega-3 fatty acid* nutritional supplements) are contaminated with mercury. To be sure, please read the label to check that your supplement has been purified to be mercury-free. But PCBs are soluble in oil, so please check that the label says "molecularly distilled" to remove contaminants (including dioxins). Tests on the top-selling fish oil supplements were found not to contain any significant amounts of mercury, PCBs, or dioxins.

> Another way to be sure is to look for the non-profit agency *United States Pharmacopeia* (*USP*) mark on the label. It means that the supplement has been checked for contaminants and cleared.

> **Note:** I don't recommend taking cod liver oil for your *omega-3 fatty acids* or for any other reason either. Cod liver oil is made from fish's livers and livers concentrate toxic substances. Stay away from liver as an organ meat or as a source of vitamins and *omega-3 fatty acids*. And besides, the amount of Vitamin A in cod liver oil is often too high.

> **Note:** *Fisol* is Nature's Way fish oil nutritional supplement containing 500mg of *EPA* and *DHA* per enteric-coated softgel. It may be absorbed better than other brands of fish oil because it is

digested in the intestines rather than the stomach. Take 2 softgels daily.

Note: Dr. Andrew Weil recommends using *omega-3 fatty acids* (in the form of fish oil capsules containing *EPA* and *DHA* for a total of 2 grams daily) to treat psoriasis. He suggests adding *evening primrose oil* or *black currant oil* (as a source of *GLA*, 500mg twice a day).

Olive oil

Olive oil, derived from the plant *Olea europaea* of the *Oleaceae* botanical family, is the major oil consumed in the healthy Mediterranean diet. *Olive oil* (as well as the olives it comes from) is predominately a *monounsaturated fat* which help to protect the coronary arteries from inflammation. Inflammation may be the root-cause of plaque build-up inside the coronaries. *Olive oil* helps to decrease LDL ("bad") cholesterol while increasing HDL ("good") cholesterol.

Olive oil has other health benefits as well. It is a rich source of the antioxidant family of *polyphenols*. This class of antioxidants acts as potent anti-inflammatory agents which is another reason why *olive oil* is beneficial for your cardiovascular system. And *olive oil* contains chemicals called *squalenes* which may interfere with cancer cell growth.

If you want the antioxidant benefits of *olive oil* without the calories, you may want to try the nutritional supplement called *Olivenol*, manufactured by CreAgri. The dose is 2 capsules daily. *Olivenol* contains the antioxidant *hydroxytyrosol*. This chemical may prevent the inflammation that is the prerequisite for the development of cardiovascular disease. It may also have anti-cancer activity.

> **Note:** *Olive oil* loses its flavor when heated to high temperatures, so you may want to use *canola oil* for cooking, reserving *olive oil* for salads, vegetables, bread dipping, and low-heat sautéing.

Note: The least processed and therefore healthiest *olive oil* is extra-virgin and cold-pressed. Extra-virgin is the highest grade because it is the least processed, preserving the high antioxidant content and containing at most 1% acid. Virgin

is more processed, containing as much as 3% acid. Cold-pressed means it is collected only from the oil that comes from the first pressing. Cold-pressed is an extraction process that crushes without heat or chemicals so as to preserve taste. However, most *olive oil* is cold-pressed these days. Extra-virgin and cold-pressed *olive oil* is also the most flavorful and the most expensive. Extra-virgin and cold-pressed *olive oil* contains *oleocanthol*, a chemical that possesses natural anti-inflammatory activity.

Note: *Olive oil* contains only a negligible amount of *omega-3 fatty acids* because it is a predominately *monounsaturated* oil. For healthy fats in the kitchen, it's wise to use several different oils for different purposes: olive, canola, and walnut, at least. The idea is to vary your fat sources. This goes for fish too, but for different reasons (please see above).

Note: *Olive oil* contains 120 calories in every tablespoon with 13 grams of fat of which 10 grams are *monounsaturated*.

Note: *Safflower oil* contains predominately *monounsaturated fats*, even more so than *olive oil*. But, when it comes to taste, *olive oil* usually wins. If you don't want to buy the more expensive *olive oil*, then use *safflower oil* instead, but understand that the medical research on the cardiovascular benefits of *olive oil* in the Mediterranean diet have not been proven using *safflower oil*.

Note: The *safflower* plant *Carthamus tinctorius* possesses anti-inflammatory activity. An ointment of concentrated *safflower* extract has been shown to provide potent pain relief for certain types of chronic pain (neck and back pain, carpal tunnel syndrome and tendonitis). The only side effect was mild rash in a very small percentage of cases which resolved after stopping the ointment. Concentrated *safflower* extract is available as *Zolacet* by NaturePath Laboratories.

Note: *Olive leaf extract* is derived from the same plant *Olea europaea*, as *olive oil* except that the leaves are made into the herbal remedy. The chemical *elenolic acid* present in *Olive leaf extract* possesses antibacterial, antiviral, and antiparasitic properties. There are *Olive leaf extract* preparations specifically for children and for pets. In addition, *Olive leaf extract* increases blood flow in the coronary arteries, making it useful in cases of high blood pressure (hypertension), angina, and arteriosclerosis. The usual dosage is two 500mg capsule once daily. It is not recommended for pregnant or lactating women.

Canola oil

Canola oil is also rich in *monounsaturated fats*. But, it is the cooking oil with the highest amount of *polyunsaturated omega-3 fatty acids (ALA)* along with a healthy amount of *omega-6 fatty acids*. *Canola oil* is among the lowest in *saturated fat*. Since it's flavorless, it's a good choice for cooking and baking.

The *Canola* plant was first produced by crossbreeding (not genetic engineering) from *rapeseed*, an herb in the mustard family. *Canola oil* is expressed from the seeds of the *Canola* plant. It belongs to the *Brassica* family of vegetables.

Note: Cold pressed *canola oil* is the least refined, healthiest, and highest in antioxidants.

Note: *Hemp oil* contains even more *omega-3 fatty acids* than *canola oil*, but it can't be used for cooking as its flavor changes unpleasantly.

Walnut oil

Walnut oil is predominately *monounsaturated* but rich in *polyunsaturated omega-3 fatty acids (ALA)*. It also contains vitamin E and other antioxidants. Walnuts and *walnut oil* ingestion tends to lower LDL ("bad") cholesterol. The FDA allows labeling of walnuts to say that they ". . . may reduce the risk of coronary heart disease."

Note: *Walnut oil* loses its flavor when heated, so you may want to use *canola oil* for cooking, reserving *walnut oil* with its distinctive nutty flavor for salads, pasta, and vegetables.

Note: Peanuts are actually members of the bean or legume family. Peanuts and *peanut oil* have a high percentage of *LA (omega-6 fatty acids)* but no *omega-3 fatty acids*. *Peanut butter* is an excellent protein source, containing 7 grams in 2 tablespoons (or one ounce). Look for organic *peanut butter* with no added sugar.

Note: *Almond butter* contains 5 grams of protein and the lowest amount of *saturated fats* of all the spreads. Buy *almond butter* made from unblanched almonds because they contain more antioxidant *flavonoids*.

Note: Sesame seeds contain almost equal amounts of *monounsaturated* and *polyunsaturated fatty acids (omega-6 only)*. Crushed sesame seeds are made into *tahini*, which together with chic peas, is used to make *humus*, an Arab-Israeli healthy "street" food, eaten inside pita bread.

Note: *Cottonseed oil*, even though it comes from a plant, contains a high percentage of *saturated fat*, similar to chicken fat! *Coconut oil*, another vegetable oil, has the most *saturated fat* of all the oils.

Note: *Enova oil* a new cooking oil, manufactured by Archer Daniels Midland, is made from an enzymatic reaction of *canola* and *soybean* oils. All other cooking oils are composed of 3 fatty acids called *triglycerides*, but *Enova oil's* are only 2, called *diglycerides* or *diacylglycerides (DAGs)*. The liver less readily stores *DAGs* as fat so *Enova oil* may be more easily burned as energy. This may be good news for weight-conscious persons, but one study found only a two-pound difference in weight in those using *Enova oil*. The calories in *Enova oil* is the same as in other healthy oils (120 calories and 14 grams of fat per tablespoon) as is the taste. It is an expensive alternative to other healthy oils. So far there are no side effects of using *Enova oil* but long-term studies are lacking.

Guidelines for Consulting Your Health Care Provider

You should consult your health care provider if:
• the patient doesn't look right or act right (trust your instincts!)
• the patient is getting worse instead of better over the course of the illness
• the patient is having trouble breathing or complaining of chest pains or there is mental confusion or lethargy or irritability
• the patient develops allergic symptoms (hives, itchy or watery eyes, runny nose, scratchy throat, asthma, shortness of breath) after taking a nutritional supplement
• after beginning a nutritional supplement the patient experiences *new onset* of any serious symptoms such as:

   paralysis, weakness, tingling, inability to focus or concentrate, blurred or double vision or blindness, slurred speech, severe headaches, seizures, irritability, dizziness, disorientation, memory loss, anxiety, depression, insomnia, blackouts, fainting, or the person complains of not feeling like himself

• the patient is taking *ANY* prescription medication
• the patient is pregnant or breastfeeding
• the patient has any serious, chronic disease which may have complications and become life-threatening, such as:

autism, cancer, HIV and AIDS, arthritis, multiple sclerosis, coronary artery disease, heart attack (myocardial infarction), blood dyscrasia, cancer (of any type), congestive heart failure, diabetes mellitus, obesity, thyroid disorders, high blood pressure (hypertension), stroke, seizures, acute and chronic kidney (renal) failure, schizophrenia, bipolar disorder, borderline personality disorder, eating disorders, fibromyalgia, chronic fatigue syndrome, Crohn's disease, ulcerative colitis, celiac disease, mental deficiency disorders, chromosomal disorders, infertility, frequent miscarriages, polyneuropathy, cystic fibrosis   [Adapted from *The Merck Manual* at www.merck.com]

Note: Do not discontinue taking any pharmaceutical medication prescribed by your health care provider unless you or your family member is under the supervision of a physician.

Note: Do not take any *fats* or *oils* as nutritional supplements without first consulting your health care provider especially if you or your family member is taking a prescription medication to treat cancer or its complications or is pregnant or breastfeeding.

In addition, it is a good idea to check with your health care provider if your family member is either very young or very old because nutritional supplements given injudiciously may overwhelm the body's defenses in those age groups.

Putting It All Together

In addition to oils and fats for their anti-inflammatory impact on immune system health (as well as for general health) in this chapter, there are other anti-inflammatory supplements that may be found in different chapters in this book.

If you are considering using *omega-3 fatty acid* nutritional supplements for their anti-inflammatory prowess or for immune system health, it is a good idea to familiarize yourself with **Chapter 22: Introduction to Nutritional Supplements**. It makes good sense to understand the role of vitamin and mineral nutritional supplements from **Chapter 23: Vitamins and Minerals**; *antioxidant* nutritional supplements from **Chapter 24: Antioxidant Phytochemicals: Natural Anti-Aging Remedies**. In addition, you will likely benefit from learning about *systemic enzymes* and *fiber* in **Chapter 25: Heart Healthy Nutritional Supplements**.

Please consider taking *prebiotics* and *probiotics* to enhance the digestive and immune systems (please refer to **Chapter 30: Prebiotics and Probiotics**). You should read about *systemic oral enzymes*, medicinal *mushrooms, modified citrus pectin,* and other immune system modulators in **Chapter 27: Nutritional Supplements to Prevent Cancer and Augment Your Immune System**.

Whenever you have decided to go ahead with using *omega-3 fatty acid* nutritional supplements, it is a good idea to consider giving the sick person's homeopathic constitutional remedy as well (please refer to **Chapter 9: Homeopathic Remedies for Constitutional Problems in Infants, Children, and Adolescents** or to **Chapter 18: Homeopathic Constitutional Remedies** if you are dealing with an adult; or **Chapter 13: Homeopathy for Elderly Persons** if you are dealing with an elderly person). Homeopathic remedies may be used in conjunction with herbal medicines and nutritional supplements as well as prescription pharmaceuticals.

Appendix

Internet Resources for Complementary and Alternative Medicine (CAM)

Organization	Website Address
Alternative Therapies in Health and Medicine (a journal)	www.alternativetherapies.com
Ask Noah About CAM	www.noah-health.org
Alternative Medicine (books and journals)	www.alternativemedicine.com
Health World Online	www.healthy.net
National Center for CAM	www.nccam.nih.gov
National Foundation for Alternative Medicine	www.nfam.org
Annie Appleseed Project	www.annieappleseedproject.org
PubMed—for scientific articles on CAM	www.ncbi.nlm.nih.gov/PubMed

Book Resources for Complementary and Alternative Medicine (CAM)

Freeman, L. W. and G. F. Lawlis. *Complementary and Alternative Medicine, A Research-Based Approach.* Mosby, Philadelphia, 2001, pp. 532.

MacBeckner, W. and B. M. Berman. *Complementary Therapies on the Internet.* Churchill Livingstone, USA, 2003, pp. 186.

Micozzi, M. S. *Fundamentals of Complementary and Alternative Medicine.* 2nd Edition. Churchill Livingstone, New York, 2001, pp. 464.

Pizzorno, L. U., J. E. Pizzorno and M. T. Murray. *Natural Medicine Instructions for Patients.* Elsevier Science, Ltd., China, 2002, pp. 374.

Rakel, D. *Integrative Medicine.* Saunders, New York, 2003, pp. 821.

Rister, R. S. *Healing Without Medication: A Comprehensive Guide to the Complementary Techniques Anyone Can Use to Achieve Real Healing.* Basic Health Publications, Inc., New Jersey, 2003, pp. 738.

Trivieri, L. and J. W. Anderson, editors. *Alternative Medicine, The Definitive Guide.* 2nd Edition. Celestial Arts, Berkeley, 2002, pp. 1231.

Yuan, C-S. and E. J. Bieber. *Textbook of Complementary and Alternative Medicine.* Parthenon Publishing, USA, 2003, pp. 404.

Internet Resources for Homeopathy

Organization	Website Address
National Center for Complementary and Alternative Medicine, National Institutes of Health	www.nccam.hih.gov
Digital Biology	www.digibio.com
Homeopathic Educational Services	www.homeopathic.com
Dr. Timothy R. Dooley's *Beyond Flat Earth Medicine*	www.beyondflatearth.com
Journal of the Homeopathic Academy of Naturopathic Physicians	www.simillimum.com
Rescue Remedy	www.rescueremedy.com www.nelsonbach.com www.bachbooks.com
Academy of Veterinary Homeopathy	www.theavh.org
Homeopathic Nurses Association	www.homeopathicnurses.org
American Instsitute of Homeopathy	www.homeopathyusa.org
National Center for Homeopathy	www.nationalcenterforhomeopathy.org
Homeopathy World	www.homeopathyworld.com
Hpathy.com	www.hpathy.com

Book Resources for Homeopathy

If you are interested in reading more about homeopathy, then I recommend that you call or email to order a catalogue from **Homeopathic Educational Services** or **Homeopathy for Health** or **WholeHealthNow** or **Minimum Price Books**. You will be dazzled by the number and quality of books, tapes, software, and homeopathic products.

Homeopathic Educational Services
2036 Blake Street
Berkeley, CA 94704
(800) 359 9051
email: mail@homeopathic.com
http://www.homeopathic.com

Homeopathy for Health
422 N. Earl Road
Moses Lake, WA 98837
(800) 390 9970
email: heath@elixirs.com
http://www.elixirs.com

WholeHealthNow
1102 Pleasant Street
Worcester, MA 01602
(250) 881-1252
email: info@WholeHealthNow.com
http://www.wholehealthnow.com

Minimum Price Books
250 H Street, P.O. Box 2187
Blaine, WA 98231
(800) 663-8272
email: orders@minimum.com
www.minimum.com

Recommended Books to Read

Allen, H. C. *Keynotes and Characteristics of Some of the Leading Remedies of the Materia Medica with Bowel Nosodes.* 8th Edition. B. Jain Publishers: New Delhi, Reprint Edition 1995, 402 pp.

Bailey, P. M. *Homeopathic Psychology, Personality Profiles of the Major Constitutional Remedies.* North Atlantic Books, Berkeley, California; Homeopathic Educational Services, Berkeley, California, 1995, 418 pp.

Coulter, C. R. *Portraits of Homeopathic Medicines.* Quality Medical Publishing, Inc., Missouri, 1998. Volume 1, 422 pp., Volume 2, 300 pp., Volume 3, 338 pp.

Dooley, T. R. *Homeopathy: Beyond Flat Earth Medicine.* Timing Publications, San Diego, California, 1996, 111 pp.

Goldberg, B. *Alternative Medicine: The Definitive Guide.* 2nd Edition. Celestial Arts, California, 2002, 1233 pp.

Gray, B. *Homeopathy Science or Myth?* North Atlantic Books, California, 2000, 190 pp.

Hayfield, R. *Homeopathy for Common Ailments.* London: Gaia Books, LDT, 1993, 95 pp.

Herscu, P. *The Homeopathic Treatment of Children.* North Atlantic Books, California, 1991, 374 pp.

Lansky, A. L. *Impossible Cure, the Promise of Homeopathy.* R. L. Ranch Press, California, 2003, 303 pp.

Lockie, A. and N. Geddes. *The Complete Guide to Homeopathy, the Principles and Practice of Treatment.* Dorling Kindersley, London, 1995, 240 pp.

PallasDowney, R. *The Complete Book of Flower Essences.* New World Library, California, 2002, 456 pp.

Ramakrishnan, A. U. and C. R. Coulter. *A Homeopathic Approach to Cancer.* Quality Medical Publishing, Inc., USA, 2001, 198 pp.

Roy, M. *A First Materia Medica for Homeopathy, a Self-Directed Learning Text.* Churchill Livingstone, London, 1994, 261 pp.

Schroyens, F. *Synthesis, Repertorium Homeopathicum Syntheticum.* London: Homeopathic Book Publishers, 1995, 1720 pp.

Shalts, E. *The American Institute of Homeopathy Handbook for Parents.* Josey-Bass/Wiley, San Francisco, California, 2005, 363 pp.

Sollars, D. *The Complete Idiot's Guide to Homeopathy.* Alpha Books, Indiana, 2001, 317 pp.

Ullman, D. *Essential Homeopathy.* New World Library, California, 2002, 112 pp.

Van Zandvoort, R. *The Complete Repertory Mind-Generalities.* Institute for Research in Homeopathic Information and Symptomatology, The Netherlands, 1994-1996, 2800 pp.

Vithoulkas, G. *Homeopathy Medicine of the New Man.* Simon and Schuster: New York, 1992, 154 pp.

Vlamis, G. *Rescue Remedy, the Healing Power of Bach Flower Rescue Remedy.* Thorsen's, London, 1994, 166 pp.

Weil, A. *Eight Weeks to Optimum Health.* Alfred A. Knopf, New York, 1997, 276 pp.

Homeopathic Remedies Supply Houses

For more information you may investigate the website:
http://www.homeopathyhome.com/directory/usa/pharmacies.shtml

The listing below is based in part on that website.

Homeopathic Remedy Supply Houses	Telephone	Website Address
Arrowroot Standard Direct Ltd.	800-234-8879 email: customerservice@arrowroot.com	www.arrowroot.com
bioAllers	800-541-1356	www.bioallers.com
Boericke & Tafel Inc.	800-962-8873	www.naturesway.com
Boiron-Bornemann Inc.	800-258-8823 (800-Blu-Tube) email: info@boironusa.com	www.boiron.com
Dolisos America, Inc.	800-365-4767 (800-Dolisos) email: dolisos@earthlink.net	www.dolisosamerica.com
Hahnemann Laboratories Inc.	888-4-ARNICA/888-427-6422	www.hahnemannlabs.com
Heel Inc.	800-621-7644 email: info@heelUSA.com	www.heelusa.com
Homeopathy Overnight	800-276-4223 (1-800-ARNICA30)	www.homeopathyovernight.com
King Bio Pharmaceutical Inc.	800-543-3245	www.kingbio.com
Luyties Pharmacal Co.	800-466-3672 (1-800-homeopathy) email: info@1800homeopathy.com	www.1800homeopathy.com
Remedy Makers	877-736-4968	www.remedymakers.com
Standard Homeopathic Company	800-624-9659	www.drugstore.com
Professional Complementary Health Formulas	503-245-2720 (for customers in Portland, Oregon), 800-952-2219 (for all others)	www.professionalformulas.com
Washington Homeopathic Products	800-336-1695	www.homeopathyworks.com
Weleda Inc.	800-289-1969 x212 email: rx@weleda.com	www.homeopathyhome.com www.weleda.com
Your Rx 4 Health	410-356-2169 888-794-4325	www.illnessisoptional.com
Treatment Options	1-800-456-7818	www.txoptions.com

Internet Resources for Herbal Remedies

Organization	Telephone	Website Address
American Botanical Council (*HerbalGram* is the Journal)	800-373-7105 512-926-4900 fax: 512-926-2345	www.herbalgram.org
American Herbal Products Association		www.ahpa.org
American Herbalists Guild	770-751-6021	www.americanherbalist.com
ConsumerLab.com	914-722-9149 reports: 201-261-5616	www.ConsumerLab.com
HerMed	301-340-1960 fax: 301-340-1936	www.herbmed.org
Herb Research Foundation	office: 303-449-2265 voice mail: 800-748-2617 fax: 303-449-7849	www.herbs.org
National Institutes of Health, Office of Dietary Supplements		www.dietarysupplements.info.nih.gov
Food and Drug Administration		www.cfsan.fda.gov

Note: You may obtain free, evidence-based, scientific reviews of many of the herbs recommended in **Chapters 20** and **21** by visiting *The Cochrane Complementary Medicine Field Registry* online at www.compmed.umm.edu/cochrane/index.html.

Evidence-based data for the general public is also freely available at HerbMed (an herbal database resource) at www.herbmed.org (please see above).

Book Resources for Herbal Remedies

Barnes, J., L. A. Anderson and J. D. Phillipson. *Herbal Medicines*. 2nd Edition. Pharmaceutical Press, London, 2002, pp. 530.

Blumenthal, M., editor. *The Complete German Commission E Monographs Therapeutic Guide to Herbal Medicines*. Integrative Medicine Communication, Boston, Massachusetts, 1998, pp. 685.

Castleman, M. *The New Healing Herbs*. Rodale Press, Pennsylvania, 2001, pp. 465.

ConsumerLab.com's *Guide to Buying Vitamins and Supplements, What's Really in the Bottle?* ConsumerLab.com, 2003, pp. 226.

Duke, J. A. *The Green Pharmacy*. Rodale Press, Pennsylvania, 1997, pp. 508.

Graedon, J. and T. Graedon. *The People's Pharmacy Guide to Home and Herbal Remedies*. St. Martin's Griffin, New York, 2001, pp. 428.

Grieve, M. *A Modern Herbal*. Dorset Press: New York, 1994, pp. 912.

Gruenwald, J., T. Brendler and C. Jaenicke, editors. *PDR for Herbal Medicines*. 3rd Edition. Medical Economics Company, Montvale, New Jersey, 2005.

Kowalchik, C. and W. H. Hylton, editors. *Rodale's Illustrated Encyclopedia of Herbs*. Rodale Press, Pennsylvania, 1987, pp. 545.

McKenna, D. J., K. Hughes and S. Humphrey. *Botanical Medicines: The Desk Reference for Major Herbal Supplements*. 2nd Edition. The Haworth Herbal Press, New York, 2002, pp. 1097.

Mindel, E. *New Herb Bible*. Fireside, New York, 2000, pp. 315.

White, L. B. and S. Foster. *The Herbal Drugstore*. Rodale Press, Pennsylvania, 2000, pp. 610.

Herbal Remedy Supply Houses

Herbal Remedy Supply House	Telephone	Website Address
Herbal Fortress	888-454-3267 fax: 208-765-5403	www.herbalfortress.com
Nature's Plus	800-645-9500 fax: 800-665-0628	www.naturesplus.com
Nature's Way	801-489-1500 fax: 801-489-1700	www.naturesway.com
Phytopharmica	800-553-2370	www.phytopharmica.com
Professional Complementary Health Formulas	503-245-2720 (for customers in Portland, Oregon), 800-952-2219 (for all others)	www.professionalformulas.com
Solaray	866-998-8855 fax: 425-869-7750	www.vitaminlife.com
The Vitamin Shoppe	800-223-1216	www.VitaminShoppe.com
TwinLabs	631-467-3140	www.twinlab.com
Weleda Pharmacy, Inc.	914-352-6165	www.homeopathyhome.com

Internet Resources for Nutritional Supplements

Organization	Website Address
American Dietetic Association	www.eatright.org
Arbor Clinical Nutrition Updates	www.nutritionupdate.org www.arborcom.com
National Academy of Sciences/Food and Nutritional Board	www.nas.edu
National Center for Alternative and Complementary Medicine	www.nccam.nih.gov
National Institute on Aging Information Office	www.nih.gov/nia
American Public Health Association	www.apha.org
American Institute for Cancer Research	www.aicr.org
President's Council on Physical Fitness and Sports	www.surgeongeneral.gov/ophs/pcpfs.htm
North American Vegetarian Society	www.navs-online.org
Consumer Reports on Health	www.consumerreports.org
National Cancer Institute	www.nci.nih.gov

Book Resources for Nutritional Supplements

Balch, L. A. and J. F. Balch. *Prescription for Nutritional Healing.* 3rd Edition. Avery Books, New York, 2000, pp. 776. This is a popular book encompassing nutritional and herbal remedies for common ailments; but it tends to neglect homeopathic remedies.

ConsumerLab.com's *Guide to Buying Vitamins and Supplements, What's Really in the Bottle?* ConsumerLab.com LLC, 2003, pp. 226.

Duff, R. I. *American Dietetic Association Complete Food and Nutrition Guide.* 2nd Edition. John Wiley & Sons, Inc., New Jersey, 2002, pp. 658.

Harvard Medical School's *The Smart Guide to Vitamins and Minerals,* available at www.health.harvard.edu. This 16-page booklet is a good resource for understanding the basics. You will refer to it again and again.

Jamison, J. *Clinical Guide to Nutrition and Dietary Supplements in Disease Management.* Churchill Livingstone, 2003, pp. 790.

Physician's Desk Reference for Nutritional Supplements. Medical Economics, New Jersey, 2001, pp. 575.

Rister, R. S. *Healing Without Medication.* Basic Health Publications, Inc., New Jersey, 2003, pp. 738.

Whitney, E. N. and S. R. Rolfes. *Understanding Nutrition.* 9th Edition. Wadsworth Group, USA, 2002, pp. 697 plus 9 appendixes. This is the book I recommend if you want the nitty-gritty, basic science of nutrition.

Willett, W. *Eat, Drink, and Be Healthy.* Simon and Schuster, New York, 2001, pp. 299.

Note: You may want to take a look at the 2 books to jump-start your odyssey to healthful nutrition for yourself and your family:

Marion Nestle's
What to Eat,
North Point Press, 2006

and for vegetarian recipies:
Goldbecks'
American Wholefoods Cuisine,
Ceres Press, 2006.

Nutritional Supplements Supply Houses

ConsumerLab.com is an independent testing laboratory. It has been certifying herbal remedies and nutritional supplements, making sure that the ingredients are present in the dosages that are claimed on the label and that the formulation is free from contaminants. You may view their results online at www.ConsumerLab.com. ConsumerLab.com reports that approximately 15% of tested supplements fail their standards for both having 1) exact correspondence of amount of active ingredients on label vs. actually determined by testing; and 2) finding that the preparation is free from contaminants. You will need to pay a fee to view their listing of brands that passed and those that failed. Or you may prefer to read the book, *ConsumerLab.com's Guide to Buying Vitamins and Supplements: What's Really in the Bottle?*

I strongly recommend that you purchase only recommended brands of nutritional supplements. If you see the *USP mark* (*United States Pharmacopeia*, a

nonprofit organization) on the label you know that the supplement has been tested for release and dissolution of its ingredients. And you are assured that label claims for potency and amount are actually true and that there is no harmful level of contaminants. In addition, the company's plant has been inspected for good manufacturing practices. You may find the list of supplement manufactures that have earned the *USP mark* of certification at www.uspverified.org.

Another nonprofit organization that certifies supplements is *NSF International*. Their certification means that the product contains what the label says it contains, is contaminant-free, and good manufacturing practices are followed. You may find them at www.nsf.org/certified/dietary.

The table below lists the brands of nutritional supplements that I most often recommend to my patients. However, it is impossible for me to guarantee with certainty that the nutritional supplements that you purchase contain the amounts of active ingredients as listed on the label or that they are free from contaminants.

Nutritional Supplements Supply Houses

Supply House	Telephone	Website Address
DaVinci Laboratories	800-325-1776	www.davincilabs.com
Life Extension	866-857-4102	www.LifeExtension.com
Moducare	877-297-7332	www.moducare.com
Nature Made	800-276-2878	www.NatureMade.com
Nature's Plus	800-645-9500	www.natureplus.com
Nature's Way	801-489-1500	www.naturesway.com
Solaray	800-669-8877	www.nutraceutical.com
Solgar	877-765-4274	www.solgar.com
The Vitamin Shoppe	800-223-1216	www.vitaminshoppe.com
TwinLab	877-297-7332	www.twinlab.com

Index

dilated pupil 167
diligent 181
dill 267
Dill seed oil 128, 221
diltiazem 203
dimensions of a symptom 25
Dimethylaminoethanol (DMAE) 327
Dimethylglycine (DMG) 327
Dioscorea villosa 131, 222
Dioscoreaceae 222
dioxin 343, 346
diplomatic 182
disability 315
disappointed love 77, 93, 96, 116, 182
discharge 61, 114, 184
discomfort 128, 129, 139
disinfectant 36, 211
disordered eating 289
disorganization 101
disorganized 103
dissatisfied 106, 184
distention 128, 129, 130, 131
distilled water 233
distractibility 101
diuretic 204, 224, 252, 296
diverticulosis 277
dizziness 167, 195, 204, 207, 218, 280, 291, 319
DNA *See:* genetic material
DNA polymerase 202
docosahexaenoic acid (DHA) 342
domineering 103, 106, 181
Dong quai 193, 219, 220
dopamine 210, 319
dramatic 183
dreams of her own death 182
dribbling 136, 138, 139, 209
driven 183
Drosera notundifolia 64, 77
Droseraceae 64, 77
drowsiness 146
drug-herb interaction 3
drug interaction 11
dry cough 63, 64
dry, cracked skin 160
dry mouth 63, 146
dry mucus membrane 144, 146
dry nose 80
dry skin 81
dryness 79
Dulcamara 66, 77, 107
duodenum 131
dyslexia 103
dysmenorrhea 115, 217, 220
dyspnea 145

ear infection 58, 64, 67, 86, 87, 199
ear, ringing 204, 329
earache 26, 38, 65, 107, 127
Earache 67
eardrum, rupture 67

easily distracted 183
eating 240
eating disorder 92, 112, 122, 158, 162, 163, 180, 198, 289, 304, 325, 326, 330
eating habit 297
eating, secret 289
eccentric 185
Echina-Spray 66, 67
Echinacea 62, 80, 192, 194, 198, 199, 200,
Echinacea angustifolia 41, 66, 80, 198
Echinacea Compound 62
Echinacea pallida 198
Echinacea purpurea 198
eczema 40, 48, 74, 78, 79, 81, 101, 106, 220, 292, 335, 336, 342, 345
edamame 222
edema 40, 68, 147
effectiveness 193
effervescent 183
egg white 77
egocentric 181
eicosapentaenoic acid (EPA) 342
elderly 2, 18, 59, 69, 89, 129, 144, 145, 148, 191, 192, 198, 216, 236, 241, 309, 326, 328, 329
electrolyte 247
electromagnetic radiation 20
elenolic acid 348
elephant yam 292
Eleuthero 205, 218
Eleutherococcus senticosus 204, 206, 217, 218, 294
ellagic acid 260
Elm 79
emaciation 146, 160, 161
embarrassment 145
Embryo suis 147
Emer'gen-C 70
emetic 76
emotion 104
emotion, inability to express 93
emotional 118, 181
emotional ailment 102, 182
emotional disorder 21, 30, 70, 75, 89, 94, 159, 325
emotional immaturity 145
emotional problem 92, 95
emotional shock 36, 38, 93
empathetic 66, 94, 96, 183
empathic 182
empathy 103
empty nest syndrome 96
end of urination 139
endangered fish 344
endocarditis 269
endocrine gland 70, 89
endometrial cancer 223
endometriosis 219
endometrium 217
endurance 258, 288, 289, 294
energetic 183
energy 102, 113, 205

energy density 286, 287
energy signature 20
English Hawthorn 207
Enoki mushroom 307
Enokitake See: Enoki mushroom
Enova oil 348, 349
Enterococcus 336
enthusiastic 183, 185
enuresis 136
enzyme 52, 202, 237, 253, 276, 277, 291, 292, 293, 306, 317, 336
enzyme deficiency 126, 201
Ephedra sinica 194, 195, 295, 296
ephedrine 194, 296
epididymis 275
epigallocatechin gallate (EGCG) 206, 296
epigastrium 131, 132
epilepsy 166, 220, 258, 325, 327
Epimedium grandiflorum 218
epinephrine 74
equilibrium 288
Equisetum 62
Equisetum hymenale 147
Equisetum verbascum 140
erectile dysfunction 139, 205, 274
erection 139, 205
Ergot of Rye 146
Ericaceae 39, 154, 219
erinacine 307
Eriodictyon californicum 81
eritadenine 308
Erpace 66
erratic 181
Erythroxylum catuaba 218
Eschscholtzia californica 169
escin 279
esophagus 131, 177
essential alternative health practice 2, 4, 10,
essential amino acid 259, 273
essential fatty acid 220, 306
essential natural alternatives 9, 10, 12
essential nutrient 229, 246
Essiac tea 306
estrogen 218, 221, 222, 223, 258, 265
ethyl mercury 325
eucalyptus 31, 41
Eucalyptus globules 81
Eupatorium perfoliatum 62
Euphrasia officinales 67, 79, 80
European Mistletoe 306
Eurycoma longifolia 218, 299
Euterpe oleracea 267, 313
evasive 182
evening 117
Evening Primrose Oil 220, 347
excess, prone to 183
excitability 101
excitable 104, 121
excretory organ 148, 186, 196, 234
exercise 13, 42
exercise-induced asthma 74

NULL

224, 234, 254, 266, 281, 295, 310, 321, 325, 329, 337, 349
Phaseolus vulgaris 293
Phellodendron amurense 298
phenobarabital 202
phenylalanine 274
phenylketonuira (PKU) 290
phenytoin 200
Phleum pratense 80
phobia 92, 94
phosphatidylcholine See: lecithin
phosphatidylethanolamine 328
phosphatidylserine 328, 329
phospholipid 183, 328, 342
phosphoric acid 63, 97, 139, 249
Phosphoricum acidum 147, 162
Phosphorus 43, 45, 65, 66, 75, 88, 97, 104, 113, 139, 161, 162, 183, 229, 247
photosensitivity 68
photosensitization 211
photosynthesis 318
phylloquinone 246
physical activity 152, 158, 160, 259, 289, 303
physical deformity 107
physical exercise 285, 288, 304
physical exercise program 289
physical fitness 289
physical fitness program 288
physical stamina 105, 205
physics of water 19
phytate 253
phytic acid 311
phytochemical 191, 229, 230, 232, 257, 262, 259, 265, 266, 273, 303, 346
phytoestrogen 221, 265, 277, 346
Phytolacca decandra 88, 120, 121, 161, 162
Phytolaccaceae 88, 120, 161
phytomedicine 191
phytonutrient 229, 230, 232, 233
phytosterol 279, 280, 309, 336
Picaridin 82
Pick's disease 325
picrotoxine 95, 167
Pilates system 289
Pine 79
pineal gland 212
pinolenic acid 298
Pinus koraensis 298
Pinus strobes 79
Piper methysticum 194, 195
piperine 262
placebo 19, 152, 204, 210, 217, 309, 315, 316
Placenta suis 147
placid 102, 181
Plantaginaceae 209
Plantago major 107, 170
Plantago ovata 209
Plantago psyllium 209
Plantain 209
plaque 248

platelet 246, 271, 273, 320, 345
platelet stickiness 203
Platina 161, 162
Platinum metallicum 115, 161
Plavix 203, 204
pleurisy 41
plodding 159
plumbago 48, 160
plussing method 176, 177, 178
PMS Relief 115
pneumonia 41, 66, 75, 88
Podophyllum pellatum 147
poison ivy 40, 78, 154, 211
Poison nut 61, 76, 117, 119, 128, 138, 183
Poison weed 79
Pokeroot 88, 120, 161
policosanol 279, 280, 281
political 182
pollutant 195
polychlorinated biphenyls (*PCBs*) 343
polychrest 25, 27, 66, 75, 77, 88, 94, 102, 104, 106, 113, 116, 129, 130, 159, 161, 176, 180, 182
polycystic ovary syndrome 112, 122, 210
polyenylphosphatidylcholine See: lecithin
Polygonaceae 64
polymorphonuclear cells 199
polymyalgia rheumatica 315
polyneuropathy 180, 198, 220, 240, 242
polyphenol 206, 207, 262, 347
Polyporus umbellatus 308
polyps 247, 271
polysaccharide 307
polyunsaturated fatty acid (*PUFAs*) 340, 342, 348
pomegranate juice 262
Poor Man's Treacle 203
Populus deltoids 79
portion size 285
possessive 104
Post-Cosmetic Procedure 45
Post-Dental Procedure 45
post-menopausal 236, 247, 251, 272
postnasal drip 64, 76
post-stroke dementia 145
post-surgical swelling 44
post-traumatic stress disorder 37, 93, 92, 97, 101, 105
potassium 229, 247, 252
potassium bisulphate 47, 66, 96, 103, 138
potassium carbonate 63, 97, 118, 130
potassium chloride 252
potassium citrate 252
potassium deficiency 252
potassium dichromate 64, 68, 76
potassium hydrate 96
potassium iodate 252
potassium iodide 80, 250, 252
potassium phosphate 63, 97
potassium tartrate 76
potency 30
potentization 19

power 182
practical 185
pragmatic 183
Prana 21
Pravachol 200
pravastatin 200
prayer 95, 96
preadolescent 104
prebiotic 303, 335, 336, 337, 338
precancerous 247
Pre-Cosmetic Procedure 45
predator fish 343, 344
pre-dementia 204
Pre-Dental Procedure 44, 45
prediabetes 250
pre-eclampsia 251
pregnancy 2, 18, 59, 112, 116, 117, 118, 122, 171, 191, 192, 198, 199, 200, 201, 202, 203, 204, 205, 207, 208, 209, 210, 211, 212, 216, 218, 219, 220, 221, 222, 223, 224, 231, 236, 241, 242, 244, 247, 248, 250, 251, 252, 253, 254, 262, 265, 266, 276, 277, 280, 281, 290, 291, 292, 294, 295, 308, 309, 311, 316, 317, 319, 325, 326, 327, 328, 329, 330, 336, 338, 343, 344, 346, 348, 349
pregnant *See: pregnancy*
prehypertension 270, 286
premature death 257
premature ejaculation 205
premenopausal 236, 298
premenstrual 116, 181
premenstrual syndrome (PMS) 114, 217, 219, 247, 251
prenatal vitamin 112, 236, 239, 254
Pre-Orthopedic Procedure 45
prepared food 13
prepubertal 103
preschooler 103
prescription medication (pharmaceutical) 32, 74, 98, 112, 166, 175, 223, 237, 270, 273, 286, 293
pressure 41, 115, 117, 132, 138, 168, 181, 184
Pre-Surgery Prescription 42, 43, 44, 49
preterm delivery 250
Primulaceae 167
Privet 79
proanthocyanidin 207, 243, 260, 263
probiotic 303, 335, 336, 337, 338
processed food 269, 302
procrastination 103
prodromal stage 60
progesterone 219, 222, 223
prohormone 299
prolapse 184
prolific interests 185
proline 274
prolonged labor 119
promiscuous 182
promote healing 40
Propolis 200, 309

Printed in the United States
133295LV00001B/31/A

9 780878 75563